Ethical Problems
in Emergency Medicine

Current Topics in Emergency Medicine

Series editor-in-chief, Peter Rosen
Associate series editor-in-chief, Shamai A. Grossman

Ethical Problems in Emergency Medicine

A discussion-based review

John Jesus, MD
Chief Resident, Department of Emergency
Medicine
Beth Israel Deaconess Medical Center
Boston, MA, USA
Clinical Instructor, Department of Emergency
Medicine
Christiana Care Health System
Newark, DE, USA

**Shamai A. Grossman,
MD, MS, FACEP**
Vice Chair for Resource Utilization
Director, Cardiac Emergency Center
Division of Emergency Medicine
Beth Israel Deaconess Medical Center
Assistant Professor of Medicine, Harvard
Medical School
Boston, MA, USA

**Arthur R. Derse, MD, JD
FACEP**
Director, Center for Bioethics and Medical
Humanities
Julia and David Uihlein Professor of Medical
Humanities
Professor of Bioethics and Emergency
Medicine
Institute for Health and Society
Medical College of Wisconsin
Milwaukee, WI, USA

James G. Adams, MD
Professor and Chair, Department of
Emergency Medicine
Feinberg School of Medicine
Northwestern University
Northwestern Memorial Hospital
Chicago, IL, USA

Richard Wolfe, MD
Chief of Emergency Medicine
Beth Israel Deaconess Medical Center
Associate Professor of Medicine
Harvard Medical School
Boston, MA, USA

**Peter Rosen, MD, FACS,
FACEP**
Director of Education
Beth Israel Deaconess Medical Center
Senior Lecturer in Medicine
Harvard Medical School
Boston, MA, USA

WILEY-BLACKWELL

A John Wiley & Sons, Ltd., Publication

This edition first published 2012 © 2012 by John Wiley & Sons, Ltd.

Wiley-Blackwell is an imprint of John Wiley & Sons, formed by the merger of Wiley's global Scientific, Technical and Medical business with Blackwell Publishing.

Registered office: John Wiley & Sons, Ltd, The Atrium, Southern Gate, Chichester, West Sussex, PO19 8SQ, UK

Editorial offices: 9600 Garsington Road, Oxford, OX4 2DQ, UK
The Atrium, Southern Gate, Chichester, West Sussex, PO19 8SQ, UK
111 River Street, Hoboken, NJ 07030-5774, USA

For details of our global editorial offices, for customer services and for information about how to apply for permission to reuse the copyright material in this book please see our website at www.wiley.com/wiley-blackwell

Library of Congress Cataloging-in-Publication Data

Ethical problems in emergency medicine : a discussion-based review / John Jesus ... [et al.].
    p. cm.
  Includes bibliographical references and index.
  ISBN 978-0-470-67347-8 (pbk.)
  1. Emergency medicine–Moral and ethical aspects.   2. Medical ethics.   I. Jesus, John.
  RC86.95.E834 2012
  174.2'96025–dc23

                                                              2011049653

A catalogue record for this book is available from the British Library.

Wiley also publishes its books in a variety of electronic formats. Some content that appears in print may not be available in electronic books.

Set in 9/11.5pt Sabon by Toppan Best-set Premedia Limited
Printed and bound in Malaysia by Vivar Printing Sdn Bhd

1   2012

Contents

Contributors, ix

Preface, xiii

Section One: Challenging professionalism

1 Physician care of family, friends, or colleagues, 3
Taku Taira, Joel Martin Geiderman

2 The impaired physician, 15
Peter Moffett, Christopher Kang

3 Disclosure of medical error and truth telling, 27
Abhi Mehrotra, Cherri Hobgood

4 Conflicts between patient requests and physician obligations, 37
Shellie L. Asher

5 Judgmental attitudes and opinions in the emergency department, 47
V. Ramana Feeser

6 Using physicians as agents of the state, 57
Jeremy R. Simon

Section Two: End-of-life decisions

7 Family-witnessed resuscitation in the emergency department: making sense of
ethical and practical considerations in an emotional debate, 69
Kirsten G. Engel, Arthur R. Derse

8 Palliative care in the emergency department, 79
Tammie E. Quest, Paul DeSandre

9 Refusal of life-saving therapy, 89
Catherine A. Marco, Arthur R. Derse

10 Revisiting comfort-directed therapies: death and dying in the
emergency department, including withholding and withdrawal
of life-sustaining treatment, 99
Raquel M. Schears, Terri A. Schmidt

11 Futility in emergency medicine, 117
Arthur R. Derse

Section Three: Representing vulnerable populations

12 The care of minors in the emergency department, 129
Chloë-Maryse Baxter

13 Chemical restraints, physical restraints, and other demonstrations of force, 139
    Michael P. Wilson, Christian M. Sloane

14 Capacity determination in the patient with altered mental status, 149
    Michael C. Tricoci, Catherine A. Marco

15 Obstetric emergency: perimortem cesarean section, 157
    Kenneth D. Marshall, Carrie Tibbles

Section Four: Outside influence and observation

16 Non-medical observers in the emergency department, 169
    Joel Martin Geiderman

17 Religious perspectives on do-not-resuscitate (DNR) documents and the dying patient, 179
    Avraham Steinberg

18 Non-physician influence on the scope and responsibilities of emergency physicians, 187
    Laura G. Burke, Jennifer V. Pope

19 Privacy and confidentiality: particular challenges in the emergency department, 197
    Jessica H. Stevens, Michael N. Cocchi

Section Five: Emergency medicine outside the emergency department

20 Short-term international medical initiatives, 209
    Matthew B. Allen, Christine Dyott, John Jesus

21 Disaster triage, 221
    Matthew B. Allen, John Jesus

22 The emergency physician as a bystander outside the hospital, 237
    Zev Wiener, Shamai A. Grossman

23 Military objectives versus patient interests, 247
    Kenneth D. Marshall, Kathryn L. Hall-Boyer

Section Six: Public health as emergency medicine

24 Treatment of potential organ donors, 261
    Glen E. Michael, John Jesus

25 Mandatory and permissive reporting laws: conflicts in patient confidentiality, autonomy, and the duty to report, 271
    Joel Martin Geiderman

26 Ethics of care during a pandemic, 287
    John C. Moskop

Section Seven: Education and research

27 Practicing medical procedures on the newly or nearly dead, 301
Ajay V. Jetley, Catherine A. Marco

28 Ethics of research without informed consent, 311
Dave W. Lu, Jonathan Burstein, John Jesus

Appendix: useful resources, 321
Alexander Bracey

Index, 325

Contributors

Matthew B. Allen, BA
Research Assistant, Department of Emergency Medicine
Brigham and Women's Hospital
Boston, MA, USA

Shellie L. Asher, MD, MSr
Associate Professor, Department of Emergency
    Medicine
Albany Medical College
Albany, NY, USA

Chloë-Maryse Baxter, MBChB, BSc MHPE
Pediatric Emergency Medicine Advanced Trainee
Sydney Children's Hospital
Randwick, NSW, Australia

Alexander Bracey, BS
Clinical Research Assistant
Beth Israel Deaconess Medical Center
Boston, MA, USA

Laura G. Burke, MD, MPH
Clinical Instructor of Medicine, Harvard Medical
    School
Harvard Affiliated Emergency Medicine Residency
Beth Israel Deaconess Medical Center
Boston, MA, USA

Jonathan Burstein, MD, FACEP
OEMS Medical Director, Commonwealth of
    Massachusetts
Assistant Professor, Harvard Medical School
Department of Emergency Medicine
Boston, MA, USA

Michael N. Cocchi, MD
Instructor of Medicine, Harvard Medical School
Attending Physician, Department of Emergency
    Medicine and Department of Anesthesia Critical
    Care
Associate Director, Critical Care Quality
Beth Israel Deaconess Medical Center
Boston, MA, USA

Arthur R. Derse, MD, JD FACEP
Director, Center for Bioethics and Medical Humanities
Julia and David Uihlein Professor of Medical
    Humanities
Professor of Bioethics and Emergency Medicine
Institute for Health and Society
Medical College of Wisconsin
Milwaukee, WI, USA

Paul DeSandre, DO
Assistant Chief, Section of Palliative Medicine
Atlanta VA Medical Center
Associate Program Director, Fellowship in Hospice
    and Palliative Medicine
Assistant Professor, Emergency Medicine and
    Hospice and Palliative Medicine
Emory University
Atlanta, GA, USA

Christine Dyott, BA
Clinical Research Assistant, Department of
    Emergency Medicine
Beth Israel Deaconess Medical Center
Boston, MA, USA

Kirsten G. Engel, MD
Assistant Professor, Department of Emergency Medicine
Feinberg School of Medicine
Northwestern University
Chicago, IL, USA

V. Ramana Feeser, MD
Assistant Professor of Emergency Medicine,
  Department of Emergency Medicine
Virginia Commonwealth University (VCU)
VCU Medical Center-Main Hospital
Richmond, VA, USA

Joel Martin Geiderman, MD, FACEP
Co-Chairman, Department of Emergency Medicine
Professor of Emergency Medicine, Cedars-Sinai
  Medical Center
Los Angeles, CA, USA

Shamai A. Grossman, MD, MS, FACEP
Vice Chair for Resource Utilization
Director, Cardiac Emergency Center
Division of Emergency Medicine
Beth Israel Deaconess Medical Center
Assistant Professor of Medicine, Harvard Medical
  School
Boston, MA, USA

Kathryn L. Hall-Boyer, MD, FACEP
CEP America, Attending Emergency Physician
Memorial Medical Center
Colonel, Army Reserve (Retired)
Modesto, CA, USA

Cherri Hobgood, MD
The Rolly McGrath Professor
Chair of Emergency Medicine, Department of
  Emergency Medicine
Indiana University School of Medicine
Indianapolis, IN, USA

John Jesus, MD
Chief Resident, Department of Emergency Medicine
Beth Israel Deaconess Medical Center, Boston, MA,
  USA
Clinical Instructor, Department of Emergency
  Medicine
Christiana Care Health System
Newark, DE, USA

Ajay V. Jetley, MD
Resident Physician, Department of Emergency
  Medicine
University of Toledo College of Medicine
Toledo, OH, USA

Christopher Kang, MD, FACEP, FAWM
Director of Research, Attending Physician,
  Department of Emergency Medicine
Madigan Army Medical Center
Tacoma, WA, USA

Dave W. Lu, MD, MBE
Acting Instructor, Department of Medicine
Division of Emergency Medicine
University of Washington School of Medicine
Seattle, WA, USA

Catherine A. Marco, MD, FACEP
Professor, Department of Emergency Medicine
University of Toledo College of Medicine
Toledo, OH, USA

Kenneth D. Marshall, MA, MD
Resident Physician, Department of Emergency
  Medicine
Beth Israel Deaconess Medical Center
Boston, MA, USA

Abhi Mehrotra, MD
Assistant Professor Emergency Medicine,
  Department of Emergency Medicine
University of North Carolina School of Medicine
Chapel Hill, NC, USA

Glen E. Michael, MD
Assistant Professor of Emergency Medicine
University of Virginia
Charlottesville, VA, USA

Peter Moffett, MD
Captain, United States Army
Medical Corps
Director of Research, Department of Emergency
  Medicine
Carl R. Darnall Army Medical Center
Fort Hood, TX, USA

John C. Moskop, PhD
Wallace and Mona Wu Chair in Biomedical Ethics
Professor of Internal Medicine, Wake Forest School
of Medicine
Winston-Salem, NC, USA

Jennifer V. Pope, MD
Clinical Instructor of Medicine, Harvard Medical
School
Assistant Residency Director
Harvard Affiliated Emergency Medicine Residency
Beth Israel Deaconess Medical Center
Boston, MA, USA

Tammie E. Quest, MD
Interim Director, Emory Palliative Care Center
Chief, Section of Palliative Medicine
Atlanta VAMC
Fellowship Director, Hospice and Palliative
Medicine
Division of Geriatrics and Gerontology
Associate Professor, Department of Emergency
Medicine
Director, EPEC-EM
Atlanta, GA, USA

Raquel M. Schears, MD, MPH
Associate Professor of Emergency Medicine,
Department of Emergency Medicine
Mayo Clinic
Mayo Graduate School of Medicine
Rochester, MN, USA

Terri A. Schmidt, MD, MS
Professor of Emergency Medicine, Department of
Emergency Medicine
Health and Science University
Portland, OR, USA

Jeremy R. Simon, MD, PhD
Assistant Professor of Clinical Medicine
Scholar-in-Residence, Center for Bioethics
Columbia University
New York, NY, USA

Christian M. Sloane, MD
Associate Clinical Professor of Emergency Medicine,
Department of Emergency Medicine
University of California
San Diego, CA, USA

Avraham Steinberg, MD
Professor and Director, Medical Ethics Unit
Senior Pediatric Neurologist
Shaare Zedek Medical Center
Jerusalem, Israel

Jessica H. Stevens, MD, MPH
Clinical Instructor, Harvard Affiliated Emergency
Medicine Residency Program
Beth Israel Deaconess Medical Center
Boston, MA, USA

Taku Taira, MD
Assistant Program Director
Assistant Clinical Professor, Department of
Emergency Medicine
Stony Brook University Medical Center
Stony Brook, NY, USA

Carrie Tibbles, MD
Instructor in Medicine at Harvard Medical School
Department of Emergency Medicine
Beth Israel Deaconess Medical Center
Boston, MA, USA

Michael C. Tricoci, MD
Resident, Department of Emergency Medicine
University of Toledo Medical Center
Toledo, OH, USA

Zev Wiener, BA
Medical Student
Harvard Medical School
Boston, MA, USA

Michael P. Wilson, MD, PhD
Clinical Research Fellow, Department of Emergency
Medicine
University of California
San Diego, CA, USA

Preface

The emergency department (ED) is a setting in which medicine is practiced with limited time and information, where relationships with patients are stressed and fleeting, and the diversity of population and the human condition is extraordinary. At once humbling and extreme, these situations are replete with ethical conflicts with which emergency clinicians continually grapple. This book is designed to consolidate the relevant literature as well as the thoughts of professionals currently working in the field into a practical and accessible reference for the emergency medical technician, student, nurse, resident, and attending emergency physician. Each chapter is divided into four sections: case presentation, discussion, review of the current literature, and recommendations. Designed to serve simultaneously as a learning and reference tool, each chapter begins with a real case that was encountered in an ED setting. The case presentation is followed by a short discussion of the case, as if at a morbidity and mortality conference, by a panel of experienced attending physicians explaining how they would approach the ethical dilemmas associated with the case, and a review of the existing literature. In the interests of convenience and ease of reading, in the discussion section, the male pronoun alone is often used when referring to a physician or patient. The concluding section contains recommendations, which, in and of themselves, may be used as a quick review and reference guide while caring for patients. Although the book is written from the viewpoint of physicians practicing in the USA, several principles would apply to physicians working in other countries as well.

The concept of this book originated from two sources: the first was a conversation with Richard Wolfe about the relative dearth of literature on ethical problems in emergency medicine. What does exist often appears to be theoretical, derived by professionals who do not practice emergency medicine and are oblivious to the nuances of making decisions in a severely time-constrained environment. The second source of inspiration came from the success of the discussion format used in the difficult airway section in the *Journal of Internal and Emergency Medicine*.

The case-based format of the book is based on the weekly morbidity and mortality conferences at the Beth Israel Deaconess Medical Center in Boston, Massachusetts, USA. This conference has been one of the most successful forms of education of our residency program in emergency medicine. We therefore felt there is educational value in presenting problems based on cases.[1] Each case is presented by the chapter author(s), and then discussed by a panel comprising the book's editors and special guests for the topic when appropriate. The editors were chosen to represent different institutions and schools of thought. We also deliberately chose editors and authors with different amounts of experience and practice, so that we could represent different generations of clinical practice. While we hoped to attain consensus on an approach to ethical dilemmas, you will quickly note that we rarely all agree. Common among all discussants, however, is a shared belief in human dignity and a respectful and collaborative approach to solving ethical problems.

Current medical literature places a heavy emphasis on "evidence" based on prior research. As one who reads any evidence-based literature knows, however, quality of evidence is hard to define, and is often referenced against the gold standard of a prospective, randomized clinical trial. Although clinical trials are possible within the field of medical ethics, generalizable answers to ethical dilemmas can be elusive. Contributing to this frustrating reality is the concept that there are no hardline principles or rules that apply to all ethical dilemmas. The often cited principles that serve as the basis for US federal regulations include respect for persons, justice, beneficence, and nonmaleficence. What is not as commonly understood, is that these principles are all equally important and should be used as a framework, rather than as strict rules, to assess moral problems in the pursuit of the "'greatest possible balance' of right over wrong."[2] We violate the principle of respect for persons when we physically and chemically restrain the agitated suicidal patient in the ED, for example, because we identify the beneficence in our efforts to protect patient safety from self-harm as more important. In addition, the value of life in and of itself is not among this list of principles obscuring what should be the fundamental tenet of ethics in medicine.

What about citing prior ethical opinions? This is, in fact, one of the foundations of medical ethics, that prior opinions are useful in helping one to decide what to do. Although useful considerations, they often will not solve a modern dilemma since attitudes change drastically on emotionally charged medical ethical issues. Although we will refer to opinions cited, we will not assign weight or term of evidence for such opinions. Instead, we hope to demonstrate realistic attitudes towards problems that are based not only on generation, but to some degree culture, and individual physician experience. This is not to provide an "answer" that will satisfy all, but rather perspective on how emergency physicians make ethical decisions.

We have tried to cover the major ethical dilemmas discussed in the emergency medicine literature over the past decade, in an attempt to make this work as relevant and useful as possible. That said, we are sure to have omitted important topics readers might deem more important than the ones we chose to discuss. Nevertheless, no book can be infinite in scope, and if our methodology works, readers may find insight herein that may better inform their decisions and approach to ethical problems not specifically discussed. The point of the book is to remember that ethical dilemmas in the ED occur on a daily basis. If one does not reflect on them and establish a coherent management strategy before they are encountered clinically, one can be paralyzed from acting appropri-ately. It is our hope that this book will help medical professionals reflect on ethical problems, and help guide their decisions before they encounter the real-life situations. We believe that while we may not have always reached a consensus about the ethical dilemmas discussed in this volume, the reader will understand that all decisions about ethical problems are not equal, that reasonable people can and will disagree over how ethical problems ought to be managed, and that there are some decisions that are clearly wrong. However, equally important during disagreements is a serious attempt at respectful resolution through reasoned argument. In the following pages, we hope to stimulate thought, discussion, and perspective on what are difficult ethical problems we all encounter in the modern practice of emergency medicine.

John Jesus, MD
Shamai A. Grossman, MD, MS, FACEP
Arthur R. Derse, MD, JD FACEP
James Adams, MD
Richard Wolfe, MD
Peter Rosen, MD, FACS, FACEP

References

1. Rosen R, Edlich RF, Rosen CL, et al. (2008) Becoming a specialist in emergency medicine. *J Emerg Med.* 34(4), 471–6.
2. Beauchamp TL, Childress JF. (2009) *Principles of Biomedical Ethics*, 6th ed. New York, NY: Oxford University Press, USA.

Challenging professionalism

Physician care of family, friends, or colleagues

Taku Taira,[1] Joel Martin Geiderman[2]

[1]Assistant Program Director and Assistant Clinical Professor, Department of Emergency Medicine, Stony Brook University Medical Center, Stony Brook, NY, USA
[2]Co-Chairman, Department of Emergency Medicine, Professor of Emergency Medicine, Cedars-Sinai Medical Center, Los Angeles, CA, USA

Section I: Case presentation

Dr. Ralph Smith is a 50-year-old emergency physician who has been practicing for 20 years. The 10-year-old son of one of the other emergency physicians, with whom Dr. Smith has worked for 15 years, is brought in by his parents for a 3-cm simple laceration on the mentum of the chin. Dr. Smith is asked by the charge nurse to see this patient. What is the proper response?

Dr. Ralph Rogers' cousin Bob and wife Joan are visiting from Texas, and their luggage is lost. The airline informs them that they have no idea where their luggage is, and cannot give them an estimate of when they will be able to locate and deliver the bags. All of Joan's medications were in her checked luggage. On the way to Dr. Rogers' house, she stops by the emergency department (ED) where he is working, asks him to come to the waiting room, and then requests him to write her prescriptions. Dr. Rogers knows Joan is a smoker and has some mild chronic obstructive pulmonary disease and hypertension, but does not know any more of her medical history. She is on an albuterol inhaler, furosemide, atenolol, sertraline, and alprazolam. How should Dr. Rogers handle this situation?

Dr. Walter St. John is the Chairman of the ED at a large metropolitan hospital, and has been on staff for 30 years. Dr. Bob Schwartz, an internist on staff for the past 25 years is brought in with vomiting, diarrhea, abdominal pain, and fever. Should Dr. St. John treat Dr. Schwartz?

Dr. Elliott Alexander is on duty at a busy ED with several physicians on duty. His brother, age 63, presents with paroxysmal atrial fibrillation with a rapid response. His vital signs are: blood pressure 80/50 mmHg; heart rate 140–150 per minute; respiratory rate 20 minute; temperature 37.2 °C. The patient would like his brother to take care of him. What should Dr. Alexander do?

Section II: Discussion

Dr. Peter Rosen: As I remember the Hippocratic Oath, it does not restrict who your patients should be. In fact, it gives special attention to the care we all owe to our physician teachers and their families. What then are the ethical issues that prevent most physicians from caring for their friends and family?

Dr. Joel Geiderman: One issue to consider is patient autonomy, and whether or not they are situated in a position to refuse care when they know their caregiver socially. Then again, there are also those patients who really want us to take care of them, because they know and trust us. Each situation requires a different approach.

Ethical Problems in Emergency Medicine: A Discussion-Based Review, First Edition. John Jesus, Shamai A. Grossman, Arthur R. Derse, James G. Adams, Richard Wolfe, and Peter Rosen.
© 2012 John Wiley & Sons, Ltd. Published 2012 by John Wiley & Sons, Ltd.

Dr. Taku Taira: The issues are definitely not black and white, but rather should be viewed as a sliding scale of what interventions are acceptable. The salient question is whether the preexisting relationship will impede good medical care. Then, a secondary consideration concerns the clinician's ability to respect patient autonomy, and to abide by all the other ethical principles by which we are supposed to practice.

PR: What is it specifically about patient autonomy that concerns you?

TT: Every patient must have the right to refuse care, and ought to expect to have an appropriate patient–physician relationship. The danger lies in the potential to consciously or subconsciously influence patients into having treatments, with which they feel uncomfortable, by nature of the shared non-medical relationship.

PR: One example of when patient autonomy may suffer is when the patient is an employee of the physician. Secondary to the mixture of relationships, the employee might not feel comfortable refusing the physician's recommendations. A similarly stressed relationship exists in professional sports, where athletes don't have the opportunity to choose their own physician, and are under an incredible amount of pressure to play, even if they have to play through injuries. One of the most prevalent situations, however, is a physician caring for their own children or spouse.

Dr. James Adams: That said, when I was growing up, our family practitioner took care of all of his own children. He would have been offended at the thought of taking his kids to another doctor. The problem, as I see it, concerns a physician's loss of objectivity when caring for friends and family. At some point, we're not able to objectively assess a child because we're too close to the situation. It's hard to be a parent **and** the doctor.

PR: It also depends on the circumstances. Attitudes towards treating your own family have changed significantly over the course of my professional lifetime. I used to work in a small town in Wyoming. The day my wife went into labor, she ruptured her membranes, but didn't progress. There were no other doctors in town that week, and after some scrambling I found a gynecologist 90 miles away. Out of necessity, I had to help perform the c-section on my wife; I would not have chosen to do this if I had any other options.

I also had a couple of nights during which I sat up all night with a child trying to decide whether the child needed to go to surgery. If I had decided that surgery was necessary, I would have been the surgeon as there were no other surgeons for 80 miles or more. Trying to write rules about what is acceptable should take into consideration what alternatives are available. Yet, I have also found in treating my family that they only respect my advice when they agree with it.

JG: One reasonable argument against physicians caring for their friends and family is highlighted by the situation in which a bad outcome occurs. I would imagine that a family death would be devastating to the treating physician. Physicians should protect themselves from this situation. This may only be possible, however, by trying to avoid caring for a truly ill family member.

Here is the other side of the story. When my son was about 5 and a half, he fell off of his bicycle and sustained a simple laceration to his chin. When we arrived home with his wrecked bike, I informed my wife that he needed to be sutured. On the automobile ride to the ED, my son said, "Daddy, I want you to do it." I turned to my wife and asked, "What do you want me to do? I want you to feel comfortable. Would you rather call a plastic surgeon?" She looked at me like I was crazy and said, "Of course, I want you to do it." At that point, I didn't feel that I was in a position to call anyone else, and sutured him myself. He will never forget it and neither will I. To us, the experience was invaluable.

PR: I've sewn up my children. Although, I will admit that one of them took out his sutures faster than I could put them in, and didn't have a great result. I really think that ethically there is nothing wrong with taking care of members of your own family. When you feel that you don't have the requisite knowledge or skill, or you feel that someone else can do a better job, then you should involve another physician.

Historically, institutions have set limits on this practice when physicians attempt to treat family members, colleagues, and friends without charging them and without documenting a record of the interaction. This is a mistake, as a physician should document the same way for any patient. I've always felt badly about having to charge other physicians. I was raised with the notion that we took care of each other without charge—but we aren't permitted to do that anymore.

Physicians must use some judgment about where to draw the line regarding what is and is not acceptable. I didn't particularly like operating on members of my own family (when I was a surgeon), and wouldn't have chosen to do so. That said, I was willing to do it when there was no other option. I agree, I would have felt terrible had any of those family members had a poor outcome, as I feel about any of my patients who don't do well.

Dr. Arthur Derse: I don't know of any legal restrictions, but the ethical problem I most identify with in treating colleagues is also the loss of objectivity. In treating colleagues and family members, you may not conduct as thorough an examination or you may avoid certain tests, and your patients may not disclose all the important information that will allow you to make an accurate diagnosis. For example, Groopman, in writing about medical error, wrote about an error he made when caring for a patient he really liked, because he deferred a buttock examination that would have allowed him to discover the abscess causing his colleague's symptoms.[1]

I will remember forever a young teenage woman I saw, the daughter of some friends, who presented with some vague symptoms and appeared a little lethargic. At the time, I thought I would pursue my infectious workup with the exception of a lumbar puncture (LP), because "that's too much." I then thought better of that decision, because I felt that I would have performed an LP on any other patient. She did, of course, have bacterial meningitis, and I have been phenomenally thankful ever since for having performed the procedure. My own objectivity and judgment were clouded, because I struggled with sparing the daughter of friends an uncomfortable procedure.

In addition, although I think most colleagues would level with us if we were to inquire about important parts of their history, there are also some people who might not disclose their sexual or psychiatric histories. There are risks to not getting the complete history.

PR: The problem I think is not with the colleague, but with the notion that special patients deserve special care (also known as VIP care). We see this with some frequency—systems seem to shut down or work less efficiently when someone of importance presents to the ED.

We should have special mechanisms for reacting to patients like these. Frequently, the professional who evaluates the patient isn't the physician who would normally evaluate the patient, but rather a chair of the division who hasn't seen a patient primarily in 10 years. We administer terrible care when we approach patients in this way. When President Eisenhower had an operation for his inflammatory bowel disease, the army surgeon who performed the procedure admitted using an approach he wasn't used to, because he thought the approach was safer, and he didn't want to perform a risky procedure on the President of the United States. This approach is wrong. We should provide the same best care for the President of the United States as we provide to the janitor of the White House.

JG: When I was growing up there was the expression "a doctor's doctor": The connotation being that you could receive no greater compliment than the opportunity to care for your physician colleagues. When a physician patient has been on staff for 15 years, as described in one of our cases, it is nearly impossible to find a physician, to treat him or his family, who doesn't know the patient. At some point, the argument that a physician should never care for a colleague becomes ridiculous, as there will be instances where that is impossible. It's my personal style to give patients a choice when I approach someone I know while I am on shift, "Do you want me to take care of you, or would you prefer someone else?"

TT: I would echo that there has to willingness on both sides to be able to recognize that one or the other isn't comfortable with the current patient–physician relationship. This is especially true of the treating physician who must respect the possible lack of objectivity, and do some introspection to determine if he is able to provide a professional service despite knowing the patient.

I had a friend of mine stop by the ED while I was working to talk to me about some upper abdominal pain he was experiencing. We didn't talk for very long before I realized that I would need to perform a rectal examination, and I said, "You know, I'm going to step out." I asked one of my colleagues to take over, letting him know the patient was a friend of mine, and I couldn't take care of him.

JG: We are also approached frequently by a technician, nurse, or a volunteer for prescriptions and medical advice which presents a dilemma. We instituted a policy dictating the need for documentation; it's not that I wanted to charge them for the visit, but we insisted on a record. In fact, I usually offer to write off their bill.

PR: There are also unknown patients who drop in, want a really minor degree of medical care, and say, "I've lost my prescriptions, and I'm here from out of town." I used to practice part time in an area where this situation occurred almost every shift. I don't see it as an ethical problem as much as I see it a logistic problem. How can you process patients like this quickly and accurately enough to be safe. If the patient can say, "This is my medicine, formulation and dose; can you fill the script for me," then I am happy to provide them with it. But when they don't know the dose, or are not sure that the indication still exists, and I can't reach a physician or get hold of their records, it's a difficult situation. What sort of legal risk does a physician expose himself to when he attempts to address this situation? Are there ways to stay out of trouble, and still provide these patients with appropriate medical care?

AD: There is no question that a physician's impulse when presented with a patient who requests prescriptions because they've forgotten their own, or their luggage has been lost, is to provide them with the necessary prescriptions. If a physician doesn't have the patient's medical record, it is much harder to defend the practice should a problem arise, or if there is a dispute as to what actually happened during the doctor–patient encounter. The situation is even more difficult when the patient requests prescriptions for controlled substances.

On the issue of prescribing a medication for someone you haven't seen or examined, I generally would not recommend the practice as it exposes a physician to tremendous legal risk, and the patient to the possibility of a bad outcome that may have been avoided had the physician performed an appropriate history and physical examination. Internists and clinicians who take call are a little more willing than are emergency physicians to prescribe medication for colleagues for whom they are covering, and for patients who they haven't interviewed or examined. I believe this too is ethically and legally problematic because, without a physical examination to assess the patient you do stand on less firm ground.

JA: There are more basic factors to consider. A basic responsibility is to be a competent doctor, and writing prescriptions willy-nilly when you're uncertain what the patient's medical problems are or what the physical examination might reveal is just bad medicine. We had one emergency medicine nurse whose husband complained of headaches for 4 months, to which she kept telling him to stop being a baby; she quickly changed her opinion and response once he was diagnosed with a brain tumor—yet another example of bad judgment and overreach. I'm very willing to write prescriptions, but I am extra cautious about those prescriptions I write for people I know well, because I don't want to make any mistakes, and I don't really want to be abused or called at all times of the night. The driving issue is providing good medical care, and recognizing when you cannot provide that care and excusing yourself when appropriate.

JG: In California, writing prescriptions for controlled substances without seeing the patient is not allowed. Physicians are routinely disciplined for violating this proscription. I'm on the credentialing committee at the American Board of Emergency Medicine (ABEM), and currently their policy requires that every license a diplomate holds be unrestricted. If a physician receives a citation and a restriction of any sort to his or her medical license, ABEM will pull the physician's certification until the restriction is corrected.

PR: Most of the clinicians who have trouble with these rules are writing controlled substance prescriptions. It's a good rule of thumb to avoid writing prescriptions for controlled substance to any family members or friends. Regarding the situation when a pharmacy calls about a patient that was seen on the previous shift—if you have the information and the record of his visit, why wouldn't you write the script for the pharmacist? On the other hand, if you don't have enough information from the record to make a good judgment, then you may have to determine a way to discover more information. I've had a couple of cases where I've actually had the pharmacist put the patient on the phone, so that I could conduct an interview on the phone, and find out exactly what was needed.

TT: This occurs at our institution on a daily basis. Most of the time, the patient has been discharged with a prescription for a medication that isn't covered by the insurance. I would argue that as a member of a group practice and being a physician with access to most patients' records, that we don't expose ourselves to any increased legal risk in participating in this practice.

PR: What I don't like to do is curbside medicine for a friend or a colleague. I'll never forget a case where one of the nurses brought a friend in for an injection of penicillin, because he thought he had been exposed to gonorrhea but didn't first ask him what his allergies were. Quite suddenly, I was called in to see a patient who wasn't even registered but was having a major anaphylactic reaction. This practice is simply bad judgment and bad medicine.

I think we all have to be very careful. I remember as a surgical resident operating on a patient who had a perforated diverticulitis. The surgeon said that he had known the patient for 40 years, and that he couldn't make a colostomy for her, because "she couldn't live with a colostomy." I was a second-year resident at the time, and said that everything I had read up until that point indicated that the appropriate intervention in a person with perforated diverticulitis was to operate and create a colostomy. He replied that he thought she would do fine. I went away from that operation thinking that he had just killed this patient, because he was afraid to inconvenience her or embarrass her. She, in fact, had a very rough postoperative course, which taught me a lesson for the rest of my professional life—when you think you might change your usual practice, you had better have some logical reason or good evidence to support your decision, because the worst thing you can do for a patient that you care about is the wrong intervention.

Section III: Review of the literature

Physician treatment of self, family, friends, and colleagues is common practice. Physicians are often asked for medical advice or treatment for a variety of conditions ranging from the simple to the life-threatening. Studies show that the majority of physicians have provided some level of medical care to family members, colleagues, or themselves.[2-4] This practice is common because there are benefits for both the patient and physician. There may be enormous psychological, professional, relationship, or familial benefits to treating patients who fall into these respective categories. By treating friends, family members, or colleagues, physicians may experience increased stature and respect, and may have improved self-esteem, gratification, confidence, and psychological wellbeing. The patients they treat, in general may thus benefit. The patient benefits from having a physician who's "deep personal investment in the patient's well-being motivates a degree of attention to detail and humanistic thoughtfulness that might otherwise be sadly lacking."[5] Close relatives may feel that they are getting something in return for the long hours the physician spends away from them.

Despite being common, the practice raises ethical concerns. Physicians intuitively acknowledge that there is a boundary between appropriate and inappropriate behavior. A physician described this as "this dangerous feeling that we all have of getting in there and doing something."[5] The American Medical Association (AMA) *Code of Medical Ethics* recommends that, "physicians generally should not treat themselves or members of their immediate families."[6] An exception is made for the treatment of emergencies, and short-term and minor problems, and when practicing in isolated settings.[6-8] The codes of ethics of the American College of Physicians and American Association of Pediatrics expand this recommendation to also advise against the treatment of friends and closely associated employees.[7] In the case of minor problems, the consensus is that "care may be given by the physician in the family without overwhelming his or her objectivity or breaching ethical principles, and with much convenience to all concerned."[9]

Although it is important that the medical societies recognize the existence of the ethical issues, their recommendations are based on consensus and anecdote, and lack concrete guidelines. There are no definitions or examples of "short-term and minor problems." These exceptions could conceivably be applied to the majority of requests. "Physicians have reportedly treated everything from hypertension to diabetes to mental disorders under the guise of minor ailments."[10]

The lack of definitions shifts the onus onto the judgment of the individual physician. Although it is reasonable to expect physicians to apply their judgment, they may be forced to do so when it is most likely to be clouded by emotions, altruism, and sometimes hubris.

Despite being a common practice with ethical concerns, this issue is rarely discussed in the journals, graduate and undergraduate medical education, nationally, or in the media. Within emergency medicine, none of the national societies have made any statements regarding the treatment of friends and family, let alone made any recommendations. Without discussions and debate among physicians, there is no way that we can build towards a general consensus that can be used to guide us. It is as if "there are rules but no rulebook."[5]

The ethical principles to consider are beneficence—the duty to do what is best for the patient; non-maleficence—to prevent the patient from being harmed; and autonomy—to do what the patients truly wishes for them. The following sections will explore the complex interplay of all of these forces as physicians are called on to treat family, friends, or colleagues. As we shall see, the path forward is not necessarily obvious.

Potential risks and benefits to the patient

For the physician who is asked to care for a family member, friend or colleague, the first inclination is to want to say yes. However, that initial reaction is often followed by unease. The physician's unease comes from acknowledgment of the difficulty in providing good medical care for those with special emotional closeness. Physicians have a responsibility to act in the best interest of the patient, even if doing so may cause the patient discomfort, pain, or embarrassment. The role of a friend or a family member is to care for that person, and to shield them from harm. When the patient is emotionally close to the physician, these two goals should be synergistic; however, in practical application these roles can be antagonistic.

The loss of objectivity leading to suboptimal care is the most commonly cited argument against the treatment of friends and family. Physicians have been known to change their usual and regular practice when evaluating a friend or family member. These changes include inadequate histories, avoiding probing into the patient's social history, or deferring intimate examinations in an effort to avoid patient and physician discomfort.[11] Incomplete physical examinations are not limited to deferring genital examinations; "performing a mental status examination on a close relative may be more difficult than examining the relative's body."[12] Although the change from standard practice is understandable, the combination of emotional closeness and the lack of perspective make it difficult to correct these errors. Ironically, the physician fails in his or her role as both physician and friend when they expose the patient to risk by their inadequate evaluation.

The potential problems from the loss of objectivity are most pronounced in the treatment of patients who are very ill. With sick patients, the potential treatments have greater risks and thus require a greater degree of objectivity. The greater need for objectivity occurs at the same time that judgment is obscured by emotional involvement. The loss of objectivity can lead to either failing to pursue risky but necessary interventions, or the pursuit of medically contraindicated or ineffective therapies thereby placing the patient's health and dignity at risk.

The exception allowing for the treatment of "minor problems" is not a shield against the dangers associated with the loss of objectivity. It is very easy for the physician to approach the care of a friend or family member with either a "wellness bias" or a "sickness bias." As emergency physicians, we are especially attuned to the possibility that a simple chief complaint may in fact be caused by a serious or even life-threatening condition. As a person close to the patient, we want to believe that the person is well. When this wellness bias is combined with incomplete history and physical examination, it can be difficult to pick up on subtle cues pointing towards a serious illness. Conversely the physician may have a desire to make a "great diagnosis" ignoring the fact that most patients with minor complaints are well. This sickness bias can lead to over-testing and over-diagnosis.

The difficult balance between the physician's role as friend or family member and as a physician is especially pronounced when the evaluation reveals that the patient has a serious or life threatening diagnosis. The role of the physician is to inform the patient of the diagnosis and medical implications, and to discuss treatment. As a friend or family member, the role is to provide caring and emotional support.

When the physician has a dual role, both the physician and the patient can suffer. The patient can suffer from either having a physician who is unable to objectively answer questions about the condition, or having a family member who is emotionally unavailable. The physician suffers from an additional psychological burden of having to give bad news to a loved one and struggling to do so.

Another barrier to developing a therapeutic physician–patient relationship when caring for friends or family is that it is difficult, if not impossible, for both the patient and physician to enter a patient–physician relationship and discard the preceding relationship. The typical patient–physician relationship is asymmetric.[13] The physician has knowledge that the patient does not have, as well as the ability to provide therapies that the patient cannot provide for himself or herself. This is in contrast to the symmetric relationship between the physician and a colleague or a spouse.

When the preceding relationship is based on equality, both the physician and the patient may have difficulty in assuming their new roles. It is hard to predict or measure the consequences of the previous relationship. The patient may have difficulty accepting the physician's authority in the medical evaluation, especially with recommendations that the patient disagrees with, leading to poor treatment compliance. On the other hand, it is possible that a patient may be **more** likely to assert his or her autonomy with a physician to whom they are close. It's possible they will be more open in expressing fears, preferences or anxieties leading to better compliance and outcomes.

The physician caring for a work subordinate, such as an employee, introduces additional potential risks and benefits. Both parties enter the relationship with the physician as the superior. The distance between the superior and the subordinate can be magnified further in the physician–patient relationship. This added distance might make it difficult for the patient to disagree with the physician's recommendation introducing the possibility of coercion. It is equally possible that the patient can build on a base of previously earned trust. The patient may be more likely to accept a difficult recommendation that is in the patient's best interest because of an accumulation of trust, which may lead to better outcomes.

Establishing a therapeutic physician–patient relationship can be especially difficult when the patient is a physician colleague. There are several barriers that exist when caring for any physician. To begin with, physicians are less likely in general to seek medical care, leading to an unfamiliarity with the patient role.[14] When the physician is a patient, there is disorientation because "the familiar aspects of the hospital are unrecognizable from a stretcher."[12] The physician as a patient may enter the relationship "unable to dissociate the individual and the new role from the previous expectations, and from vestiges of the former identity in the old role."[15] This applies to the difficulty for the physician accepting the new relationship with the treating physician and the medical staff, as well the medical system.

Both physician and patient anxiety and frustration may be exacerbated if the illness or complaint falls within the expertise of the physician patient.[16] Such a situation can lead to therapeutic and diagnostic negotiations that lead to over- and under-testing and treatment. It can increase the treating physician's anxiety, leading to timidity. The converse is equally dangerous. The treating physician may falsely assume that the physician patient has the same level of knowledge and expertise with regards to the medical complaint. As a result, the physician may fully explain the risks and benefits as would be done for a non-physician patient, leading to poor choices by the patient and physician.

When the physician patient is a colleague, there are additional potential barriers. Physicians often choose a personal physician on the basis of a previous relationship, and not on objective factors.[17] The patient may have chosen the physician because of the previous collegial relationship, and a desire to maintain that collegiality in the patient–physician relationship. Choosing a physician on the basis of social interactions can "further compound the development of a working doctor–patient relationship."[18]

Risks and benefits to the physician

The potential risks are not limited to the patient. Physicians who take care of friends or family are exposed to personal risk. Medical involvement can "provoke or intensify intrafamilial conflicts . . . [as the physician is] thrust into the lead as hero or scapegoat, depending on the course of the family member's illness."[9] The risks to interpersonal relationships exist regardless of the physician's choice about involvement. Patient, family, and colleagues may be hurt because the physician was "not willing" to help them, even if the physician refuses for noble reasons. Different expectations from different family members can lead to conflicts, no matter what the physician decides to do.

The greatest risk to the physician is psychological. In treating friends, family, or a colleague, the physician may experience a great deal of anxiety, mostly from a desire to "get it right." The psychological impact of the death, disability or even morbidity (due to complications) of a friend or family member may be devastating if the physician had a direct role in or responsibility for the poor outcome.

Physicians should consider the legal risks they expose themselves to by providing informal care. Regardless of the physician's or the patient's perception of a request for medical care, providing medical advice to a person constitutes the establishment of a patient–physician relationship. As a result, the physician is legally liable for the consequences of the advice. In addition, the majority of casual medical interactions have no documentation, making the practice difficult to defend when there is a negative outcome.

Refusal of care

Both the physician and the patient may experience a difficult time saying "no," when it comes to a patient being cared for by a person with whom they enjoy a special relationship. Both parties must be free to acquiesce or not, and the choices should be independent, not reciprocal. The sense of duty and a desire to be a good colleague or family member plays a role in the physician's willingness to provide care, but may lead to the provision of care against one's better judgment.[3]

Even though the majority of physicians have provided some degree of medical care to friends and family, a majority of physicians have also refused requests.[4] It is rare that a physician would agree to all requests for treatment. Common causes for physician refusal include: requests for care outside of one's area of expertise, inadequate ability to follow up, inadequate opportunity for examination, absence of medical indication for the request, and lack of objectivity.[4]

It is clear that there is a sliding scale of appropriate and inappropriate treatments. In examining the char-

acteristics of physician treatment of family members, La Puma et al. find that the majority of physicians have provided some degree of medical care for family members. Moreover, 22% of physicians honor a request for treatment by a family member with which they felt uncomfortable, and 33% of physicians observe another physician who was "inappropriately involved" in a family member's care. Physicians report performing elective invasive surgeries and procedures such as angiography, colectomy, and pacemaker placement.[4] Although these procedures may be routine for the physician they can hardly be called minor.

The practical question remains, for any given situation, when should a physician refuse to perform medical treatment for family or friends? "Is this ethics, etiquette, or just sound judgment?" Whether family members will receive high quality care from a related doctor, or whether they would be better off seeing someone else, probably depends on the judgment of the physician, the medical urgency of the case, and the availability of medical colleagues."[4] Several authors have proposed self-reflective questions to guide physicians considering treating a friend or family member (Box 1.1). In addition to self-reflections, the physician should consider several characteristics of the request itself. These include: the chief complaint, the setting, the person making the request, and patient expectation.

The physician should first consider the chief complaint. There are complaints that have a predictable workup and a low risk of a poor outcome. These include problems such as mild ankle pain, or rhinorrhea during allergy season with no constitutional symptoms. However "family members may also request care that requires a complete history and physical examination, new knowledge, or facilities that are unavailable, thus sometimes embarrassing and frustrating the physician relatives."[4] The physician should be wary when the chief complaint has a less predictable diagnostic workup or clinical course, or if there is a possibility of a serious underlying condition.

The request for medical care in the informal setting, or the "curbside" evaluation, can be problematic. Although it may be convenient for the patient, the curbside evaluation may magnify some negative aspects of the treatment of friends and family. By its informal nature, there is a tendency for the physician

Box 1.1 Self-reflective questions to guide physicians in the treatment of friends and family

- Am I trained to meet my patient's medical needs?
- Am I too close to probe my relative's intimate history and physical being and to cope with bearing bad news?
- Can I be objective enough to not give too much, too little, or inappropriate care? To do or order necessary procedures that may cause pain?
- Will my relatives comply more readily with medical care delivered by an unrelated physician?
- Am I willing to be accountable to my peers and to the public for this care?[9]
- Can I maintain an appropriate doctor–patient relationship or is an inappropriate collegial rapport likely to ensue?
- Do I have excessive anxiety that may jeopardize my ability to care for family, a colleague or friend?
- Can I maintain the patient's confidentiality?
- Can I always act for the good of the patient even if it means making decisions that may jeopardize the friendship?[18]
- Can I anticipate and negotiate family conflicts?[4]

can ensure alignment of the patient and physician expectations, desires, as well as affording both parties the ability to terminate the relationship without guilt or anxiety.

When a physician makes a decision about providing care, he or she should remember that responsibility of the physician is first and foremost to protect the health of the patient. The physician should "act for the good of the patient even if it means making decisions that may jeopardize the friendship."[18] Even though physicians are more highly motivated to help those who are closest to them, greater emotional distance may afford greater objectivity and a better medical outcome.[3]

Although physicians may feel pressure to be involved, refusing to be directly involved does not equate to an unwillingness to help. The physician is still available for love, caring, and emotional support. The physician can aid the medical care through access to the medical system through direct referral to a trusted colleague, or advocacy within the hospital.

Special circumstances

Under most circumstances there is no ethical obligation to treat a patient. However when "no other physician is available, as is the case in some isolated communities or when emergency treatment is required . . . the physician is morally bound to provide care."[7] This situation would be common in rural areas, and in times of disaster and war. If the patient has a life-threatening emergency, it would be prudent to reevaluate the appropriateness of the relationship as circumstances allow.

The emergency medicine perspective

The practice of emergency medicine has many unique aspects to it, yet, as previously noted, there is little available to specifically guide emergency physicians through this dilemma. None of the literature that was reviewed was published in an emergency medicine journal; we could find no emergency medicine book chapters that addressed this; and the organized emergency medicine groups are silent on the issue. Some hospital bylaws address the issue, but often in vague terms that lack specificity for the emergency physician.

to be overly casual in the evaluation. Even if the physician wanted to perform a complete evaluation it is impossible in an informal setting. This is especially true if the request is for a third party person who is not the actually consulting the physician. In such a situation, there is an increased risk for incorrect diagnosis, improper treatment, and medication-related risks. Further the informal nature of the request may increase the social pressure to "help" the person.

The physician should consider requests made by the patient, and requests made by staff or the patient's family member differently. When the patient has not made the request, they may not truly want to be treated by that physician, and should be allowed to exert autonomy. Upfront discussions with the patient

11

Most policies that do exist have exceptions allowing for care of family during emergencies and for short-term and minor ailments. The terms "emergency," "family," "minor," and "short term" are all open to interpretation. No literature or policies specifically address treatment of friends or colleagues. In point of fact, these groups are different and require different approaches.

Family

Some policies that proscribe treatment of family members specifically confine this to immediate family members, but other polices, including those adopted at one of the authors' hospitals (JMG) is much more expansive and includes aunts, uncles, in-laws, and even ex-in-laws. However, there are still exceptions for emergencies and minor conditions. It is clear that there is a sliding scale rather than hard and fast rules. For reasons outlined above, emergency physicians should avoid treatment of serious illnesses or performing complicated procedures on family members to whom they are emotionally close, unless absolutely necessary. Rendering minor care may be acceptable.

In fact, drawing a line on treating family members that begins at the ED entrance is somewhat arbitrary. If the spouse of an emergency physician awakens him or her because their child has fever, who would expect that the doctor would not look at the child, and render an opinion as to whether or not they needed to go to the hospital? The examination might even include looking in the ears with an otoscope or checking the neck for meningismus. There is always the chance that the initial decision may be wrong, but how does one separate oneself from the fact that he or she is a family member and a doctor at the same time? Further, rendering an opinion that precludes taking the child to a doctor or the hospital could help avoid unnecessary tests or treatment. Taking the child to the hospital, where caregivers are likely to know that the parent is a doctor, might bias them into thinking the child is sicker than actually is the case. There are biases and risks associated with any course.

Friends

It is similarly hard to draw hard and fast rules regarding friends. Similar to the interaction with family, for many friends of the emergency physician, the physi-

cian's advice (which constitutes the practice of medicine) is often rendered well before they ever get to the ED. In some cases, friends will prefer that they or their family are taken care of by the emergency physician they know, and they may even expect it or be upset if the physician demurs. It is not always clear if such care will be better, worse, or the same, as could be rendered by another physician. Some doctors might feel compelled to over-test while others, because they understand the human nature of their friend and may be able to provide close personal follow-up, may save the patient from needless tests.

For emergency physicians who have lived and worked in the same neighborhood and hospital for many years, it is likely they will see friends, acquaintances, fellow religious organization members, etc., often, perhaps even on a daily basis. It is hard to avoid treating these patients, and in many cases they will expect it, and desire it. It may make them feel special. There is little downside in providing such care in routine circumstances.

It is probably best to avoid rendering care to very sick friends to whom one is emotionally close (or their very sick immediate family members) for reasons that have been previously discussed, unless there is no other choice. The physician can then be free to serve as a friend and confidant, and is free to offer advice and counsel.

The emergency physician may be called on by friends to write or refill prescriptions. This is fraught with dangers, both legally and from a regulatory standpoint.[10,18] In addition, prescribing controlled substances to persons a physician has not examined may result in licensure problems. It is best for the emergency physician to adopt a firm policy against writing prescriptions for friends (and for that matter family or colleagues) unless they are formally seeing them in the ED setting.

Colleagues

Physicians who work in the same hospital regularly for many years are likely to know many of the medical staff, nurses, and others fairly well. Similarly, particularly for active medical staff members, they are likely to know all the emergency physicians. Therefore, if a physician colleague presents to the ED for care, some colleague will have to be the one to render care. This arrangement should not present any major ethical problems as long as the emergency physician maintains objectivity and professionalism, and does not alter what would be done for another patient in a similar situation Moreover, an emergency physician choosing to be cared for at their own institution by another specialist is likely to choose a colleague for care. There are always risks of hard feelings or a spoiled relationship if things do not go well, but these are risks a physician always is subject to when practicing the profession.

The colleague presenting to the ED, may have a preference for one emergency physician over another. Some attempt should be made to assure that the colleague can make as autonomous a choice as possible, but since it an emergency visit, it may not be possible to accommodate the wish. Traditionally, physicians have treated colleagues and their families free of charge, in some ways influenced by the Hippocratic Oath, the writings of Thomas Percival, and the rich traditions of the profession. Nowadays, compliance (anti-kickback) laws place limits on our ability to do this. Physicians should neither waive a payment as an inducement, nor decide to treat a colleague purely for financial gain.

Confidentiality

Confidentiality is almost always a primary duty of physicians. In treating family, friends, or colleagues, human nature may tempt physicians even more than usual to violate this duty. Nevertheless, unless confidentiality can be completely assured, and the integrity of the EP is known to be above reproach, patients may be reluctant to disclose necessary information to physicians. This is another danger in entering into a therapeutic relationship with these individuals. Physicians who do not adhere to expected confidentiality in these situations are committing an even greater ethical breach than when they violate the same duty with strangers; in addition to violating a professional duty, they have disregarded a personal trust.

Section IV: Recommendations

• Objective research should be done on the actual positive and negative effects of caring for family, friends, and colleagues in the emergency setting.
• Professional emergency medicine societies and other influential bodies should promulgate policies to guide emergency physicians.

• Emergency physicians should avoid treating first-degree relatives in the hospital setting, except for minor, routine situations, unless there is no alternative. The decision to treat other relatives should be based on the complexity of the situation, emotional distance, and the estimated ability to remain objective.
• Treating friends and colleagues in the emergency setting is mostly an acceptable practice.
• In deciding to treat family, friends, or colleagues, an earnest attempt should be made to ascertain their true autonomous choice as to physician.
• Confidentiality must be adhered to except in extraordinary circumstances, e.g., in order to save a life or to prevent bodily harm.

References

1. Groopman J. (2007) What's the trouble? How doctors think. *The New Yorker*, January 29.
2. Fromme EK, Farber NJ, Babbott SF, et al. (2008) What do you do when your loved one is ill? The line between physician and family member. *Ann Intern Med.* 149(11), 825–31.
3. Aboff B, Collier V, Farber NJ, et al. (2002) Residents' prescription writing for nonpatients. *JAMA.* 288, 381–5.
4. La Puma J, Stocking C, La Voie D. (1991) When physicians treat members of their own families. Practices in a community hospital. *New Engl J Med.* 325, 1290–4.
5. Chen FM, Feudtner C, Rhodes LA, et al. (2001) Role conflicts of physicians and their family members: rules but no rulebook. *West J Med.* 175(4), 236.
6. American Medical Association. (2006) Self treatment or treatment of immediate family members. Section 8.19. In: *Code of Medical Ethics: Current Opinions with Annotations.* Chicago: American Medical Association (updated 2006).
7. Snyder L, Leffler C, Ethics and Human Rights Committee ACoP. (2005) Ethics manual: 5th edition. *Ann Intern Med.* 142(7), 560–82.
8. Bioethics Co. (2009) From the American Academy of Pediatrics: Policy statements—Pediatrician-family-patient relationships: managing the boundaries. *Pediatrics.* 124(6), 1685–8.
9. La Puma J, Priest E. (1992) Is there a doctor in the house? An analysis of the practice of physicians' treating their own families. *JAMA.* 267, 1810–2.
10. Krall EJ. (2008) Doctors who doctor self, family, and colleagues. *WMJ.* 107(6), 279.

11. Wasserman RC, Hassuk BM, Young PC, et al. (1989) Health care of physicians' children. *Pediatrics.* 83(3), 319.

12. Spiro HM, Mandell HN. (1998) When doctors get sick. *Ann Intern Med.* 128(2), 152.

13. Oberheu K, Jones JW, Sade RM. (2007) A surgeon operates on his son: wisdom or hubris? *Ann Thorac Surg.* 84(3), 723–8.

14. Latessa R, Ray L. (2005) Should you treat yourself, family or friends? *Fam Pract Manag.* 12(3), 41–4.

15. Glass GS. (1975) Incomplete role reversal: The dilemma of hospitalization for the professional peer. *Psychiatry.* 38(2), 132–44.

16. Schneck SA. (1998) "Doctoring" doctors and their families. *JAMA.* 280(23), 2039–42.

17. Bynder H. (1968) Doctors as patients: a study of the medical care of physicians and their families. *Med Care.* 6, 157–67.

18. Capozzi JD. (2008) Caring for doctors. *J Bone Joint Surg Am.* 90(7), 1606–8.

2

The impaired physician

Peter Moffett,[1] Christopher Kang[2]
[1]*Captain, United States Army, Medical Corps, Director of Research, Department of Emergency Medicine, Carl R. Darnall Army Medical Center, Fort Hood, TX, USA*
[2]*Director of Research, Attending Physician, Department of Emergency Medicine, Madigan Army Medical Center, Tacoma, WA, USA*

Section I: Case presentation

A 30-year-old physician is trying to park at a local supermarket, and another driver pulls into a spot for which the physician was waiting. The physician is enraged, and starts a verbal altercation. While the other driver is apologizing, the physician punches him in the face. The physician then gets back into his car and drives away, hoping not to get caught. Another customer reports the incident, and the physician is arrested by the police. He claims that he was so concerned about some of his patients that he acted abnormally, and apologizes. When the story is published in the daily newspaper, many of the other physicians at the hospital appear skeptical. This particular physician has been known for many years as someone with whom it is difficult to work, and to have substantial anger management issues.

Section II: Discussion

Dr. Peter Rosen: In dealing with an impaired physician, we first must understand our legal and moral responsibilities. When encountering a colleague in this scenario, what would one need to do legally and institutionally to address the situation?

Dr. Richard Wolfe: Actions required by law differ significantly based on the specifics of the situation and variability from state to state. In this case, the physician has been arrested and the incident is in the press. An administrator should meet with the physician to ensure that he had the opportunity to receive counseling, attend an anger management course, or enter into a remediation program. In addition, the physician may be subject to an investigation of potential substance abuse. The physician also has the option to resign, or he could lose his staff privileges if he is found guilty of a felony.

Dr. James Adams: There are some subtleties that we may want to consider: For example, the location of the incident is an important factor. This event occurred outside the hospital, which blurs the lines of responsibility more so than if the event had taken place in the hospital setting. If it occurs in the workplace, it is the responsibility of the physician's senior administration to address the situation. If the event takes place outside the hospital, however, it raises the question of how precisely the event would have an impact upon the physician's work in the hospital, and to what extent the hospital's senior administration should take action against the physician that would affect his career. The nature of the legal classification may also influence how the situation is handled.

Ethical Problems in Emergency Medicine: A Discussion-Based Review, First Edition. John Jesus, Shamai A. Grossman, Arthur R. Derse, James G. Adams, Richard Wolfe, and Peter Rosen.

In my contract, for example, there are two different clauses: a moral turpitude clause and a felony clause. As a result, how the situation is addressed will depend on whether the physician is convicted of a crime, and if that crime is classified as a misdemeanor or a felony.

It is also important to address lesser events that are commonly overlooked. For example, a physician yelling and screaming in the clinical setting will often irritate and have a negative impact upon peers around the physician; all too rarely, however, is this behavior addressed. When we do nothing, we permit this type of behavior and overlook potentially serious problems that underlie this behavior. Once we acknowledge a behavior is inappropriate, how should we address an infraction that may be relatively minor? I would suggest an approach that is initially supportive and non-judgmental. For instance, someone could take the physician aside and ask how everything is going? When we engage in this kind of scenario, we should acknowledge that the physician is also a person who may be under extraordinary stress, who may be struggling with addictions, and may be in need of help.

PR: I would like to present a second case, which might also be illustrative of the issues surrounding the impaired physician. Many years ago, I received a call from a colleague of mine who wanted to report that paramedics had brought in a mutually known young surgical subspecialist the night before after he had suffered an overdose of heroin. My colleague said he wouldn't ordinarily share sensitive patient information, but he was concerned by the fact that the physician had simultaneously been on call at his own hospital. Obviously some kind of intervention was necessary, but what exactly are our moral and legal obligations?

Dr. Arthur Derse: The case might be complicated by the possibility that the physician had a medical diagnosis for which he was prescribed a narcotic medication. Though it would be important to find another subspecialist to take over the responsibility of being on call, it might be more prudent to gather more information in a timely manner before taking any actions against the physician that have long lasting consequences.

PR: The key issue in this scenario concerns the ethical and clinical responsibility of the physician while he is on call. Had the subspecialist not been on call, the reporting physician would likely have advised the patient and wife about seeking help for his drug abuse. Because he had clinical responsibilities, however, patient safety was an immediate concern.

I advised the reporting emergency physician to call the Chief of Service of the hospital where the surgeon had clinical responsibilities, and report that an event occurred that suggested that this person had a drug abuse problem that required intervention.

RW: Most states have a law protecting you if you report suspicions of substance abuse to a person's employer. You would be acting in the best interest of protecting not only the physician's patients, but also protecting the physician himself.

AD: In fact, many medical examining boards and state boards of medicine have a "positive duty to report" those individuals with whom you are concerned about impairment. This duty requires a report be made to the medical board, not necessarily to his employer. Depending on your state's regulations, you may have a separate responsibility to report to state boards in addition to questions of disclosing information to employers.

Though I believe drugs and alcohol present a larger problem than does anger management, the case initially presented for discussion is fascinating, in particular because it resembles an event that occurred in Los Angeles last summer. An emergency physician on his way to work felt he was purposefully slowed down by two bicyclists. Once he was able to pass them, he slammed on the brakes and caused them to crash through his rear window.

Anger management is an important issue, particularly when it affects a physician professionally. I would question, however, whether anger management necessarily impairs a physician's judgment in a manner comparable to the influence of drugs and alcohol. When considering how to handle cases of physicians who abuse drugs and alcohol, one must consider the duty to prevent harm to third parties. If the surgical subspecialist's supervisor is aware of the overdose event, for instance, the supervisor would share legal responsibility for subsequent harm caused by the physician's drug abuse. To some extent, both scenarios highlight the conflict between the duty to report knowledge of physician impairment and the duty to preserve doctor–patient confidentiality.

Returning to the case concerning the physician with anger management problems, there's no question that anger management can impair judgment, and can also represent unprofessional behavior. Disciplinary strategies may stem more from the concerns about professionalism than concerns about patient safety. It may be more difficult to draw a clear connection between anger issues and danger to patients than with drug- or alcohol-induced impairment.

JA: There have been attempts to make the connection between anger management problems and patient safety, but the relationship is tenuous at best. The concept behind these attempts is the association of anger management issues with an unsafe work environment. Angry staff members make it less likely that their colleagues will share information and work as a team, which may contribute to an increased rate of error and has the potential to harm patients. Though this conclusion is intuitive, it is difficult to differentiate between a person who has a difficult personality and a person who has an actual anger management problem? When is a physician truly impaired by anger as opposed to being "a little rough around the edges"?

PR: It is easier to recognize the need to address situations during which physicians behave inappropriately secondary to drug use. Other physicians, however, are simply hard to get along with or may be having a particularly tough day. When is it acceptable to allow a physician leeway, and when is it necessary to say, "This behavior is unacceptable, and this is somebody who can't continue to work in our institution?"

JA: We can identify two possible forms of danger resulting from a physician's anger management problem. The first form of danger relates to how a physician's anger affects his own judgment and behavior in a clinical setting. For example, anger can cloud judgment during an important phase in the patient's care, and may manifest itself in more physical ways such as throwing scalpels, posing obvious risks for trauma and spread of infection. The second form of danger is the negative impact a physician's anger can have on communication and on a functioning team dynamic. Communication between team members is a key element of reducing errors and

improving patient safety. Behavior that creates these dangers must be addressed. If the staff of a particular institution does not address physician impairment, then the joint commission or the liaison committee on medical education responsible for accreditation may hold the institution accountable.

Dr. John Jesus: If a clear line of documentation of patient harm or medical mistakes is not available, one might differentiate between physicians who pose real danger, and those who don't, by establishing a critical mass of opinions from colleagues and medical personnel, or patient complaints that clearly report a trend in a physician's behavior demonstrating a more tangible link between violations of standards of conduct and patient safety compromise.

PR: There is a wonderful book called *To Forgive and Remember* written by Bosk.[1] It is a sociologic study of surgical training at the University of Chicago in the early 1970s. The author highlights the distinction between normative and technical errors. Technical errors are failures in performance that can be improved upon through better training and education. Normative errors, on the other hand, are a more intractable problem. People with anger management problems tend to make normative errors. These errors cannot be easily fixed, because the source of the problem lies in the clinician's personality and disposition. Clinicians prone to this behavior frequently act outside the norm with a certain arrogance that leads them to feel entitled to behave in a way that most people would not think is acceptable. Just as it is difficult to prove the link between anger management and impairment, it is also hard to punish or change the behavior. Difficulties in definitively identifying and managing problematic behavior likely fuel the trend of ignoring the issue of physician impairment.[2,3]

Dr. Peter Moffett: It is also important to consider patients' perceptions of physician behavior. When I was in medical school, I would tell my family that similar behaviors were part of a normal day at the hospital. Their reaction was one of disbelief, and they frequently questioned me as to how someone could get away with acting so unprofessionally. There are a certain number of individuals who will respond to direct constructive feedback and change their behavior accordingly. There are others who will not change their behavior, and who would necessitate further action.

PR: This is a much more common problem than we are willing to admit. A big part of the problem is the inherent difficulty of confronting someone who is misbehaving, particularly if the person is angry. We are far more likely to walk away not having addressed the behavior in any productive way. Codes of social and professional behavior are important, but codes alone will not overcome the impediments to confronting unprofessionalism and enforcing standards of what is acceptable. Interventions frequently require a senior figure who has the power to do something to affect the physician's career, and who has the potential to intervene in a way that places more pressure upon the physician to change his behavior. If improvements in behavior prove ineffectual, then the senior figure should be empowered to remove the physician from the institution.

JJ: If you are a witness to physician impairment at an early stage, to whom should you express your concerns?

RW: Those who observe or suspect physician impairment should first go to the chief of service who has an obligation both to patients and to the staff member, and may be in a good position to provide the impaired physician with resources and assistance. If the problem is not resolved at that level, then the next step would be to present the problem to the hospital chief of staff, who could strip the physician of his clinical privileges. The board would be the last option as they may apply an abstract standard of behavior and punishment that does not resolve the issues on every level.

JA: There are two issues I would like to draw out. The first is that changes in behavior can take place over a long period of repeated conversations about the issue. In the volatility of the confrontation at hand, it may be important to deescalate the situation. It may be more productive to help the physician express a calmer attitude before addressing the negative behaviors and suggesting better methods of dealing with frustration and stress. Though temperament modification is an important skill, even more important are conflict resolution skills and the ability to deal with inevitable frustrations in the setting of exhaustion and stress. We can condition better behavior with good role models and consistent constructive feedback throughout a physician's medical education. Many people who may seem to have an inflexible temperament can learn better strategies for dealing with stress and frustration—it just takes time. [The second is that] passive aggression is more difficult to identify than aggressive behavior, but is equally damaging to a work environment, and also constitutes a failure of professionalism.

PR: We end up being responsible for people's personalities, and depending on the situation these might be unlikely to change. Though we owe our colleagues a chance to improve their behavior and performance, there is also a time when we must accept that it may not happen despite our best efforts. At this point, we must have the courage to undertake the painful and distasteful task of dismissal.

Section III: Review of the literature

Physician impairment is a significant and discomforting issue for the medical community that continues to grow in scope, definition, and complexity. Since 1973, physician impairment has been traditionally associated with alcohol and drug dependence.[4] Over the past 40 years, multiple studies suggest that substance abuse has been a major disabling condition for physicians, with at least 10% of all healthcare providers developing a substance abuse disorder sometime during their career.[5–7] Emergency physicians may be up to three times more likely to experience a substance abuse disorder than the general population of healthcare providers.[8] With the maturation of the practice of emergency medicine, additional causes of physician impairment have been considered, including depression, burnout, and disruptive behavior.[9–14] When all factors are considered, one-third of all physicians will experience a period during which they have a condition that impairs their ability to practice medicine safely.[14] This chapter will review the evolution of the definition and types of physician impairment, and present strategies to manage and assist the impaired physician.

Definition and diagnosis of physician impairment

Since the rise of the guild system in the Middle Ages, professional societies have monitored and regulated their members and associated practices. In 1958, the Federation of State Medical Boards recognized alcohol and drug addiction as a disciplinary problem. In 1973, the American Medical Association (AMA) formally recognized physician impairment as a significant problem in a policy paper entitled, "The sick physician: impairment by psychiatric disorders, including alcoholism and drug dependence."[4] In response to this policy paper, each state medical society established a physician health committee and a physician health program (PHP) to assist impaired physicians.

The AMA and other medical professional organizations have since amended their definitions of physician impairment. Current AMA policy defines physician impairment as, "any physical, mental or behavioral disorder that interferes with the ability to engage safely in professional activities."[15] In addition, the American College of Emergency Physicians (ACEP) states that impairment exists "when a physician's professional performance is adversely affected by mental or physical illness, aging, alcoholism, chemical dependence or any other circumstance that interferes with his or her ability to engage safely in patient care."[16]

Despite the evolution of the definition of physician impairment, the diagnosis of impairment remains imprecise and problematic for three reasons. First, impairment is no longer considered "an all-or-none phenomenon."[9] Regular alcohol consumption may occur for years before possibly evolving into abuse and dependence. Second, physicians are reluctant to report their suspicions for professional, financial, and social reasons. Concerned physicians usually believe that a potentially impaired colleague is simply "under a lot of stress" and will "work it out." Third, physicians are adept at hiding signs and symptoms of impairment at work through a variety of coping mechanisms. Although healthcare professionals would easily recognize an acutely intoxicated colleague on duty as impaired, how many of them would consider the same colleague who has recently appeared fatigued, missed several appointments, and fallen behind on patient charting as impaired?[17] Unfortunately, deterioration in clinical performance is usually one of the last signs of impairment.[6]

In light of the revised, expanded definitions of physician impairment, some experts advocate the need for greater recognition of the role and impact of stress and burnout on physician performance.[9-14] In light of recent renewed emphasis on improving patient care and safety, some experts have also logically suggested disruptive behavior as another cause of physician impairment.[18-20]

Types of physician impairment

Alcohol and substance abuse

Alcohol and substance use disorders represent the most commonly recognized type of physician impairment. For many physicians, alcohol and substance misuse may be traced back to medical school and residency.[21-23] After completion of residency, alcohol remains the leading drug of abuse.[24] Recreational drugs, such as marijuana, are superseded by opioids and benzodiazepines. A 2008 study of 16 state PHPs reports that alcohol is the leading drug of abuse in 50% of physicians, followed by opioids in 36%, and stimulants in 8%. Fifty percent of participants also report misusing more than one substance.[25] Physicians in different specialties tend to abuse different classes of drugs, with alcohol, marijuana, and cocaine more prevalent among emergency physicians.[6,7]

Psychiatric disorders and burnout

Psychiatric disorders represent the second type of physician impairment. Physicians have a 16%–18% lifetime incidence of depression; at least equal to that of the general population.[26-28] This incidence may be attributed to several causes. The stresses associated with practicing medicine have continued to increase, resulting in greater job dissatisfaction and vulnerability to maladaptive coping strategies, such as alcohol and substance use.[14] Alcohol is the drug of choice for the self-medication of depression, and those who abuse alcohol often have a depressive disorder.[29,30] If unrecognized or untreated, depression and substance use may lead to suicide. With nearly 400 physician deaths each year, the suicide rate for physicians is greater than that of the general population, with a relative risk ratio of 1.1 to 3.4 for male physicians and 2.5 to 5.7 for female physicians.[28,31-33]

Stress and burnout represent the third type of physician impairment. With the increasing complexity of healthcare, physicians have been subject to a growing number of escalating work-related stressors, including considerable educational debt, decreasing reimbursement, conflicts with colleagues and administrators, mounting bureaucracy, and greater pressure to see more patients in a shorter amount of time.[10,12,14,34–36] First introduced in 1975, burnout represents the culmination of these long-term work-related stressors.[37] Although emergency physicians may not be more prone to burnout than other physicians, when physicians do suffer from burnout, they can become more vulnerable to growing job dissatisfaction, which may result in decreased productivity at work, medical errors, and, ultimately, diminished patient care. Burned out physicians may also experience a variety of affective changes, such as anxiety, depression, and hostility.[11]

Disruptive behavior

Disruptive behavior has recently been suggested as an additional type of physician impairment.[10] Traditionally tolerated as "eccentric," disruptive behavior has been recently recognized by a number of healthcare organizations.[38–42] The Federation of State Medical Boards currently defines disruptive behavior as behavior that "interferes with patient care or could reasonably be expected to interfere with the process of delivering quality care."[39] Disruptive behaviors may manifest in different forms, including passive aggression and poor anger management. From 1995 to 2000, a PHP report notes that 4% of referred cases were related to disruptive behavior, with more than half of the cases reported in 2000.[13] Although still deliberated, recent studies have started to demonstrate a connection between disruptive behavior and patient care.[18] A 2002 survey of over 4500 healthcare workers reports that over 50% of respondents believe that there is a link between disruptive behavior and medical errors. Fourteen percent of respondents report that disruptive behavior caused a specific adverse event.[10,43] Further study in this area is needed to validate the effects of disruptive physician behavior on patient care and safety.

Age impairment

Advanced age has also been suggested as another type of physician impairment, and is notoriously difficult to define and monitor.[44] Several recent reviews of the topic have suggested that increasing age is linked to decreasing performance as measured by patient complaints and disciplinary measures.[44,45] Further investigations suggest that although aging physicians may experience a decline in analytical ability and increased

difficulty incorporating new knowledge, they are often better able to utilize non-analytical abilities, such as experience-based decisions.[45] Further confounding the issue is that the impact of aging on various technical and cognitive abilities does not occur uniformly. Some aged physicians possess cognitive abilities and can function at higher levels as compared with many junior colleagues. This conundrum suggests that age is a factor in cognitive decline, but that indiscriminate use of age alone to judge a physician's ability is unreliable.[44,45]

Management of the impaired physician

Preparation and organizational structure

One of the most important considerations in the management of the impaired physician is to have established, accepted, and well-known protocols and resources already in place. Most hospitals have a structure where individual physicians report to the chair of the department, who in turn reports to the chief of the medical staff. All medical staff must abide by hospital bylaws in order to be granted clinical privileges.[41] This system is endorsed and monitored by The Joint Commission, which also requires a process at the medical staff level to objectively define standards for granting such privileges.[41] It is at the level of the medical staff that a code of conduct should be implemented to help objectify the definitions of impairment. A code of conduct should define specific behaviors that are considered unacceptable for physicians, and protocols for managing any transgressions.[6,14,38,46,47] All providers should recognize and formally acknowledge in their contracts that such a code of conduct exists, and is part of their responsibilities at the hospital.[14,38,46,47] Violations of hospital bylaws may lead to counseling, restriction of privileges, and dismissal, as well as reporting to the state medical board. The state medical boards are reactionary in that they require formal notification of transgressions and punitive actions prior to taking action. These actions are then reported to the National Practitioner Databank.[7,14,41,48] The hope is that by preparing a code of conduct, and quickly responding early to even minor transgressions, the individual and hospital can be prepared to intervene to protect patients, assist the impaired physician, and maintain the well-being of the hospital community.

The physician impaired by alcohol or substance use

Any reasonable suspicion of a physician impaired by alcohol or substance use must be immediately reported to the most appropriate hospital authority. Conclusive proof is not required to initiate an inquiry, as patient safety is paramount. When correctly identified, physicians impaired by alcohol or substance use may be in the advanced stages of the addiction process.[6,9] A practical first step when concerned that a colleague has an alcohol or drug problem is to speak to with the physician's co-workers, friends, and family to confirm or refute one's suspicions.[7,9] While some experts suggest directly confronting the physician, other experts advocate immediately involving the chair of the department and approaching the impaired provider in numbers.[7,9] An important distinction is when the impaired provider is intoxicated at work or on call, in which case immediate action is necessary. An obviously intoxicated provider should be immediately confronted by a group, and escorted to employee health or the emergency department for evaluation and testing.[9] This process must be clearly detailed in the hospital bylaws. Hopefully, and preferably, the provider should acknowledge that a problem exists. After these steps, the provider should then be referred to the hospital employee assistance committee, and if necessary, the state PHP.

PHPs are an outstanding resource for both the impaired provider and the involved hospital.[6,7,9,13,14,24,48,49] Each state has a PHP that is focused on the assessment and therapy of the impaired provider. Although often managed by the state medical board, PHPs are non-punitive. A provider is referred to the PHP as a way of forgoing disciplinary action in favor of rehabilitation. Most PHPs have an extensive testing and assessment component. They then typically refer a provider directly to several inpatient substance abuse rehabilitation centers specialized for physician treatment. Upon successful completion of inpatient treatment, the impaired provider is typically enrolled in outpatient therapy. These revolve around mandatory meetings at Alcoholics Anonymous, or Narcotics Anonymous. During this phase of treatment, the PHP facilitates the physician's reintegration into the work environment. Perhaps the most important component of these programs is that the impaired provider is followed for at least 5 years with random drug screens to monitor compliance. Upon successful completion, the provider may forego dismissal and

reporting to the state medical board. Refusal to participate in the PHP, or failure to successfully complete treatment directed by the PHP may result in formal reporting to the state medical board for consideration of loss of licensure and reporting to the National Practitioner Databank. While up to 25% of impaired providers may experience one relapse during treatment, the PHP programs are very successful, with up to 92% of providers making a complete recovery, and up to 85% of them returning to work.[6,7] Providers experiencing a relapse are typically reassessed, recycled, and rehabilitated.

The physician impaired by mental illness

Management of the physician impaired by mental illness is a straightforward but delicate process. Meeting with the colleague one-on-one and discussing your concerns may be a helpful first step. A number of programs are designed specifically for healthcare providers suffering from depression and anxiety, and frequently a psychiatrist in the hospital will specialize in treating physicians.[50] In addition, employee assistance programs may help locate and facilitate appropriate psychiatric referrals. The privacy of the provider must be respected, and a minimum number of people should be involved.[50] Perhaps the most useful strategy is to help providers avoid stress, depression, and the development of burnout. This preventive measure may be instituted through a variety of organized wellness and education events as well as workplace modification such as: providing adequate lighting, flexible scheduling, providing adequate staffing, and ensuring direct communication between providers and hospital management.[11]

The physician impaired by behavioral problems

In some ways, the provider impaired by anger or disruptive behavioral issues can be more difficult to deal with than the provider impaired by drugs and alcohol. This is due to the insidious nature of the problem, and the difficulty in objectively identifying the problem. As mentioned above, a well-defined code of conduct can greatly assist the management of this type of physician impairment.

Many experts agree that an effective first step in dealing with a disruptive provider is the initial "coffee talk", or a one-on-one meeting.[13,14,38,46,47] During this meeting, the provider should be offered an opportunity to explain the negative actions, and in addition, should be made to acknowledge the disruptive behavior as wrong, even if the provoking action seems justified. Although some providers may attempt to rationalize their actions, especially if it is an isolated event, they should still recognize that other more professional means of addressing the situation are available. Certain behaviors such as sexual harassment, racism, and overt personal threats should not be handled at the "coffee talk" level, but prompt more immediate and direct disciplinary action.

If required, the next level of response should be a formal documented conversation with the chair of the department.[13,14,38,46,47] Before this meeting occurs, the chair should gather all available information and solicit evaluations, assessments, and opinions from the co-workers of the disruptive physician. Some hospital systems have developed anonymous surveillance systems whereby patients and employees can submit concerns about providers.[44] The chair of the department should then present the information to the disruptive provider and allow for an opportunity to respond. A plan should then be laid out that can involve assessment by a psychiatrist or behavioral health provider, anger management courses, or referral to a PHP that provides behavioral health support. If this level of response does not remedy the problem, the matter should then be brought to the medical staff and hospital administration for revocation of privileges and dismissal. During this final level of management, it is essential that the provider fully comprehend the gravity of the situation (Figure 2.1). For an institution to be successful, the policy and punishments for disruptive behaviors must be applied consistently

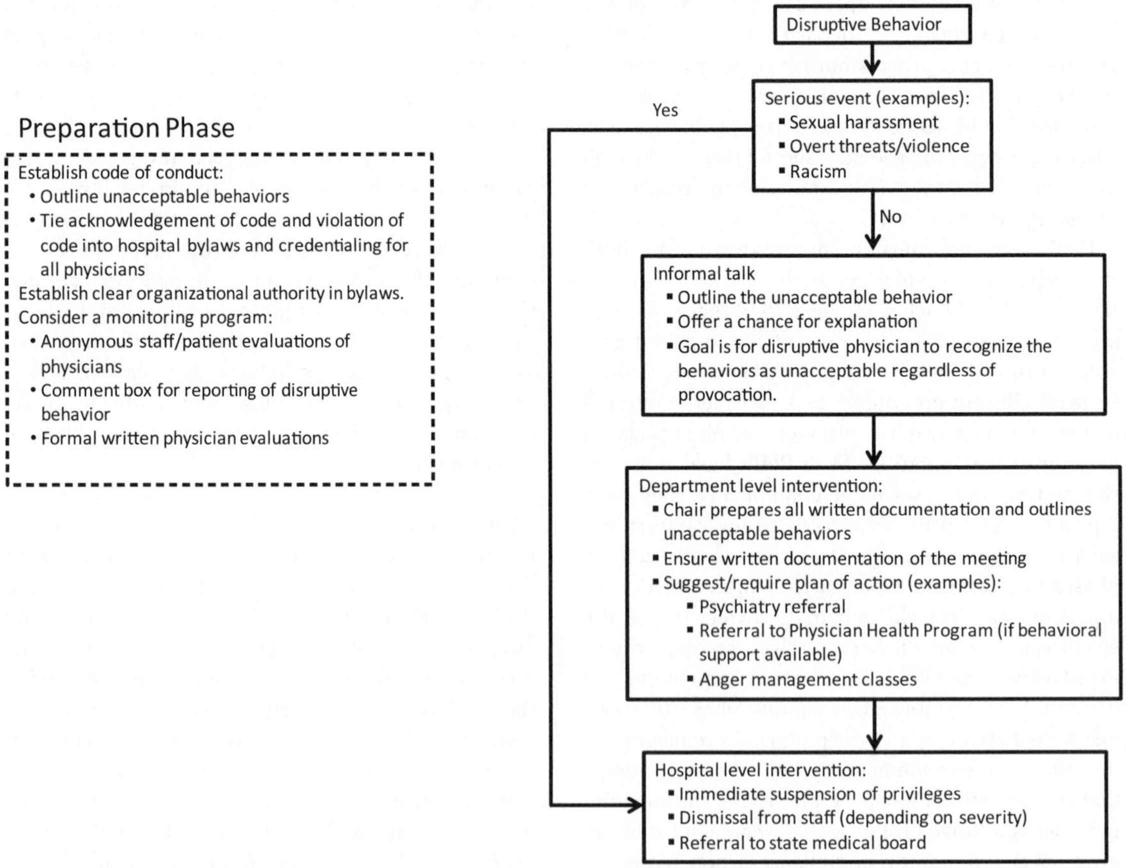

Preparation Phase

Establish code of conduct:
- Outline unacceptable behaviors
- Tie acknowledgement of code and violation of code into hospital bylaws and credentialing for all physicians

Establish clear organizational authority in bylaws.

Consider a monitoring program:
- Anonymous staff/patient evaluations of physicians
- Comment box for reporting of disruptive behavior
- Formal written physician evaluations

Disruptive Behavior

Serious event (examples):
- Sexual harassment
- Overt threats/violence
- Racism

Yes

No

Informal talk
- Outline the unacceptable behavior
- Offer a chance for explanation
- Goal is for disruptive physician to recognize the behaviors as unacceptable regardless of provocation.

Department level intervention:
- Chair prepares all written documentation and outlines unacceptable behaviors
- Ensure written documentation of the meeting
- Suggest/require plan of action (examples):
  - Psychiatry referral
  - Referral to Physician Health Program (if behavioral support available)
  - Anger management classes

Hospital level intervention:
- Immediate suspension of privileges
- Dismissal from staff (depending on severity)
- Referral to state medical board

Fig. 2.1 Management of the disruptive provider.

and without exception even for the most clinically proficient or financially successful physicians. Unfortunately, it is often these very physicians who become disruptive providers out of a sense that others are below them or that excellence in performance excuses poor behavior.[38]

The provider impaired by age

It is important to mention again that age alone is not sufficient to screen physicians for impairment. A more accurate description of the problem is to characterize the issue as diminished physician cognition. Recognizing this event can be problematic as family, friends, and colleagues of the aging provider may be reluctant to report perceived cognitive decline. Although, it has been suggested that a mandatory retirement age for physicians may mitigate this issue, this criteria may be difficult to enforce as it could be challenged as "age discrimination" under the Americans With Disabilities Act.[44] As noted previously, an arbitrary age cut-off would undoubtedly remove some very high-functioning physicians from practice. Several programs for monitoring for cognitive decline of aged physicians have been suggested. One suggestion is basic cognitive screening for dementia just like that used in the general patient population; however, physicians may score higher on these tests based on education and higher-functioning status. Another suggestion is periodic reviews of physicians starting at a predefined age.[44,45] In Canada, the Physicians' Achievement Review is an evaluation of the provider by patients, peers, and non-physician colleagues. If the provider scores in the lower third of the sample, additional evaluation of the provider is conducted. Another program that has been successful in determining cognitive decline is the Canadian Physician Review and Enhancement Program.[44,45] Once the problem has been confirmed, the affected physicians should retire or be removed from practice. If the problem is advanced, the state medical board will need to be notified to take action to protect the public. Unfortunately, other proposed strategies, such as reducing the number and complexity of patients, cannot be easily applied to emergency physicians. This evolving problem merits additional study as well as agreement among state medical boards and credentialing committees on appropriate courses of action.

Legal and ethical responsibilities

Few legal standards mandate what must be done with an impaired provider. In the United States, individual state governments are responsible for the health and welfare of their constituents, and therefore applicable laws may differ among states. Only 20% of states have laws that mandate reporting of providers suspected to be impaired by drugs and alcohol.[6] Reporting to the National Practitioner Databank only occurs when a disciplinary action against a provider is reported by the state medical board. The latter may actually benefit the impaired provider willing to undergo treatment, in that the PHP will only report a provider to the state medical board after rehabilitation has failed.

Individuals and hospitals often worry about falsely accusing an individual of being impaired, and thereby becoming named in lawsuits. Most states have laws that protect against a civil suit for reporting a reasonable concern about a provider.[6] Hospitals may consider consultation with their legal departments to ensure that records and other documentation collected in internal investigations of a provider are non-discoverable in court. This measure may facilitate more open reporting of a potentially impaired physician without fear of "ruining" a provider's career.

While law dictates what must be done, the ethical physician considers, "What should I do?" The AMA asserts that, "Physicians have an ethical obligation to report impaired, incompetent, or unethical colleagues . . ."[51] While sometimes difficult to approach or report a disruptive or impaired colleague, it is often the first and most important step in helping the affected provider. Finally, the duty to protect the patients or future patients of the impaired provider is paramount. As Edmund Burke noted, "All that is necessary for evil to triumph, is that good men do nothing."

Conclusion

Physician impairment is a significant, well-known problem that continues to grow in scope, definition, and complexity. Although substance abuse has been long identified as a cause and sign of an impaired physician, mental health conditions, behavioral issues, and cognitive decline are increasingly recognized as additional causes of physician impairment. Although acknowledging and managing an impaired physician can be awkward and difficult, physicians must remember that they have a collegial responsibility to assist the impaired physician as well as professional and ethical duties to protect patients and the general public.

Section IV: Recommendations

• Physician impairment can be broadly recognized as "any physical, mental or behavioral disorder that interferes with the ability to engage safely in professional activities."[15]

• Types of impairment include alcohol and substance abuse, depression, stress, burnout, disruptive behavior, and cognitive decline.

• All institutions should have preestablished policies and procedures to include a code of conduct that governs employee conduct.

• PHPs are excellent resources in helping impaired providers and while traditionally associated with non-punitive management of alcohol and substance abuse, these programs may also provide assistance for the depressed or disruptive physician.

• While few laws exist that require reporting of the impaired provider, there is an ethical responsibility for all physicians to report the impaired provider through proper channels.

References

1. Bosk CL. (2003) *Forgive and Remember: Managing Medical Failure*, 1st ed. Chicago, IL: University of Chicago Press.

2. Rosen P, Markovchick V, Dracon D. (1983) Normative and technical error in the emergency department. *J Emerg Med*. 1(2), 155–60.

3. Rosen P, Edlich RF, Rosen CL, et al. (2008) Becoming a specialist in emergency medicine. *J Emerg Med*. 34(4), 471–6.

4. American Medical Association Council on Mental Health. (1973) The sick physician: Impairment by psychiatric disorders, including alcoholism and drug dependence. *JAMA*. 223, 685–7.

5. Talbott G, Wright C. (1987) Chemical dependency in healthcare professionals. *Occup Med*. 2, 581–91.

6. Baldisseri MR. (2007) Impaired healthcare professional. *Crit Care Med*. 30(2), S106–16.

7. Berge KH, Seppala MD, Schipper AM. (2009) Chemical dependency and the physician. *Mayo Clin Proc*. 84(7), 625–31.

8. Mansky PA. (1996) Physician health programs and the potentially impaired physician with a substance use disorder. *Psychiatr Serv*. 47, 465–7.

9. Boisaubin EV, Levine RE. (2001) Identifying and assisting the impaired physician. *Am J Med Sci*. 322(1), 31–6.

10. Boisaubin EV. (2009) Causes and treatment of impairment and burnout in physicians: The epidemic within. In: Cole TR, Goodrich TJ, Gritz ER. (eds) *Faculty Health in Academic Medicine*. Totowa: Humana Press, pp. 29–38.

11. Goldberg R, Barnosky AR. (2010) Wellness, stress, and the impaired physician. In: Marx J. (ed.) *Rosen's Emergency Medicine: Concepts and Clinical Practice*, 7th ed. Philadelphia, PA: Mosby Elsevier, pp. 2158–61.

12. Garmel GS. (2008) Conflict resolution in emergency medicine. In: Adams JG. (ed.) *Adams: Emergency Medicine*, 1st ed. Philadelphia, PA: WB Saunders/Elsevier, pp. 2171–85.

13. Kaufmann M. (2001) Recognition and management of the behaviorally disruptive physician. *Ontario Med Rev*. 53–55.

14. Leape LL, Fromson JA. (2006) Problem doctors: Is there a system-level solution? *Ann Int Med*. 144, 107–5.

15. American Medical Association (AMA) Policy Finder Database. H-95.955. *Substance Abuse Among Physicians*. Chicago, IL: AMA. Available at: www.ama-assn.org/ad-com/polfind/Hlth-Ethics.pdf. Accessed May 21, 2010.

16. American College of Emergency Physicians (ACEP). *Practice Resources. Physician Impairment*. Dallas, TX: ACEP. Available at: www.acep.org/practres.aspx?id=29630. Accessed May 21, 2010.

17. Talbot GD, Gallegos KV, Angres DH. (1998) Impairment and recovery in physicians and other health professionals. In: Graham AW, Schultz TK. (eds) *Principles of Addiction Medicine*, 2nd ed. Chevy Chase: American Society of Addiction Medicine, pp. 1263–79.

18. Rosenstein AH, O'Daniel M. (2008) Managing disruptive physicians: Impact on staff relationships and patient care. *Neurology*. 70, 1564–70.

19. Institute of Medicine Report. (2000) *To Err is Human: Building a Safer Health System*. Washington, DC: National Academy Press.

20. American College of Physician Executives (ACPE). *On Target: Managing Disruptive Physician Behavior*. Tampa, FL: ACPE. Available at: http://net.acpe.org/resources/publications/OnTargetDisruptivePhysician.pdf. Accessed May 26, 2010.

21. Clark DC, Eckenfels EJ, Daugherty SR, et al. (1987) Alcohol-use patterns through medical school: A longitudinal study of one class. *JAMA.* 257, 2921–6.

22. Baldwin DC, Hughes PH, Conrad SE, et al. (1991) Substance use among senior medical students: A survey of 23 medical schools. *JAMA.* 265, 2074–8.

23. McNamara RM, Margulies JL. (1994) Chemical dependency in emergency medicine residency programs: Prospective of the program directors. *Ann Emerg Med.* 23, 1072–976.

24. Johnson BA. (2009) Curbside Consultation: Dealing with the impaired physician. *Am Fam Phys.* 80(9), 1007–8.

25. McLellan AT, Skipper GS, Campbell M, et al. (2008) Five year outcomes in a cohort study of physicians treated for substance use disorders in the United States. *BMJ.* 337, a2038.

26. Gallery ME, Whitley TW, Klonis LK, et al. (1992) A study of occupational stress and depression among emergency physicians. *Ann Emerg Med.* 21, 58–64.

27. Schernhammer E. (2005) Taking their own lives—The high rate of physician suicide. *N Eng J Med.* 352, 2473–6.

28. Andrew LB. *Physician Suicide. eMedicine.com.* Available at: http://emedicine.medscape.com/article/806779-overview. Accessed May 29, 2010.

29. Regier DA, Farmer ME, Rae DS, et al. (1990) Comorbidity of mental disorders with alcohol and other drug abuse: Results from the Epidemiologic Catchment Area (ECA) Study. *JAMA.* 264(19), 2511–8.

30. Barclay L. *Confronting Physician Depression and Suicide: A Newsmaker Interview with Morton M. Silverman, MD.* Medscape.com June 17, 2003. Available at: http://medscape.com/viewarticle/457429. Accessed May 29, 2010.

31. Lindeman S, Laara E, Haako H, et al. (1996) A systematic review on gender-specific suicide mortality in medical doctors. *Br J Psychiatry.* 168, 274–9.

32. Wilson A, Rosen A, Randal P, et al. (2009) Psychiatrically impaired medical practitioners: An overview with special reference to impaired psychiatrists. *Austr Psychiatry.* 17(1), 6–10.

33. Schernhammer ES, Colditz GA. (2004) Suicide rates among physicians: A quantitative and gender assessment (Meta-Analysis). *Am J Psychiatry.* 161, 2295–302.

34. Chapman DM. (1997) Burnout in emergency medicine: What are we doing to ourselves? *Acad Emerg Med.* 4, 245.

35. Cunningham W, Cookson T. (2009) Addressing stress-related impairment in doctors. A survey of providers' and doctors' experience of a funded counselling service in New Zealand. *J N Z Med.* 122(1300), 19–28.

36. Brown SD. (2009) Beyond substance abuse: Stress, burnout, and depression as causes of physician impairment and disruptive behavior. *J Am Coll Radiol.* 6(7), 479–85.

37. Freudenburger H. (1975) The staff burn-out syndrome in alternative institutions. *Psychother Theory Res Pract.* 75, 12.

38. Piper LE. (2003) Addressing the phenomenon of disruptive physician behavior. *Health Care Manag.* 22(4), 335–9.

39. Federation of State Medical Boards of the United States. (2010) *Report of the Special Committee on Professional Conduct and Ethics.* Dallas, TX: Federation of State Medical Boards of the United States.

40. College of Physicians and Surgeons of Ontario. (2005) *CPSO Task Force on Disruptive Physician Behaviour.* Ontario: College of Physicians and Surgeons of Ontario.

41. Youssi MD. JCAHO standards help address disruptive physician behavior. The Physician Executive; Nov–Dec 2002. In: American College of Physician Executives. *On Target: Managing Disruptive Physician Behavior.* Tampa, FL: American College of Physician Executives, pp. 47–8. Available at: http://net.acpe.org/resources/publications/OnTargetDisruptivePhysician.pdf. Accessed May 26, 2010.

42. Weber DO. Poll results: Doctors' disruptive behavior disturbs physician leaders. The Physician Executive; Sep–Oct 2004. In: American College of Physician Executives. *On Target: Managing Disruptive Physician Behavior.* Tampa, FL: American College of Physician Executives, pp. 9–17. Available at: http://net.acpe.org/resources/publications/OnTargetDisruptivePhysician.pdf. Accessed May 26, 2010.

43. Rosenstein A, O'Daniel M. (2005) Disruptive behavior and clinical outcomes: Perceptions of nurses and physicians. *Am J Nurs.* 105, 54–64.

44. LoboPrabbu S, Molinari V, Hamilton J, et al. (2009) The aging physician with cognitive impairment: Approaches to oversight, prevention, and remediation. *Am J Geriat Psychiatry.* 17, 445–54.

45. Eva K. (2002) The aging physician: Changes in cognitive processing and their impact on medical practice. *Acad Med.* 77(10), S1–6.

46. Hickson G, Pichert J, Webb L, et al. (2007) A complementary approach to promoting professionalism: Identifying, measuring, and addressing unprofessional behaviors. *Acad Med.* 82(11), 1040–8.

47. Kaufmann M. (2005) Management of disruptive behavior in physicians: A staged, rehabilitative approach. *Ontario Med Rev.* 59–64.

48. DuPont R, McLellan A, White W, et al. (2009) Setting the standard for recovery: Physicians' Health Programs. *J Subst Abuse Treat.* 36, 159–71.

49. DuPont R, McLellan A, Carr G, et al. (2009) How are addicted physicians treated? A national survey of physician health programs. *J Subst Abuse Treat.* 37, 1–7.

50. Rosen A, Wilson A, Randal P, et al. (2009) Psychiatrically impaired medical practitioners: Better care to reduce harm and life impact, with special reference to impaired psychiatrists. *Austr Psychiatry.* 17(1), 11–8.

51. American Medical Association (AMA). *Opinion 9.031—Reporting Impaired, Incompetent, or Unethical Colleagues.* Available at: www.ama-assn.org/ama/pub/physician-resources/medical-ethics/code-medical-ethics/opinion9031.shtml. Accessed May 26, 2010.

Disclosure of medical error and truth telling

Abhi Mehrotra,[1] Cherri Hobgood[2]

[1]Assistant Professor Emergency Medicine, Department of Emergency Medicine, University of North Carolina School of Medicine, Chapel Hill, NC, USA
[2]The Rolly McGrath Professor and Chair of Emergency Medicine, Department of Emergency Medicine, Indiana University School of Medicine, Indianapolis, IN, USA

Section I: Case presentation

A 63-year-old female patient was brought to the emergency department (ED) by prehospital care providers (emergency medical services) with a chief complaint of dizziness and nausea. She was recently started on a β-blocker by her primary care physician. The paramedics found her hypotensive and bradycardic. She was administered atropine, glucagon, and calcium gluconate on arrival at the ED. During her workup in the ED, she was also found to be hyperkalemic, and in acute renal failure. Blood sugar in the ED was normal. The electrocardiogram had peaked T-waves, but was otherwise unremarkable. She was alert and oriented. The hyperkalemia was treated with calcium, albuterol, kayexalate, and glucose, as well as intravenous insulin. Eight units of regular intravenous insulin were ordered. The nurse drew up the insulin, obtained verification with a second registered nurse, as per protocol, and proceeded to administer the medication. The attending physician caring for the patient signed her out to the oncoming attending. Shortly after sign-out, the attending was called into the room as the patient was somnolent, and had sonorous respirations. A fingerstick blood glucose determination was performed, and the patient was found to be severely hypoglycemic. Dextrose was infused intravenously with recovery of mental status

and the patient was stabilized. The attending physician reviewed the chart and medications administered. It was discovered that while the order was written for 8 units of regular insulin, the patient was administered 80 units of regular insulin. Serial blood sugar checks were instituted, the patient was started on a continuous dextrose infusion and admitted to the intensive care unit. This error was discussed with the patient, her family, and the inpatient team taking over care of the patient.

Section II: Discussion

Dr. Peter Rosen: We have a clear ethical problem, and that is—what to do when we make a mistake during the care of a patient. What do you feel are the ethical constraints for the management of error in the ED?

Dr. James Adams: There's a certain core ethic that we shouldn't forget, which is fulfilling the role of being a trusted caregiver. I've seen people realize they made a mistake, walk in to introduce themselves to the family and immediately start talking about the error. That's an absolutely terrible way to do it. Error disclosure has to occur in the context of a trusting relationship. The first conversation should be to introduce yourself, talk about the patient, talk about the clinical circumstances, and eventually you'll get to the error.

Ethical Problems in Emergency Medicine: A Discussion-Based Review, First Edition. John Jesus, Shamai A. Grossman, Arthur R. Derse, James G. Adams, Richard Wolfe, and Peter Rosen.
© 2012 John Wiley & Sons, Ltd. Published 2012 by John Wiley & Sons, Ltd.

The interaction shouldn't be solely about error disclosure.

PR: One aspect that makes error disclosure difficult is that we are often given conflicting advice by physicians and risk managers or attorneys. I had a case in Denver where we made a clear-cut error in management, and I wanted to simply call the family and apologize. Our city attorney, however, said that under no circumstances should I do that, because it would harm the subsequent lawsuit. I called the family anyway, and I believe it prevented a lawsuit altogether.

Dr. Arthur Derse: For many years the standard recommendation was to never say you're sorry, because it can be used against you as implication of guilt. For the most part that is no longer true. When an error has occurred, disclosing that error may not have implications for any kind of legal liability, because not all errors can be shown to fall short of providing the standard of care within the local community. Sometimes, however, there is a serious management error that results in patient harm, about which the attorney doesn't want you to take immediate responsibility. Many people say disclosure of errors actually decreases the likelihood of liability. Similarly, many believe that if a family finds out there has been an error and you haven't disclosed it, they are more likely to sue than not.

The results of studies about errors in the ED demonstrate that errors occur more frequently than we recognize. A number of studies show errors, whether or not they have resulted in serious injury, in one out of every 10 pediatric visits, and one out of every 10 adult visits.[1] In any given case, it is less likely that you'll be sued if you disclose the error rather than if the patient or family discovers the error. If you disclose all errors, paradoxically, because errors happen so frequently, disclosure increases the cumulative risk of lawsuit.[1]

PR: While error disclosure may or may not prevent a suit, the reality is that it's going to depend on the degree of damage. Should every error be disclosed, or should disclosure occur only if there is actual harm or the potential for real damage?

Dr. Cherri Hobgood: Not all errors are the result of negligence, and not all errors cause harm. There are some clear-cut cases where harm occurs, and the patient's future care depends on the open acknowledgment of what happened. There are several levels of disclosure. The first is disclosure of the error to the patient and family. There is also error disclosure within the healthcare team, including attending physicians, residents, and nurses. Errors that cause bad outcomes and result in needed treatments to repair them require honest disclosure. If, on the other hand, a patient is given 25 mg of promethazine when the order was written for 12.5 mg, and there is no adverse outcome, that error may not be worthy of disclosure to the patient. Participants in patient care must understand why an error occurred, in order to prevent the error from occurring in the future. Furthermore, there needs to be open disclosure within the healthcare team without fear of shame or condemnation, and with the clear understanding that the purpose is to promote increased patient safety.

PR: It's easy to discover errors when there is a bad outcome, and the cause is immediately apparent. A seizure induced by too much insulin, for example. How does one discover that the wrong dose of a medication has been given when there is no outcome change? I agree that our system for checking on dosing administration is important, but how do we discover mistakes when the outcome is unchanged?

Dr. Abhi Mehrotra: If an environment and culture existed that valued open communication and promoted patient safety, where people can disclose an error without blame or ridicule, then many of the barriers to disclosure would evaporate.

Dr. John Jesus: The basis of our ethical requirement to tell the patient the truth is based on human dignity and mutual respect. Without this ethic being operative, I believe patients become more suspicious of our actions, and begin to believe that their caregiver doesn't have the patient's best interest at heart. If we recognize an error, it should be communicated either to the medical team or to the patient when it has an appreciable effect. If we promote an environment of trust and mutual respect through our pursuit of truth telling, even if it is uncomfortable, the practice will eventually become an expectation. Attending physicians are role models to their residents, and can teach by living by the principles they attempt to teach residents.

PR: Kant once said that there was no condition in which it was ethically permissible to lie. Do you agree with that position, or are you like most of us who feel that Kant had no appreciation of the real world?

Dr. Shamai Grossman: Our primary goal as physicians is to take care of our patients, but that doesn't mean we disclose to them every minute detail of their care. In some instances, telling the patient about a minor error would not benefit the patient, and would instead create an aura of uncertainty around their care. Although the ideal is to be as honest as possible, one must be very careful about disclosing everything to everyone.

JA: Sometimes patients are strangely reassured by a strong and confident presence. They can see your commitment to doing what's best for them in your body language, and hear it in your tone of voice. That's the best and really the only way to build trust. Then, in the right context, in the right way, with the right confidence and competence, you can say, "Look, we're doing a lot of things that you need, but something went awry in the management of your conditions. We're fixing it, however, and this is how." In a strange way that can be reassuring, because they believe that you are simultaneously trustworthy and competent. Learning to inspire trust in the patient is really one of the critical but unspoken tasks of our training programs.

CH: A critical part of communication is demonstrating integrity to a patient through your willingness to engage a patient on a difficult topic in a way that is caring, honest, compassionate, and to approach the issues from the patient's perspective. Bringing the patient onto the care team as a partner is very important to our efforts to engender trust.

PR: There are two other issues of importance I would like to discuss. The first concerns what physicians should do when there occurs an obvious error with disastrous consequences, such as operating on the wrong breast or the wrong limb? Secondly, in my view of error disclosure, I also take responsibility for the error. As part of that responsibility, I would attempt to ensure the patient doesn't have to pay for my error. It has been extraordinarily difficult in my experience to coax the hospital administration to waive charges for care that was induced by error.

JA: When the error is catastrophic, the first thing I would suggest is to find help. In such a situation nobody has the poise to be objective. Call for backup, a program director, or nursing administrator who can help navigate the error disclosure and provide support for all of parties involved—the patient, families, as well as the caregivers.

JJ: Is there a suggested approach for managing the situation legally?

AD: Physicians should seek out a systems-based approach, because disclosure of a major error shouldn't be managed by a single person. If there is someone on call from risk management or the legal department, try to involve them as soon as possible. That said, you should be careful about how that is perceived by the family. If the people for whom you work are used to error disclosure and promote being transparent with families, are willing to offer immediate compensation for serious error, and are willing to make sure that charges are waived for the current care of the patient, you are in a much better position.

CH: What patients in this situation often want to know is how the error will have an impact upon them, and what will happen moving forward. It's important to anyone disclosing an error to be able to tell them about this. It is also incumbent upon the department leadership to address what should be done when errors occur before they actually happen. With preparation, a team could be assembled on short notice that is able to provide support to the providers who have committed the error, as well as assist in the disclosure. This includes addressing all the significant issues that you can anticipate patients will have in this situation. In cases where the physician has performed a procedure on the wrong leg or the wrong breast, the discussions with the family will be devastating. It is essential to have a member of your team who can communicate how the situation will be managed, and how it is going to impact them financially.

JJ: I'd like to share an anecdote about an error I witnessed in the hospital. I was the resident working in an adjacent ICU [intensive care unit], and learned that a patient diagnosed with septic shock required a central venous line. The resident taking care of the patient along with the attending of record appropriately prepped and draped the patient for the sterile procedure. Ultrasound was used to identify the vessel and lidocaine was used to anesthetize the skin. The resident had some difficulty puncturing the vessel, and made two or three passes. On the third pass, however, instead of the flash of venous blood, there was a flashback of air. She had punctured the apex of the lung. Over the course of the next 10 minutes, the patient became more tachypneic and tachycardic, developed hypotension, and went into cardiac arrest. Despite the medical team's attempts to revive her, the patient expired. The resident and attending spoke with the family about what happened, however, the resident involved in the case was completely distraught, because of her role in causing the complication that led to the patient's death. How we can better support our residents, and teach them to disclose errors especially when they feel a sense of responsibility?

PR: This is a different class of error than operating on the wrong side of someone's body. This represents a complication that any physician could have in performing a complex procedure, and it represents a risk of performing lifesaving invasive inventions. I don't believe that this should be presented to the family as a medical error so much as it is an unfortunate complication. I understand the resident's feeling of responsibility, but the resident should be counseled about the difference between a true medical error and a complication, and that she is **not** responsible for the underlying disease or the patient's death.

CH: "Medical error: the second victim by Albert Wu," published in *JAMA* a number of years ago, describes the author's angst around a similar event he witnessed a fellow resident experience.[2] We need to begin talking about such events in ways that acknowledge our own fallibility as humans, and we should be more supportive of each other as we negotiate the complexity of medical care.

The HEEAL mnemonic is the methodology I've developed for teaching residents how to do this. It is a very simple teaching tool that we use as the foundation for a dialog with patients and their families. The residents practice HEEAL using role play and by working through actual cases. We then video tape residents working through cases with standardized patients, and debrief to discuss their entire approach, recognizing that it's not just about the words you say. The HEEAL mnemonic stands for some simple concepts. First is honesty—one needs to be as completely honest as possible, being clear to disclose what you know and being honest about what you don't regarding the

error event. Second, one needs to explain, the events that led up to the error, and the impact the event will have on their health. Third, one must have empathy for the patient and project this through one's tone, word choice (free of medical jargon if possible), and through one's physical presence. Fourth, one should offer a sincere apology based on your responsibility as a physician leader of the healthcare team. Finally, one should then tell the patient what one has learned from the incident and what one's plan is to lessen the chance for future errors. The HEEAL mnemonic provides a quick structure for a stressful conversation with a substantial amount of content [see also Section III].

JA: That's extremely valuable both as a tool and as a way to change the culture around thinking about error disclosure. Attending physicians at an academic institution must recognize that residents are in a program to learn, and part of that learning process is making errors. It is natural for students and residents to make mistakes. In order to learn from their mistakes, they need to face them in a constructive environment without fear or intimidation or ridicule.

SG: Ultimately we need to change the environment to one where truth-telling is valued and medical mistakes are routinely communicated to the patient. To do so, we should have support systems and protocols in place for residents as well as for faculty and nursing.

JA: This requires the leadership not only from our training programs, but also from departments, and hospital administration, in order to create a culture that fosters a supportive environment.

JJ: Error disclosure is an issue relevant to every physician; if you haven't already found yourself in the position of having made an error, you will at some point in your career. It is crucial for every physician to consider truth disclosure before the error occurs, in order to prevent making a decision that he might regret, or worse, be paralyzed by indecision and avoid the discussion altogether.

Section III: Review of the literature

"Despite the cost pressures, liability constraints, resistance to change and other seemingly insurmountable barriers, it is not acceptable for patients to be harmed by the same health care system that is supposed to offer healing and comfort."[1] The Institute of Medicine (IOM) made this statement in its report *To Err Is Human—Building a Safer Health System*. The publicity stemming from the release of that report has led to a dialog between the public and medical community regarding medical errors. Why should we, as providers, care about this issue? Not only is the subject of error within the healthcare arena a focus of discussion, the ED is one of the highest risk hospital locations for an error as well as being notable for the highest percentage of adverse events related to negligence.[3] Fordyce et al. demonstrate a rate of 18 errors reported per 100 registered patients in an academic ED.[4] This is not unexpected given the environment in which we practice, where there are multiple factors contributing to the cognitive load. The setting frequently is rife with multiple interruptions of care delivery, crowded conditions, and noisy with frequent distracters. Adding to this are patient-related dynamics of diagnostic uncertainty, management of multiple patients (frequently critically ill), and limited knowledge of prior medical history. The physician-related factors also must be considered, taking into account the transitions of care and fatigue as well as circadian dysynchronicity.[5]

In order to maintain consistency, we will utilize the IOM definition of error and adverse event. There can exist an error of execution—defined as the failure of a planned action to be completed as intended. An alternative is an error of planning—the use of an inappropriate plan to achieve an aim.[6] This is in contradistinction to an adverse event: an injury caused by medical management rather than the underlying condition of the patient.[7] Thus, an adverse outcome may occur without an underlying error. An idiosyncratic drug reaction in a patient who had not previously been exposed to the medication is an adverse event, yet no error may have occurred in the administration of the drug.

An adverse event that is attributable to error is defined as a preventable adverse event. An adverse event related to the administration of a drug is classified as an adverse drug event (ADE). For example, a drug reaction that occurs in a patient with a known allergy to the class of medication would be an ADE that is due to an error. This can be further delineated to include negligent adverse events, which satisfy legal criteria used in determining negligence. In this situation, the etiology of the error is due to the failure of the care provided to meet the prevailing standard of care.[8]

Our patients' perception of healthcare delivery is of a system that is safe and when errors occur, it is a provider issue.[1] It is not perceived to be a failure of the process of delivering care in a complex system. Patients expect accurate information about their medical care and treatment alternatives, which allow informed treatment choices.[9] Providers should feel a duty to provide care consistent with their training and reflected in professional guidelines. The American Medical Association's *Principles of Medical Ethics* includes the principle that "a physician shall uphold the standards of professionalism, be honest in all professional interactions, and strive to report physicians deficient in character or competence, or engaging in fraud or deception, to appropriate entities."[10] Further guidelines specific to emergency physicians have been published by the American College of Emergency Physicians (ACEP), in policy statement, unless the urgency of the patient's condition demands an immediate response.[11] They also speak to the need for education on effective communication of errors. Physician training tends to focus on individual responsibility and accountability, thus the physician expectation of error disclosure may vary from the patient expectation. From this conflict arises the dilemma of what to disclose? Informing patients of every aspect of their care, while truthful, is not practical for expedient care delivery. The disclosure of technical aspects of care delivery may be disadvantageous to both the patient and the physician. Moskop et al. suggest that one guiding principle in disclosing information to patients is the legal doctrine of informed consent.[9] Most physicians are familiar with this concept and have become accustomed to the discussion with regard to specific, invasive procedures. There is usually a discussion held with the patient regarding the risks and benefits of the procedures that includes potential complications, as well as an opportunity to query potential alternatives. Importantly, this sort of dialog is not commonplace prior to every action performed on the patient, for instance, the obtaining of intravenous access or placement of oxygen via nasal cannula. The legal standard of a "reasonable person" is applicable here—"what a reasonable person in the patient's position would want to know to make an intelligent and informed treatment decision."[12] They argue that the same standard could be extended beyond the consent process to frame the communication between patient and physician. In other words, what would a reasonable person want to know about all aspects of the care: diagnosis, treatment options, prognosis, and errors. Thus, many physicians would agree that written informed consent is required prior to performing an invasive procedure such as a lumbar puncture or a high risk treatment, such as a blood transfusion.

As noted above, the physician and patient attitudes towards error vary. Gallagher et al. conducted focus groups of physicians, of patients, and a combination of both.[13] They found that the patient definition of error was quite broad, and included deviations from standard of care, some non-preventable adverse events, poor service quality, and deficient interpersonal skills of practitioners. This was despite being given a definition of error that was quite narrow: failure of a planned action to be completed as intended, or the use of a wrong plan to achieve an aim. Patients associated long waits for routine radiography, exposure to unknown drug allergies and rude physician behavior with unsafe care. On the other hand, physicians had a narrower definition of error, consisting of only deviations from the standard of care, and appeared frustrated that patients had such a broad view. Patients wanted full disclosure of all errors that harm, while physicians noted that they may not disclose errors when the harm is trivial, the patient cannot understand error, or the patient does not want to know about the error.[13] This is inconsistent with the growing body of evidence that patients want all error disclosed. This is from a systems perspective, as demonstrated in Mazor et al.'s survey of a New England health maintenance organization. Mazor et al. find that 91% of the respondents to a survey on medical errors agree with the statement "Patients should always be told if an error is made— even if the patient is not injured or harmed."[14] This attitude has also been demonstrated in ED patients. Hobgood et al. find that 88% of ED patients want full disclosure of all errors, and 76% prefer that the disclosure be performed immediately upon discovery of the error. This attitude is prevalent regardless of the patient's healthcare utilization.[15] In fact, the desire for full disclosure is generalizable to all patients, regardless of their background—there is no relation

with race/ethnicity, gender, age, and education, with the exception of an increased desire for reporting in younger patients and those with less education.[16] This also holds true for parents of pediatric patients seen in the ED. Not only do they want disclosure, they want reporting to an authoritative body, and are less likely to sue if there is disclosure.[17] The same trend is seen in pediatric patients admitted to the hospital, where 99% of parents want disclosure if there is potential or actual harm to the child.[18] While there may be some agreement about disclosure between physicians and patients when an error actually occurs, there is no consensus regarding disclosure with a near-miss. Patients have mixed opinions about near-miss events while physicians seem to disfavor their disclosure. Most physicians felt that this is impractical and would diminish trust.[13]

The gap between patient and physicians extends beyond the error disclosure—the method and content of the information requested versus that which is delivered is incongruent as well. While patients want an open discussion and an apology, physician training and attitude have been to be a "spin doctor" in the delivery of the message. "I think you have to be a spin doctor all the time and put the right spin on it. . . . I don't think you have to soft pedal the issue, but I think you try to put it in the best light."[13] Physicians choose their words carefully, and are variable in their attitudes toward error disclosure, regardless of their practice environment.[19] While we now know that patients are interested in the disclosure of errors, there continue to be barriers to implementation of a systematic process of identification, disclosure and investigation of errors. These can be attributed to our healthcare system and environment, our patients, our legal system, and ourselves.

The healthcare system in general and the ED in particular are rife with opportunity for error (as discussed above). Most hospitals have legal counsel and risk management departments that are integrally involved in error disclosure. While systems to disclose error may be institutionalized by risk managers, physicians are not always aware of their presence. Compounding this problem is the fact that risk managers support error disclosure, but not a full apology, which is what our patients want.[20] Witnessing this attitude from risk managers, physicians may conclude that acknowledging or disclosing errors is not of import to the healthcare system. The ED clinical environment itself is a systemic barrier to addressing medical errors. The nature of the care provided: acute, episodic, with limited background information and the frequent need for rapid decision-making with multiple priorities makes EDs prone to error, as discussed by Croskerry and Sinclair.[5] The hazards of frequent transitions of care lead to an increased risk of medical error as well. These can include a failure to reevaluate a patient at sign-out as well as a faulty transfer of information—delayed, inaccurate, incomplete, or poorly organized.[21] Finally, the nature of the ED visit itself, the lack of a pre-existing relationship or any continuity of care can lead to limited opportunity for the identification of an error.

The patient population frequenting the ED also contributes to the complexity of error identification and disclosure. These factors can range from logistical issues such as language barriers and lack of resources to clinical presentation. The lack of a phone, verifiable address, immigration status can all lead to patients giving ED providers incorrect information. Obviously, this will lead to difficulty in follow-up and patient contact to discuss an error that may have occurred.

The medical training and culture in which physicians are indoctrinated lead to significant barriers in the disclosure of errors. The edict of *primum non nocere*, "first do no harm," is given such paramount importance that the occurrence of an error leads to significant complications for the healthcare team as well as its leader. Kaldjian et al. have derived a taxonomy to categorize physician barriers to disclosure. The four areas identified are: attitudinal barriers, helplessness, uncertainties, and fears/anxieties.[22] Attitudinal barriers perpetuate the culture of silence by denying errors, doubting the benefits of disclosure, externally placing blame for errors, and advancing self-interests. Helplessness may result due to perceived or actual lack of institutional support, as well as feeling a loss of control after the information is disclosed. Lack of education regarding disclosure of errors and adverse events or disagreement with a supervisor or trainee leads can be classified as uncertainties. Finally, there are many sources of fear (founded or not) that can be a barrier to disclosure: legal and financial liability, professional reputation, personal failure, and patient/family anger. All of these factors can lead to a multitude of emotions, including guilt, shame, and professional inadequacy.[2] This can

be particularly troublesome for trainees, and may help explain the findings that while 90% of house officers admit to committing an error with serious adverse outcomes, only 24% had discussed the error with either the patient or the patient's family.[23] Many physicians, both residents and attending, may wish to disclose errors, but cite a lack of training and the communication skills to adequately convey the message. In fact, only 12% of a sample of an academic medical center residents and attending emergency physicians report any instruction on error disclosure.[24] Physicians also fear the loss of trust that a patient may undergo after an error is disclosed. This may lead to further patient harm by decreasing adherence to treatment or deterring them from seeking care in the future.[25] The converse argument is also made by others—the truth-telling of full disclosure enhances patient trust and encourages communication.[15]

The last barrier to disclosure relates to legal concerns. Identified as a contributor to healthcare system and physician barriers, the threat of malpractice liability is a significant factor in its own right. Defense attorneys frequently counsel against speaking with patients about medical errors for fear of revealing that patient injury was the result of error, or admissibility of the error and apology as evidence against the physician.[26] There is evidence mounting that disclosure and apology may reduce the likelihood of litigation,[17,27] or at the very minimum, have no effect on the patient's desire to sue.[28] Recognizing this barrier to error disclosure, many states have enacted statutes making error disclosure and apology inadmissible in civil suits. For example, North Carolina's statute provides that "statements by health care providers apologizing for an adverse outcome in medical treatment, offers to undertake corrective or remedial treatment or actions, and gratuitous acts to assist affected persons shall not be admissible to prove negligence or culpable conduct by the health care provider. . . ."[29] Concern still exists that these statutes will not provide complete protection to the physician.

What do patients want in a disclosure? The key content items include: **honesty, explanation, empathy, apology,** and the chance to **lessen the chance of future errors.**[13] We have created a mnemonic that addresses these concerns "HEEAL":

• Honesty—patients prefer an open statement of error that allows for a full disclosure of the care delivered and the events leading to the error. They need and want to feel that their physician is open with the information, and that they do not have to pry the information from the doctor.[13,14]

• Explanation—patients want physicians to provide an open acknowledgement and acceptance of responsibility. They believe this should be provided by the leader of the healthcare team. The explanation should entail facts about the event and events leading up to the event. Their fear needs to be addressed with the knowledge that the results of the error will be mitigated (if harm occurred). They need to understand implications in terms of future treatment, additional procedures, monitoring, increased length of stay, and expense. They want to know if temporary or permanent disability will occur. Finally, they want to know what will be done to help them recover from the error.

• Empathy—the disclosure should demonstrate empathy towards the patient, giving the patient permission to express any fear and emotion, as well as acknowledging these as being legitimate. Once identified, the issues need to be addressed—questions as well as the potential desire to change providers.

• Apology—A vital component of the disclosure is the apology. A complete apology that accepts responsibility and is sincere is the goal. While hospital risk managers may prefer a partial apology,[20] it may do more harm than good. In fact, it has been demonstrated with groups of litigants offered settlement that a full apology that is authentic increases the acceptability of an offer. A partial apology was worse than no apology at all.[13]

• Lessen the chance for future errors—finally, patients want to ensure that the chance for future errors has been lessened. Ensuring that others are not harmed in the same manner is a frequent motivation. The physician should provide reassurance, and potentially follow up the event in regard to this need. This can include discussion at educational or morbidity and mortality conferences, creation of new policies, system change, as well as reporting the event to regulatory bodies.

Section IV: Recommendations

• Error disclosure should become a standard part of medical practice.
• Disclosure protocols should be in place and vetted through ED and hospital administration.

• Students, residents, and attending physicians should be taught specific methods of error disclosure to ensure that patients' needs are met.
• All patients deserve our honesty, empathy, reassurance, and an apology when errors occur in the delivery of healthcare.

References

1. Kohn LT, Corrigan JM, Donaldson MS. (2000) In: *To Err Is Human: Building a Safer Health System.* Washington, DC: National Academies Press.
2. Wu AW, (2000) Medical error: the second victim: the doctor who makes the mistake needs help too. *BMJ.* 320, 726–7.
3. Thomas, EJ, Studdert DM, Burstin HR, et al. (2000) Incidence and types of adverse events and negligent care in Utah and Colorado. *Med Care March.* 38(3), 261–71.
4. Fordyce J, Blank FS, Pekow P, et al. (2003) Errors in a busy emergency department. *Ann Emerg Med.* 42(3), 324–33.
5. Croskerry P, Sinclair D. (2001) Emergency medicine: a practice prone to error. *CJEM.* 3, 271–6.
6. Reason JT. (1990) *Human Error.* Cambridge: Cambridge University Press.
7. Brennan TA, Leape LL, Laird NM, et al. (1991) Incidence of adverse events and negligence in hospitalized patients: Results of the Harvard Medical Practice Study. *N Engl J Med.* 324, 370–6.
8. Leape LL, Brennan TA, Laird NM, et al. (1991) The nature of adverse events in hospitalized patients: results of the Harvard Medical Practice Study II. *N Engl J Med.* 324, 377–84.
9. Moskop JC, Geiderman JM, Hobgood CD, et al. (2006) Emergency physicians and disclosure of medical errors. *Ann Emerg Med.* 48(5), 523–31.
10. American Medical Association (AMA). (2001) *Principles of Medical Ethics.* Chicago, IL: AMA. Available at: http://ama-assn.org.libproxy.lib.unc.edu/ama/pub/category/2512.html. Accessed June 2011.
11. American College of Emergency Physicians. (2011) Principles of ethics for emergency physicians. Available at: www.acep.org/Content.aspx?id=29144. Accessed June 2011.
12. Brock DW. (1987) Informed consent. In: VanDeVeer D, Regan T (eds) *Health Care Ethics: An Introduction.* Philadelphia, PA: Temple University Press, pp. 98–116.
13. Gallagher TH, Waterman AD, Ebers AG, et al. (2003) Patients' and physicians' attitudes regarding the disclosure of medical errors. *JAMA.* 289(8), 1001–7.

14. Mazor KM, Simon SR, Yood RA, et al. (2004) Health plan members' views about disclosure of medical errors. *Ann Intern Med.* 140, 409–18.

15. Hobgood C, Peck CR, Gilbert B, et al. (2002) Medical errors: what and when: what do patients want to know? *Acad Emerg Med.* 9, 1156–61.

16. Hobgood C, Tamayo-Sarver JH, Weiner B. (2008) Patient race/ethnicity, age, gender and education are not related to preference for or response to disclosure. *Qual Saf Health Care.* 17(1), 65–70.

17. Hobgood C, Tamayo-Sarver JH, Elms A, et al. (2005) Parental preferences for error disclosure, reporting, and legal action after medical error in the care of their children. *Pediatrics.* 16(6), 1276–86.

18. Matlow AG, Moody L, Laxer R, et al. (2010) Disclosure of medical error to parents and paediatric patients: assessment of parents' attitudes and influencing factors. *Arch Dis Child.* 95(4), 286–90.

19. Gallagher TH, Garbutt JM, Waterman AD, et al. (2006) Choosing your words carefully: how physicians would disclose harmful medical errors to patients. *Arch Intern Med.* 166(15), 1585–93.

20. Loren DJ, Garbutt J, Dunagan WC, et al. (2010) Risk managers, physicians, and disclosure of harmful medical errors. *Jt Comm J Qual Patient Saf.* 36(3), 101–8.

21. Beach C, Croskerry P, Shapiro M. (2003) Profiles in patient safety: emergency care transitions. *Acad Emerg Med.* 10, 364–7.

22. Kaldjian LC, Jones EW, Rosenthal GE, et al. (2006) An empirically derived taxonomy of factors affecting physicians' willingness to disclose medical errors. *J Gen Intern Med.* 21(9), 942–8.

23. Wu AW, Folkman S, McPhee SJ, et al. (1991) Do house officers learn from their mistakes? *JAMA.* 265, 2089–94.

24. Hobgood C, Xie J, Weiner B, et al. (2004) Error identification, disclosure, and reporting: practice patterns of three emergency medicine provider types. *Acad Emerg Med.* 11, 196–9.

25. Rosner F, Berger JT, Kark P, et al. (2000) Disclosure and prevention of medical errors: Committee on Bioethical Issues of the Medical Society of the State of New York. *Arch Intern Med.* 160, 2089–92.

26. Robbennolt JK. Apologies and legal settlement: an empirical examination. *Mich Law Rev.* 102, 460–516.

27. Kraman SS, Hamm G. (1999) Risk management: extreme honesty may be the best policy. *Ann Intern Med.* 131, 963–7.

28. Wu AW, Huang IC, Stokes S, et al. (2009) Disclosing medical errors to patients: it's not what you say, it's what they hear. *J Gen Intern Med.* 24(9), 1012–7.

29. North Carolina General Statutes. (2004) Ch. 8C, Art. 4, Rule 413.m.

4 Conflicts between patient requests and physician obligations

Shellie L. Asher

Associate Professor, Department of Emergency Medicine, Albany Medical College, Albany, NY, USA

Section I: Case presentation

An 82-year-old man presents to the emergency department (ED) complaining of "pain all over." The patient has prostate cancer with multiple bony metastases, and he has a do-not-attempt-resuscitation and do-not-intubate order. His pain has not been able to be controlled with oral medications at home. The patient tells the physician that his suffering is unbearable, and requests "enough medicine to end it all." The physician is willing to treat the patient's pain, but is concerned that if he uses significant amounts of pain medicine, it may inhibit the patient's drive to breathe, causing his death. The physician believes it would be morally wrong to intentionally shorten the patient's life. The patient's pain is subsequently managed successfully in the ED, and the department social worker is able to find the patient a placement in hospice care.

Section II: Discussion

Dr. Peter Rosen: Many ethical questions seem to hinge upon whether or not we have the right medical facts. In this case, we are faced with an ethical dilemma, in which we possess adequate medical facts, but do not possess an ethical interpretation of how to use those facts. I'm referring to the fear of taking away the patient's respiratory drive through efforts to relieve his pain. This approach fails to recognize the three missions of the practice of medicine. The first involves curing disease when possible, the least frequent occurrence we encounter. Disease management with the intent of prolonging life is the second and much more common mission. Finally, the third is to give comfort. When the first two objectives are impossible, either because of the ravages of disease or because of an incurable, quickly progressing pathology, we are then obligated to meet the third objective— to give comfort, and cease to concern ourselves with the complications associated with our ability to give comfort.

Dr. Arthur Derse: I think there is a misunderstanding here; it is well-accepted in ethics and in law that narcotic administration to the terminally ill that may shorten the patient's life is ethically permissible if the intent of the medication administration is to reduce the patient's suffering. The concept in play here is called the principle of double effect. This principle has also been recognized by the United States Supreme Court in cases dealing with physician-assisted suicide, where the court itself recognized that there is no legal responsibility for the death of a patient that results from the unintended consequences of therapy administered in the attempt to relieve pain. The physician and the potential treatment in this case clearly meet the principle of double effect, and are therefore legally and ethically acceptable.

Ethical Problems in Emergency Medicine: A Discussion-Based Review, First Edition. John Jesus, Shamai A. Grossman, Arthur R. Derse, James G. Adams, Richard Wolfe, and Peter Rosen.
© 2012 John Wiley & Sons, Ltd. Published 2012 by John Wiley & Sons, Ltd.

Dr. Shamai Grossman: Religious law tends to agree; administration of analgesics is appropriate and virtuous, as long as the goal is to lessen pain and not hasten death. Unexpectedly, the palliative disease literature suggests that giving an analgesic to the terminally ill may paradoxically extend their life. Regardless, opiates in the terminally ill at most have a 1% chance of respiratory depression.[1]

PR: Are you taught in medical school that the complications of your treatments have to be considered no matter what the aim of your drug administration should be?

Dr. John Jesus: We do have an increasing presence of medical ethics within medical education, but I don't recall specific attention paid to this topic. Though medical education is in need of a focus on medical ethics, it is also impossible to address every issue a physician will face during a career. Many medical schools are attempting to provide their students with the tools to analyze moral problems, so that they can extrapolate to situations and dilemmas not specifically addressed.

Dr. Shellie Asher: The overlying principle taught, at least in our current education, is that before administering any medications to a patient you need to explain to them the risks, benefits and alternatives, as part of the informed consent process. This is also part of the Center for Medicare and Medicaid Services survey guidelines, assessed through information gathered from patients after discharge, which includes whether a patient had received any medications, and if the patient had been told what the medication was for and what the possible side effects were.

PR: We frequently encounter patients with whom we do not have a longstanding relationship so it is difficult to know where they stand on the curve of the quality of life; we rarely know what they are willing to tolerate, or if they are at a point of suffering they no longer feel is bearable. On the other hand, I have encountered many patients who would have been perfectly happy to have me help end their life. In my experience, however, ending their life wasn't their primary goal either. Rather, they simply wanted to have a quality of life that was not so full of suffering that they could once again enjoy their existence. I began to understand that it isn't just an ethical splitting of hairs to say that "I don't care what amount

of pain medicine I'm giving to terminally ill patient. I want to use the amount that will give some quality to their life, and if, at the same time it happens to shorten their life, then so be it." A clinician needs to arrive at the position where he can say the goal is to comfort, and not to try to preserve the ideal medical therapy with medications in patients who have no ideal outcome.

There are other situations in which ethical conflicts between patients and physicians are probably as problematic. For example, we are all aware of the conflicts between a teenage Jehovah's Witness on chronic renal dialysis and the physician's responsibility: when his clinical assessment concludes with the need to transfuse the patient. At what point are those patients going to be forced to take blood transfusions as they inevitably develop their chronic anemia? When I was in San Diego I reviewed such a case as a member of the hospital's ethics committee. In San Diego, physicians treating Jehovah's Witness patients with renal failure couldn't obtain a court order that gave them the authority for more than for a single administration of blood. We ended up suggesting that the treating physicians submit to those patients an optimal treatment protocol, and ask them to comply with it or find another physician. You shouldn't demean your standards of when it is appropriate to transfuse a patient simply to avoid interpersonal conflict. Are there other instances in which you have ethical conflicts with your patients?

SA: One case which comes to mind is the physician who fundamentally opposes the use of postcoital contraception, but who is faced with a patient requesting it in the ED.

PR: If we presume the physician works in an institution that is not affiliated with a particular religion, and a patient presents requesting abortion advice or postcoital abortion therapy, how should the physician proceed? I suppose one solution is to turn to another member of your team and request that your colleague write the prescription. What if the physician is in a single-coverage ED?

AD: This is one of the more challenging ethical and legal situations that exist, in my experience. The physician would like to stand on his or her own ethical principles. Certainly, emergency physicians have a certain amount of autonomy to be able to refuse certain actions based on their autonomy as a physician and their religious beliefs. At the same time, the patient retains the right to be referred or directed to someone who can accomplish what is seen to be within the realm of legal medical choices for a patient.

While I don't think a physician should be required to do something that contravenes deeply held ethical principles, if those principles conflict with certain essential elements of emergency care, they shouldn't have pursued a career within emergency medicine. On the other hand, I believe that physicians do retain the right to refuse certain interventions as long as it is not going to harm the patient. For example, an individual physician cannot both refuse to participate in a particular medically appropriate procedure, because of moral qualms, **and** refuse to refer the patient to another physician who could provide the intervention. The responsibility of a physician is to respect a patient's choice, even if they don't participate in those choices, which is a concept that ought to trump a physician's protestations of complicity.

PR: I heard of a case not too long ago, in which a pharmacist refused to fill birth control prescriptions because it was against his moral beliefs. Do you have the right to impose your own moral understandings and moral principles on patients who are dependent on your services? Part of the problem we face is that there are no ethical absolutes that apply to all situations. Just as Gödel suggests that there are mathematical theorems that can't be proved, there are ethical principles that can't be extended and generalized to every situation. Having said that, the postmodernists added that all ethical principles are therefore equivalent, which I also think is wrong. I think when you are living in a pluralistic society as we do, you have to give space to moral opinions that you find morally repugnant, even though you think they are wrong, especially if you are holding yourself out as a representative of that pluralistic society as opposed to a representative of the group ethics to which you belong. How would you resolve this dilemma?

JJ: John Rawls in his book *Political Liberalism* argues that coercive public policy ought to be based upon a comprehensive doctrine, or a worldview, that all reasonable people can accept.[2] In order to achieve this, he goes on to argue that the principles of justice for the basic structure of society should be decided upon by rational, risk averse individuals under a "veil of ignorance," which obscures their religious affiliation, socioeconomic status, and other factors that might sway them to choose unfairly. Similarly, James Childress and Tom Beauchamp argue in their book *Principles of Biomedical Ethics* that the four ethical principles (non-maleficence, beneficence, respect for persons, and justice), derive from a "set of moral norms that bind all [morally serious] persons in all places."[3] These principles form the medical ethics that guide our federal regulations governing the treatment of human subjects. In their text, the authors recognize the four ethical principles as "prima facie obligations." Accordingly, each of the obligations must be fulfilled unless an equally important competing obligation outweighs it in the pursuit of the "'greatest possible balance of right over wrong.'" The authors of these two works both argue persuasively that though there are no absolute principles to guide us in all situations, we can derive principles upon which most of us can agree to guide us through most situations. I think this is a much better way of thinking about ethical problems, and also gives a clue into why ethical problems can be difficult.

SG: Ultimately, a physician does have a right and perhaps an obligation to stay true to a personal moral and ethical value system. If this belief system cannot be balanced with the obligation to care for the patient, the physician can, and perhaps should, withdraw from caring for this patient so long as this does not create a life threat to the patient by so doing.

JJ: When we become physicians we sign up for a job that necessitates interaction with patients who have a variety of beliefs. We should act in ways that stay true to the fiduciary relationship that we have with them. We have a responsibility to protect patient interests, and if we have a moral quandary with regard to a particular decision that they would like us to make or with a particular intervention that they would like us to facilitate, I think that we should be transparent and openly communicate that moral quandary. We must not prevent the patient from obtaining more information about a particular intervention by proactively hiding such information. Such an act would be a lie of omission, dishonest, and a blatant infraction of the basic principle of respect for persons with no other more important competing obligation.

39

PR: I think that this case is an excellent example of another ethical dilemma in which there are perhaps medical compromises that can be made that will help relieve the physician's anxiety, as well as to help the patient acquire the comfort and outcome the patient wants. You were able to establish an admission to a hospice where there may be physicians at that hospice who are more comfortable administering larger quantities of analgesics than the emergency physician. There existed a medically appropriate outcome to help address the ethical dilemma, which should always be sought out. I don't know how to help the physician who feels the action that he is being asked to perform is so morally repugnant that he cannot, in good conscience, advise the patient where the intervention can be performed, in addition to not performing the intervention himself. I believe there are attitudes that are right and wrong, which may leave you morally confused. For these conflicts it helps to consider them before you find yourself in the position to make decisions that affect the lives of your patients. If you feel so strongly that you refuse to advise people on alternatives to what you personally are unwilling to do, then perhaps you shouldn't be in this position in the first place. Instead of being an emergency physician at the only county hospital in your community, for example, perhaps you should work at the hospital in your community that is consonant with your ethical position, and clearly identified with it, where patients can expect and understand that the hospital operates under such an ethical doctrine. Is there a legal obligation to advise patients about procedures that you feel are morally repugnant?

AD: You have a legal obligation to tell the patient what your objection is, and to explain all reasonable or viable alternatives to a particular intervention as part of informed consent. You also risk abandoning a patient if a patient is injured or harmed as a result of your withholding of information. The legal ramifications may be more apparent in particularly egregious situations, such as when an abortion is necessary to save the life of the mother or prevent serious morbidity, and the physician is unwilling to arrange its performance.

Whether or not the physician in our case felt that the patient's request for enough medication to "end it all" were morally permissible, however, was not the only issue highlighted by our case. Appropriately the emergency physician didn't take the request at face value, because the statement may not have accurately reflected the patient's true wish. It could be that the patient is in so much pain that taking enough medication to end life was desired as a convenient way to end the suffering. The patient's true wish is for pain relief. It may be that more questions, more analysis, and a little bit more understanding of what the patient is truly asking for, may help in realizing that the conflict is not between what the patient wants and what the doctor wants, but rather that there isn't a conflict at all, as both can be aligned behind the goal of alleviating the patient's pain.

JJ: Emergency physicians are often judged to be ignorant or unwilling to adequately treat pain. We certainly are medically and morally responsible to give patients analgesics. However, there are pressures against prescribing pain medicines at will. In 2010 the Massachusetts Supreme Court upheld a suit against a physician who prescribed an analgesic to a person who then drove after taking it, and had an accident. The physician was found guilty for not giving adequate instructions to the patient about not driving while on the analgesic. Although appropriate discharge instructions are important, they cannot detail every action that might impair a patient, and endanger someone around them. Though we want to relieve suffering, there are also other legal risks and ramifications that emergency physicians think about that perhaps contribute to inadequately addressing patients' pain.

AD: The understanding I had years ago when I was going through my emergency medicine residency was that emergency physicians couldn't get in trouble for prescribing too little analgesic; they only could get in trouble for prescribing too much, too easily or for unintended consequences such as the car accident. Because we do not have long-term relationships with our patients, we tend to err on the side of undertreatment of patients. With the advent of palliative care, emphasizing an understanding of the importance of pain relief, the pendulum is finally swinging back toward the middle, recognizing pain as the "fifth vital sign." Keep in mind that the likelihood of getting in trouble is far less likely with patients who are at the end of life, have a terminal condition, or are in such severe pain that they won't be driving. The danger that you can get into prescribing narcotics is one in which you don't differentiate between the patient in the case here who has a terminal condition and other ED patients who are less critically ill. Even if the patient should have a respiratory arrest, and had a do-not-resuscitate/do-not-intubate (DNR/DNI) code status, and you are unable to sustain the patient's life by bag, valve, mask ventilation, you would be able to justify your action by saying: "I was trying to relieve pain, I knew that this was an unintended side effect, and, yes, the patient died as a result of my giving him this narcotic, but in addition to and mainly of the ravages of the underlying disease that I was trying to alleviate."

PR: The fact that we've gotten into trouble for over-prescribing analgesic medications doesn't justify our not prescribing them where they are indicated. The justification for giving an analgesic, no matter how appropriate, doesn't justify our giving it in a negligent fashion. Whether we use an adequate dose of opiate or an inadequate dose, the reality is that in the ED, you don't send people out to drive when you've just given them sedatives or analgesics. If they don't have someone who can accompany them, then you can't discharge them until there's somebody to safely get them home. We need to separate the purposes of what we're trying to do therapeutically from the mechanics of doing this.

An example of being punished for doing something appropriate is as follows: I worked as a surgeon in a small town in Wyoming for a number of years, and at the time I made house calls. I was on call at the time for the entire town every third or fourth night. It was a mechanism to provide some work relief for solo physicians. The downside, however, was that you frequently made house calls on patients who were followed by another practice and of whose medical details you knew little. I was called to make a house call on a man with chronic back pain on the nights that I was on call. In a month, I saw him two or three times for significant back pain, and this particular night, I ended up giving him a shot of narcotics so he could sleep through the night. I later received a letter from the medical license board in Wyoming saying that I and four other doctors were pandering to this man's narcotic habit, and that we should be more cognizant of how we're writing pain prescriptions or we could lose our licenses. It turned out that the patient actually had a large aortic aneurysm, which was not detected on physical examination, and he

ended up dying from its rupture. His back pain was likely the aneurysm enlarging and leaking. There is an impulse to be unwilling to give pain relief when you are going to be blamed for writing a narcotics prescription, and I think we just have to accept, ethically, that it's part of our job.

AD: Appropriate use and practices within the standard of care are important. Furthermore, regulatory oversight may or may not be in accord with good medical care, but you must still do the right thing for your patients. Neither the frequency nor the amount of narcotic use by patient should be, in and of itself, the determinant of whether the patient is abusing it. There has been a change in the federation of state medical boards approach to narcotic prescriptions, but the federal drug enforcement administration has been slower in coming around to this viewpoint. This is where the best medical practice and your medical judgment may be second guessed, and regulatory oversight may or may not comport with what's ultimately good for the patient. The appropriate action here is to use your best medical judgment, and to provide sound ethical treatment.

PR: The criticisms of the emergency physician and our reputation of not treating pain in an adequate fashion are perhaps less justified than they were 20 years ago. Today, we have better education about the correct dosage, and I think we have managed to succeed in overturning some of our consultants' views. I remember for years having to fight with surgeons about giving analgesics to patients with abdominal pain because it "masked their examination," yet they were not quick to respond to the call for consultation. Here again we have a case where medical data have enabled us to stop arguing about ethics, and say there are data that show that adequately treating a patient's abdominal pain doesn't interfere with the diagnosis or mask the disease course, and we are therefore justified in administering analgesics.

Section III: Review of the literature

The practice of emergency medicine requires the ability to interact with and treat patients from many cultures in myriad medical situations. In the course of practice, emergency physicians may find themselves in a situation where fulfilling the need or request of a patient conflicts with the physician's own ethical beliefs. In such cases, the physician must examine several aspects of the situation to determine the most appropriate course of action. Examples of common scenarios that may cause conflict include those involving end-of-life care, resource utilization, and treatments in the setting of pregnancy or potential pregnancy. Studies of US physicians across multiple specialties demonstrate that a significant number of practicing physicians are ethically opposed to some of the medical interventions legally available to various populations of patients in the United States. Of physicians surveyed, 69% object to physician-assisted suicide, 18% to terminal sedation, and 5% to withdrawal of artificial life support. Most physicians (63%) believe that it is ethically permissible for doctors to explain their moral objections to patients; 86% believe that physicians are obligated to present all options, and 71% believe that the physician must refer the patient to a non-objecting clinician.[4,5]

In light of the significant number of physicians who relate ethical qualms with procedures they may be asked to perform, individual physicians must be aware of their own ethical beliefs, cognizant of possible areas of patient care that may cause conflict between the patient and physician, and have a plan in place for determining the most appropriate course of action based on ethical principles. The purpose of this chapter is to illustrate the ethical sources of these conflicts, and to propose mechanisms for amelioration supported by the ethical principles of respect for persons, non-maleficence, beneficence, and justice.

Specific ethical considerations

In the case discussion, Dr. John Jesus lays out a framework for ethical decision-making using Childress and Beauchamp's argument that there are four ethical principles (non-maleficence, beneficence, respect for persons, and justice) that function as "prima facie obligations" on the part of physicians toward their patients, which must be fulfilled unless an equally important competing obligation outweighs them in the pursuit of the "greatest possible balance of right over wrong."[3] Though inadequate to provide resolution in all situations, these principles can be agreed on as an initial basis for decision-making and utilized to guide most situations. Conflicts between the prin-

ciples can be a common source of ethical conflict in the patient–physician relationship.

The American College of Emergency Physicians' code of ethics addresses the actions and responsibilities of emergency physicians based on the foundations of moral pluralism, unique duties of emergency physicians, and virtues in emergency medicine, noting that "emergency physicians must be tolerant of people of different races, creeds, customs, habits, and lifestyle preferences . . . [practicing] impartiality by giving emergency patients an unconditional positive regard, and treating them in an unbiased, unprejudiced way."[6]

Physician conscience

Arguments for and against allowing physicians to limit interventions offered based on their own moral compass are typically set in the context of physician conscience. But what does "conscience" really mean? Conscience can be defined as "the sense or consciousness of the moral goodness or blameworthiness of one's own conduct, intentions, or character together with a feeling of obligation to do right or be good,"[7] or "an individual's faculty for making moral judgments together with a deep commitment to acting on them."[8] In order for conscience to function, the physician must have a developed sense of what is good or blameworthy, and be able to apply that sense to decision-making processes. Conscience, suggests Thomas Aquinas, is simply "knowledge applied to an individual case."[9] Conscience may be thought of as having two intertwined parts: a commitment to acting and choosing morally to the best of one's ability, and the activity of judging whether an act would violate that commitment.[10] Conscience arises from a fundamental commitment to morality, to upholding one's deepest moral beliefs, discerning the moral features of individual situations and acting upon "what one discerns to be the morally right course of action."[10] Conscientious refusal, therefore, may be defined as "refusal to perform an action or participate in a practice that is legal and professionally accepted, but which the individual professional believes to be deeply immoral."[8]

To determine the most ethical course of action in any given situation, a variety of sources of ethical guidance are available to emergency physicians, including professional oaths and codes of ethics, general cultural values, social norms embodied in the law, religious and philosophical moral traditions, and professional role models.[6] While all of these sources can provide useful guidance, problems arise when they come into conflict with one another. The individual physician must be able to understand, interpret, and weigh conflicting sources to guide beliefs regarding the moral or ethical framework in which they will live and practice.

Some authors have argued that a physician's right to make judgments based on a personal conscience or moral framework is limited by the duties of their profession, as "entering into a profession in the public realm imposes some level of duty that may at times conflict with one's personal moral ideals."[11] Since the patient is dependent on the physician for information regarding treatment options, the physician is obligated to provide information regarding all options to the patient—even those options which the physician may find morally objectionable. Refusal to give information would "supplant one person's moral judgment with another's, it would also allow professional standing to be used as a justification for imposing one person's moral views on another."[11] Others argue that duty to patients trumps individual belief, and "doctors cannot make moral judgments on behalf of patients" concluding that "if people are not prepared to offer legally permitted, efficient, and beneficial care to a patient because it conflicts with personal values, they should not be doctors." Since "the primary goal of a health service is to protect the health of its recipients," physicians must set aside their own values in deference to those of the patient.[12]

Alternatively, it has been argued that it must be recognized that healthcare providers are independent moral agents, and that protection of the individual's right to act according to his or her conscience is fundamental. "While the patient has the right to pursue care, it cannot be done at the cost of liberty to a fellow citizen. Patient pursuit and preference should not trump the liberty of others. Making exceptions of healthcare professionals makes them second-class citizens."[13] The author also argues that the character and convictions of the healthcare provider are necessary for ethical patient care and protection.[13]

Acting conscientiously is the heart of the ethical life, and to the extent that physicians give it up, they are no longer acting as moral agents. Conscientious practice in a pluralistic world is messy even when peaceable. Yet the alternative is a society in which physicians are required to forfeit conscience in order to join the profession. Patients will not be well served by moral automatons who shape their practices, without struggle or reflection, to the desires of patients and the dictates of whatever regime is currently in power.[4]

Just as there are varying philosophical approaches to balancing the views of the physician with the views of the patient, legal statutes surrounding provider conscience vary by state, with some states giving broad protections. For example, the Illinois Health Care Right of Conscience Act protects a healthcare provider from all liability or discrimination that might result as a consequence of "his or her refusal to perform, assist, counsel, suggest, recommend, refer or participate in any way in any particular form of health care service that is contrary to the conscience of such physician or health care personnel."[14] A complete listing of US federal and state-specific statutes can be found at www.consciencelaws.org/laws/usa/law-usa.html and www.consciencelaws.org/laws/usa/law-usa-01.html.

Respect for persons

Respect for persons, self-determination, or patient autonomy is a prominent concept in modern medical ethics. Emergency physicians often must weigh and balance autonomy with other ethical principles. This is the case when a physician must weigh patient autonomy with physician beneficence in the setting of a patient who wishes to sign out against medical advice (AMA). In most cases where a patient has capacity to make decisions, the patient's autonomy is respected even if the physician disagrees with the patient's decision. While patients have a right to self-determination, there is a difference between the negative rights (right to non-interference) usually applied in the case of an AMA decision, and positive rights (the right to be assisted in some way). Also, there is a distinction between moral and legal rights. Put another way, a patient's (negative) right to self-determination does not necessarily confer a moral obligation on the part of a medical provider to provide a requested service (positive right).[15]

Respect for persons is typically carried out in the process of informed consent—a legal term which includes physicians' recommendations that encompass risks, benefits, and alternatives to treatment.

To choose and act autonomously, patients must receive accurate information about the medical conditions and treatment options. Emergency physicians should relay sufficient information to patients for them to make an informed choice among various diagnostic and treatment options.[6]

Medical care in the United States has rapidly moved away from a paternalistic approach to patients and toward an emphasis on patient autonomy. On the one hand, strong paternalism favors beneficence over autonomy, with the physician making decisions based on an interpretation of what is best for the patient. On the other extreme, autonomy can be weighted too heavily, with the physician presenting the patient with all the options but withholding the physician's own recommendations, allowing the patient "a free choice." A more balanced model would encourage patients and physicians to exchange ideas, negotiate differences, and come to a mutual conclusion in the interest of the patient's health and wellbeing. This type of collaboration would respect the views of the patient and physician, utilizing the physician's experience, and maintaining the patient's autonomy, with the final choice belonging to the fully informed patient.[16] Unfortunately, this process can be very labor intensive and time-consuming, making it difficult to carry out in practice in the ED.

Beneficence

Physicians assume a fundamental duty to serve the best interests of their patients by treating or preventing disease or injury, and by informing patients about their conditions. Emergency physicians respond promptly to acute illnesses and injuries in order to prevent or minimize pain and suffering, loss of function, and loss of life. In pursuing these goals, emergency physicians serve the principle of beneficence, that is, they act for the benefit of their patients.[6]

Unfortunately, the "best interest" of the patient can be the source of conflict between patient and physician, as physicians who have ethical objections to certain interventions often have the good of the patient in mind. In the case discussion, for example, the conflict occurs because of the patient's expressed desire to "end it all," which the physician does not believe is the best outcome for the patient. While

physicians must practice with beneficence, keeping the best interests of the patient in mind, they must also be mindful of the patient's perspective on the patient's own best interest.

Non-maleficence

Physician refusal to offer or provide a specific treatment should not leave the patient worse off than when they started.[17] As in the case of beneficence, this may be a difficult determination, and might vary depending on the perspective of the physician and the patient. In our case example, the patient may consider that to go on suffering is an untenable outcome, whereas the physician may believe death to be so. Where the physician sincerely believes that preventing the patient's death will be beneficent, the patient may consider it to be maleficent, if it leads to continued suffering.

When refusing to fulfill a request, the physician should reveal the moral reasons for the refusal, lest the patient think there were medical reasons for the objection, which may influence future decision-making and leave the patient worse off than from where the patient began.[17]

Another essential virtue of emergency physicians is trustworthiness. Sick and vulnerable emergency patients are in a dependent relationship, forced to trust that emergency physicians will protect their interests through competence, informed consent, truthfulness, and the maintenance of confidentiality.[6]

Failure to provide complete information regarding the medically acceptable options available to the patient may also cause harm, violating the principle of non-maleficence.

Justice

The fourth basic ethical principle is the fair treatment of patients and distribution of resources, or justice.[3] Based on this principle, some argue that while individual physicians may refuse treatments on the basis of moral integrity, the profession as a whole is required to meet its social obligations to provide "all legal and beneficial medical interventions sought by patients."[8] This requires: the physician to provide all relevant clinical information to the patient; the physician to refer the patient to a willing clinician; and that this process should not be unduly burdensome to the patient.[8]

Summary and analysis

In the case above, the patient's request for "enough medicine to end it all" conflicts with the physician's moral belief that it would be wrong to intentionally shorten the patient's life. While the physician in this case was able to successfully treat the patient's pain and refer him to hospice care, the emergency physician may encounter cases where it is impossible to fulfill the request of a patient due to beliefs that to do so would be morally wrong. In this particular case, the physician may need to be educated with respect to the principle of double effect—that if the intent is to treat the patient's pain, the unintended consequence (in this case, potentially shortening the patient's life) may not be morally wrong, even in the physician's moral framework. Clarifying the goals of care—curing disease, prolonging life, or treating suffering—is key to determining the right approach in end-of-life care. In other cases, the conflict may not be as amenable to education or compromise, as in the case of the physician who will not provide postcoital contraception on the basis that it is an abortifacient.

In practice, most physicians in a large survey report that when faced with an ethical conflict, it is acceptable to explain the nature of the physician's objection to the patient, but that the physician must also provide information about the alternatives and refer the patient to another provider if the physician has personal objections to the patient's choice. A sizable minority (14%), however, do not believe there is an obligation to disclose information regarding objectionable choices, and 29% do not believe the physician is obligated to refer the patient to another (non-objecting) provider.[4] The authors conclude that most physicians attempt to balance paternalism and autonomy, providing full disclosure about options and maintaining a bidirectional dialog between patient and physician.[4] Transfer-of-care requirements may "represent a compromise (albeit imperfect) between the fundamental rights of persons to practice both their desired profession and their religious belief system, while protecting patients from denial of access to services because of the religious or moral beliefs of another."[11] As stated in the case discussion above, "ultimately, a physician does have a right and perhaps an obligation to stay true to a personal moral and ethical value system. If this belief system cannot be balanced with the obligation to care for the patient, the physician can, and should, withdraw from caring for this patient so long as this does not create a life threat to the patient by so doing."[11] It helps to consider such conflicts before you find yourself in the position to make decisions that affect the lives of your patients. If you feel so strongly that you refuse to advise people on alternatives to what you personally are unwilling to do, then perhaps you should not be in this position in the first place.

Published models for medical decision-making recommend doctor–patient relationships that acknowledge room for independent moral beliefs on the part of the physician and the patient, encouraging open communication on the part of all parties and negotiation to a mutually acceptable solution.[16,18–20] Physicians must keep in mind that by virtue of their profession, there is an imbalance of power in the decision-making process. They must place close attention to patient vulnerability, and use their power responsibly in the best interests of the patient. With this in mind, physicians are still free to make their own informed decisions and must do so with integrity and a healthy respect for moral ambiguity. In order to balance autonomy and beneficent paternalism, the physician must use the same judgment and communication skills in making ethical judgments that they use in making medical judgments.[20]

In summary:

When we become physicians we sign up for a job that necessitates interaction with patients who have a variety of beliefs. We should act in ways that stay true to the fiduciary relationship that we have with them. We have a responsibility to protect patient interests, and if we have a moral quandary with regard to a particular decision that they would like us to make or with a particular intervention that they would like us to facilitate we should be transparent and openly communicate that moral quandary. We must not prevent the patient from obtaining more information about a particular intervention by proactively hiding such information. Such an act would be a lie of omission, dishonest, and a blatant infraction of the basic principle of respect for persons with no other more important competing obligation. (Dr. John Jesus, case discussion)

Section IV: Recommendations

• Individual physicians must be aware of their own ethical beliefs, cognizant of possible areas of patient care that may cause conflict between the patient and physician, and have a plan in place for determining the most appropriate course of action based on ethical principles.

• One proposed framework for determining a course of action mirrors the clinical decision-making process with which most physicians are familiar: (1) a plain statement of the problem; (2) a careful gathering of data; (3) a differential diagnosis; and (4) an articulation of a reasoned plan.

• The physician must pay close attention to the goals of care, which may include curing disease, prolonging life, or providing comfort, and determine whether or not the goals of the physician are the same as those of the patient.

• The physician must address whether the primary problem is medical, ethical, or some combination, as in the case discussion.

• The plan should be based on sound medical and ethical principles and be agreed on by all parties.[15]

• If the physician and patient are unable to come to an agreement, then the physician should facilitate transfer of care to another provider.

References

1. Wilson WC, Smedira NG, Fink C, et al. (1992) Ordering and administration of sedatives and analgesics during the withholding and withdrawal of life support from critically ill patients. *JAMA*. 267, 949–53.

2. Rawls J. (1996) *Political Liberalism*. New York, NY: Columbia University Press, pp. 6–46.

3. Beauchamp T, Childress J. (2009) *Principles of Biomedical Ethics*, 6th ed. New York, NY: Oxford University Press, pp. 1–25.

4. Curlin FA, Lawrence RE, Chin MH, et al. (2007) Religion, conscience, and controversial clinical practices. *N Engl J Med*. 356, 593–600.

5. Curlin FA, Nwodim C, Vance JL, et al. (2008) To die, to sleep: US physicians' religious and other objections to physician-assisted suicide, terminal sedation, and withdrawal of life support. *Am J Hosp Palliat Care*. 25(2), 112–20.

6. American College of Emergency Physicians. *Policy Compendium, 2010*. Dallas, TX: American College of Emergency Physicians. Available at: www.acep.org/workarea/downloadasset.aspx?id=9104. Accessed July 10, 2010.

7. Merriam-Webster. Dictionary entry: conscience. Available at: www.merriam-webster.com/netdict/conscience. Accessed July 10, 2010.

8. Brock D. (2008) Conscientious refusal by physicians and pharmacists: who is obligated to do what, and why? *Theor Med Bioeth*. 29, 187–200.

9. Aquinas, T. (1948) *Summa Theologica*, vol. I, Q. 79, A. 13 (trans: Fathers of the English Dominican Province). New York, NY: Benziger Bros.

10. Sulmasy DP. (2008) What is conscience and why is respect for it so important? *Theor Med Bioeth*. 29, 135–49.

11. May T, Aulisio M. (2009) Personal morality and professional obligations: rights of conscience and informed consent. *Perspect Biol Med*. 52(1), 30–8.

12. Savulescu J. (2006) Conscientious objection in medicine. *BMJ*. 332, 294–7.

13. Rudd G. (2007) Healthcare without conscience—unconscionable! *Ann Pharmacother*. 41, 1903–5.

14. *Health Care Right of Conscience Act*, 745 Ill. Comp. Stat. § 70/1–14.

15. Kaldjian LC, Weir RF, Duffy TP. (2005) A clinician's approach to clinical ethical reasoning. *J Gen Intern Med*. 20(3), 306–11.

16. Quill TE, Brody H. (1996) Physician recommendations and patient autonomy: finding a balance between physician power and patient choice. *Ann Intern Med*. 125, 763–9.

17. Davis JK. (2004) Conscientious refusal and a doctor's right to quit. *J Med Philos*. 29, 75–91.

18. Emanuel EJ, Emanuel LL. (1992) Four models of the physician-patient relationship. *JAMA*. 267, 2221–6.

19. Siegler M. (1981) Searching for moral certainty in medicine: a proposal for a new model of the doctor-patient encounter. *Bull N Y Acad Med*. 57, 56–69.

20. Thomasma DC. (1983) Beyond medical paternalism and patient autonomy: a model of physician conscience for the physician-patient relationship. *Ann Intern Med*. 98, 243–8.

5 Judgmental attitudes and opinions in the emergency department

V. Ramana Feeser

Assistant Professor of Emergency Medicine, Department of Emergency Medicine, VCU Medical Center-Main Hospital, Virginia Commonwealth University (VCU), Richmond, VA, USA

Section I: Case presentation

A 22-year-old male patient with sickle cell disease presents to the triage area of the emergency department (ED) complaining of pain in his back and legs. He is wearing baggy, low-hanging jeans and a hooded sweatshirt, and is listening to loud music on his iPod. The triage nurse instructs him to turn down the music. His pain is typical of previous sickle cell crisis pain and he has been using his home narcotic medication without adequate relief. He reports that he is having 10 out of 10 pain. The nurse looks at him and explains the pain scale to him again and asks what level of pain is he really having. The patient repeats the same answer. The nurse directs him to the waiting room and after 4 hours, he is taken to the back to see the emergency physician (EP). Once in the treatment area, he tells the physician that hydromorphone is the only thing that works for him and requests the specific dose that works for him. The physician recognizes the patient from his past visit just a few days back, and attempts to treat his pain. His complete blood count shows chronic anemia and reticulocyte count is similar to previous values. After three rounds of medications, the physician tells the patient that he cannot offer further narcotics in the ED, and that he was just recently hospitalized and does not meet criteria for hospitalization again. The patient is discharged but he returns 3 days later with fever, cough,

and sickle cell pain crisis, and is diagnosed as having pneumonia. He is admitted to the inpatient medical service, where he develops respiratory failure and sepsis and is then transferred to the intensive care unit for antibiotics, blood transfusions, and ventilator management.

Section II: Discussion

Dr Peter Rosen: As an introduction, I believe the single most difficult area of patient assessment and treatment in the ED is pain management. It is an area filled not only with judgmental prejudice, but has led to numerous reports that emergency physicians don't know how to treat pain, frequently undertreating patients in pain. In truth, we are afraid of the addicted patient, and of supporting the addict's habit. We are also hurt by the many complaint letters written to the hospital authorities by people who didn't get the amount of analgesic they wanted. What can we do to solve these conundrums?

Dr. James Adams: The pain-seeking patient, broadly speaking, makes life extraordinarily difficult for the EP just as life is extraordinarily difficult for the patient in pain. Historically, EPs were repeatedly accused of inadequately treating pain. In recent years, however, EPs have been accused of contributing to narcotic addiction, as well, because we are now prescribing a

Ethical Problems in Emergency Medicine: A Discussion-Based Review, First Edition. John Jesus, Shamai A. Grossman, Arthur R. Derse, James G. Adams, Richard Wolfe, and Peter Rosen.

lot more narcotics than we did 10 years ago: so we can't win, we can't break even, and we can't get out of the game. In fact, it is impossible to tell who is having pain, or who is not. The situation is further complicated by our own human judgmental attitudes that rarely help the situation. We could just surrender and start giving out narcotics, but that doesn't make us happy. Furthermore, if the patient is seeking analgesics because of an opiate addiction, it simply enables and exacerbates the addiction. The first step is to recognize and acknowledge our own frustration. The second step is to have a consistent approach to the patient complaining of pain. In this case, for example, after 3 rounds of medication the physician tells the patient he will not offer further narcotic medication, which suggests that he has a systematic approach to the treatment of sickle cell patients complaining of pain.

PR: How does a consistent approach help the emergency physician and the patient?

JA: With a consistent approach the physician doesn't have to present personal negative emotional judgments. Moreover, it gives the EP a clear plan and mitigates the frustration of trying to guess who is and is not in pain, and how best to treat them. We have to calm ourselves and recognize that we may be expressing a negative reaction. It is useful to think about what you would do if the patient was a friend or family member.

Dr. John Jesus: I would emphasize the importance of recognizing and acknowledging our frustration before we attempt to address patients with complaints of pain that we are not sure is real. There are lots of examples of patients with chronic pain syndromes who also have "real" disease that we can more easily identify with objective measures and data. In the back of our mind, we know that one day they will present with a true health crisis. We just hope that we're not working when the event occurs because these patients are frequently cast aside, and their complaints downplayed. When these events do occur, I have observed that physicians and nurses feel a lot of guilt at having missed the crisis event, especially when they made the incorrect conclusion that the patient was simply pain pill seeking. I believe these feelings of guilt are reflective of an underlying compassion we have for these patients, and a realization that any prior disrespect

we may have directed toward them was an expression of an impotent frustration born out of our inability to address the patient's fundamental problem. Often this frustration is expressed by creating pejorative nicknames and placing similar problem patients in "special spaces" where we can more easily ignore them. Acknowledging our frustration and the various ways we express that frustration may help practitioners better manage pain and resist the impulse to belittle and make fun of these patients with chronic pain syndromes.

PR: It's clear that we underestimate the degree of pain patients have in the management of sickle cell disease. This is true despite literature that supports the notion that patients with true sickle cell disease have real pain, and are not just addicted to pain medications. The management of patients with sickle cell disease is much easier in those institutions that see a lot of them. Many institutions have a sickle cell clinic and a relationship with hematology outside of the ED that can help draw up pain management protocols with which both the patient and physician are comfortable. With other patients who have chronic pain syndromes as well as with those patients who are true narcotic-seeking addicts, the situation becomes much more difficult.

PR: I've been struck over the years in reading the pain literature, that we're expected to give analgesics to patients even when they don't want it, and that our failure to do so is judged as hypoanalgesia. The reality, however, is that every patient may not need pain management, even for painful injuries like fractures.

Dr. Richard Wolfe: A lot of the pain literature tries to create objective data from a subjective problem in a way that just doesn't capture the individuality of each case, and tries to eliminate clinical judgment. As a result, we're given guidelines that lack clinical judgment and may even be incorrect due to the subjective nature of pain. This makes me suspicious of the validity of the current literature. That said, I suspect we do undertreat patients in the case of chronic pain syndromes. This is particularly true of the recurrent visitor. Recently, I had the opportunity to sit and speak to a group of 100 sickle cell patients and their family members. It was an eye-opening experience to listen to the horror and fear they used in their descriptions of ED visits, largely due to inadequate pain management. I would argue that what is lacking in cases similar to these is an established process of what to do with the patient who repeatedly presents to the ED. With the introduction of electronic medical records, every patient with chronic pain can, and perhaps should, have a pre-established pain protocol that is shared with the patient and medical team, clearly delineating the suggested parameters of management to the patient and medical team. In our case, the patient sat in the waiting room for 4 hours before being seen. Though the ED may have been severely crowded, one suspects that his appearance, the loud music on the iPod, and the triage nurse's judgmental attitude were the true reasons the triage nurse tormented him by prolonging his wait time. A pain protocol may have lessened the frustration of all parties involved, and expedited the management of his pain.

PR: The patient in our case demanded hydromorphone. It has been my experience that many sickle cell patients do have a preference for a certain kind of analgesia. In fact, many patients seem to get benefit from meperidine, which is a drug that we are trying not to prescribe anymore due to the metabolic breakdown products that accumulate with repeated dosages. Do you think that part of the judgmental response from the medical team was stimulated by the patient's demand of a particular drug rather than being dutifully servile, and leaving it up to the nurse and physician?

Dr. Ramana Feeser: When patients come in specifically asking for a certain medication and dictating the dosage, practitioners often quickly conclude that the patient is drug seeking. I do believe that was the situation in this case, as I see this frequently in the ED. I often hear nurses and other staff say "Oh, this patient was seen recently in several EDs," and "Oh, this patient was just here, they must be a drug seeker." Labeling patients in that manner, however, often clouds your judgment, clinical assessment, and management.

PR: I think those are very real issues. There was an article that was published in JEM [the *Journal of Emergency Medicine*] about an institution that developed a policy stipulating that they would no longer give opiate analgesia for headache patients. I wrote an editorial in response because I think this practice

lacks any data to support the policy.[1–3] We are frequently led astray by our triage personnel. When the nurse comes to you and says, "Don't bother with Mr. Jones, he's been here 7 times this week, and he's just pain pill seeking," we're likely to respond differently than when the nurse describes the same patient by saying, "I have a patient with 10/10 pain, can you come and see him?" Clearly we have to be very careful of the attitudes with which we work. If we do create policies to manage patients with pain, they should be more patient oriented and less physician oriented. How do you develop a method for dealing with patients who are addicts and seeking narcotic medication? How do you deal with these patients, without expressing rage and disgust, and a wish that you hadn't come to work that day?

JJ: How young physicians perform is largely based upon on how we observe our attending physicians and mentors perform. One of the key points to address in this conversation is the importance of having the leaders in the department, those who educate medical students and residents, treat these kinds of patients with respect and refrain from demeaning them or referring to them with pejorative nicknames. Just as residents will place a chest tube based on the techniques they have observed, they will also treat their patients with sickle cell disease with disrespect if they observe their attending physicians doing the same. Though every patient requires a slightly different individualized approach, the constants in my approach are an attempt to treat them with compassion and respect.

PR: As mentors, however, we're often too passive about addressing inappropriate behavior that we encounter in our colleagues. We have to be a little more up front in our unwillingness to accept that behavior. If we hear a triage nurse say, for example, "You damn niggers all have this fake anemia, go sit in the waiting room," we should step in and voice our disapproval. I don't think any of us would tolerate that, but it is essentially what this triage nurse did. There comes a time when it is appropriate and imperative to say to the triage nurse, "It's inappropriate for you to put someone with 10/10 pain in the waiting room. I don't care how much experience you've had and whether or not you judge the patient's pain to be real or fake; 10/10 pain has to be addressed, and I expect you to do so." It's very hard for most of us to be confrontational. It's easier to be passive and say, "Boy, I don't want that nurse triaging me when I come in." The same is true of physician behavior. Take the physician in our case, for example, who says "You don't meet criteria for admission." Well, in fact, the patient did meet the criteria for admission. Even though we don't have a cure for sickle cell disease we can always provide comfort. It is incumbent upon senior physicians to refuse to allow a lack of idealism to diffuse throughout the department. Because we are subject to responding to our own culture, we have to be very careful of what we allow to develop in our departments. In the past we have spoken about a tendency to make ethical dilemmas out of misunderstood or mismanaged medical decisions. I think that this is yet another example of this phenomenon. The physician in our case tells the patient that he doesn't meet criteria for admission, but in fact, a sickle cell patient's failure to respond to analgesics is one of the indications for admission. Could you comment on whether you think patients with sickle cell disease have a particularly difficult time getting appropriate treatment because of hidden racial prejudices, or because we've become frustrated by treatment failure, and inappropriately conclude that they really aren't sick?

Dr. Shamai Grossman: As I read this case, what bothers me most is the lack of compassion with which the patient was treated. The physician attending to the patient sees him after 4 hours, gives him three rounds of medications and then says, "Ok, we're done." He won't admit the patient to the hospital, which we could argue is simply unethical, and he doesn't give the patient any other options. He doesn't contact the patient's primary care physician, and he doesn't arrange a good follow-up plan. It's certainly possible that the outcome may have been different if there had been better follow-up and a plan for outpatient treatment after discharge. There are no good indicators to distinguish between patients having a true sickle cell crisis from those patients who are seeking narcotic medications. Attempts to use hematocrit and reticulocyte counts to better identify patients in a true crisis have been made without success. Therefore, the only evidence you have is a patient telling you "I'm in pain, and my outpatient medication is just not adequate for me." Consequently, you must use this evidence rather than allow yourself to be jaded and ignore it.

PR: Even in those cases where we're quite convinced we're dealing with addiction and narcotic seeking, it's easier for the physician to assume the patient is having real pain than to assume he's faking pain. In the long run, it's a better position from which to argue. My personal approach to the narcotic addicted patient is to remove any personal confrontation between the patient and physician, and place the conversation within third party rules, under which both physicians and patients must live. Accordingly, when a patient says I want a boxcar full of Vicodin [acetaminophen and hydrocodone], I say, "I'd love to give you one, but **they** won't let me". It's not that I'm refusing to give the patient medication; it's that I don't have the power to grant the patient's wish. In this way we can work together, maintaining a positive patient–physician relationship, rather than in breaking down the relationship with conflicting goals. With diseases like sickle cell disease, which have chronic exacerbations, the best policy is to take the patient at his word, even if he doesn't quite meet our overall observations of how we think sick people should look.

JA: I would emphasize the importance of assuming patients are telling us the truth. The consequence of failing to believe our patients is the default assumption that we're being manipulated. This leads one to negatively judge all patients in similar circumstances. Constantly anticipating that patients are out to manipulate you is exhausting. Not only are patients likely to be undertreated, but it's also corrosive for our happiness, our health, our well-being as EPs. It benefits both patients and ourselves to assume patients' pains are real. Secondly, this case is fascinating, in part, because every EP can relate to it. The negative reaction we have against this scenario is strikingly universal. The only thing worse to irritate the staff that this guy could have been doing was to have been eating a bag of chips. Given the situation, I would put forth the question "Is the nurse who made him wait 4 or 5 hours, happy?" There's a norm of human reciprocity that occurs during these interactions. If the patient presents and acts with a great deal of frustration, and the nurse responds with similar frustration, the suffering is shared.

JJ: I frequently hear our nursing staff and other physicians express a reluctance to administer pain medications to patients when they are sleeping, or who are listening to music, or eating, but these are all methods of distraction. We often use these same techniques to distract children on whom we perform procedures. We should not be surprised when adults attempt to use the same techniques to distract themselves.

JA: What we should do as caregivers beginning to feel frustrated, is recognize and acknowledge our feelings, and then reframe the situation. Sometimes we have to talk to ourselves to make it happen. "This is a fatal disease and the pain can be real. Yes, the patient might be manipulated me, but it's better to err on the side of treating the pain." When a patient says, "Hey, I'm in pain," I respond by saying, "You know, I know you're suffering." Even if they are drug addicted, I believe they are suffering and that it is appropriate to acknowledge it. How I address and manage that suffering is a different question. This approach to the patient in pain is important in our discussion regarding judgmental attitudes, which we all experience at some point.

RW: One problem we are faced with, however, is that you can't transplant compassion. Fatigued EPs working in highly stressful conditions may have a hard time reaching out to that particular emotion. Viewing the problem from the standpoint of EM [emergency medicine] leadership, the answer comes down to having protocols in place in the ED that gives physicians a method to help intervene downstream as well as during that initial visit. Having an established process by which a patient's case can be referred to a committee that would then set in place limits or rules under which the patient would live may be helpful. This committee could also find ways to care for patients as outpatients as opposed to a repeat ED visitor, in order to begin to address long-term patient needs, in addition to the immediate needs on any particular shift.

PR: Although some of our decisions are based on our own negative judgmental attitudes, they are not necessarily bad medical decisions. The natural course of sickle cell disease is that it gradually worsens over time. Simply because one physician didn't adequately treat a patient's pain once, does not mean the patient will develop a complication. We should be careful in the ways we criticize each other. We're often accused of treating certain groups of people differently in EM. For example, we have been accused of not treating women properly or minorities. Yet, my own anecdotal experience as I've worked in a multitude of EDs

across the country is that this phenomenon does not exist. Perhaps I'm just naïve.

SG: It is human nature to have biases and prejudices, and naïve to believe that we are so enlightened to be free of them. Clearly, some of that baggage will be brought into the ED. Our goal as emergency physicians is to mitigate how they affect medical decisions and our approach to patient care. If we are not able to communicate with our patients, however, they will not receive the same level of care. This is why we mandate having translators, and why we initiate very broad diagnostic plans in the unresponsive, mentally disabled, or those otherwise unable to better describe their symptoms and history.

RW: I've been in two EDs that have studied wait times and treatment decisions of different groups of people. In those studies, African Americans had longer waiting room times and were placed in hallway beds rather than in rooms more frequently. How much of that was linked to the acuity of disease versus actual discrimination is hard to say.

PR: I think this case superbly illustrates the importance of judgmental attitudes in EM, what warning signs we must watch for, and some of the behaviors we must work to avoid. The "frequent flyer" induces great rage in emergency personnel. The goals of medicine are hard to meet when we attend to patients with chronic pain syndromes that we are unlikely to resolve in the ED. We should set up procedural structures or administrative bodies that can support physicians, and help us avoid our all too human failings. Perhaps in this way we can provide the kind of care and humane concern we all believe ought to be a norm for the emergency physician.

JJ: As a final point on this discussion I would point out that the ED is a unique space in which we witness public drunkenness, disorderly and inappropriate conduct, and attend to patients who are otherwise not experiencing their proudest moment. Maintaining this space as a safe place where anyone can take refuge is one of our more important responsibilities. Judgmental attitudes threaten this safe space. It's important for us to protect it because it engenders mutual respect and trust not only in specific EDs, but also in our profession. Trust and mutual respect, in turn, allows us to have greater effectiveness as EPs.

PR: That is an excellent summary of what is a type of behavior we're all guilty of at times, and all need to control. The message for our readers should not be that we're better or any different than they are, we all are subject to our own judgmental attitudes, and we all have to find ways to address them. One of the methods of doing so is to constantly sit down and ask yourself, "Who are the patients who make me angry? Who are the patients that disgust me? Who are the patients that I would prefer not to see or treat?" Then sit down and find a methodology for taking care of that very group of patients. Only by so doing can we avoid negative repercussions of judgmental attitudes and preserve the safe haven concept of EM.

Section III: Review of the literature

Judgmental attitudes and opinions are made on every patient that enters the ED. Experienced emergency physicians form opinions on whether a patient looks "sick" or "toxic" and in the majority of patients, even without diagnostic tests, make judgments to determine which patients need to be admitted to the hospital. These kinds of judgments are an integral process in the care of the emergency patient. They have a positive impact on patient care. Yet, emergency physicians need to be cognizant of those times when our judgments have a negative impact on patient care. Deciding a patient is a "drug seeker" or "frequent flyer" are judgments that we all make or observe others make in the ED. How do these types of judgments have a positive impact on patient care? In the majority of cases, these types of judgments have a negative influence and we need to recognize this and eliminate or at least minimize their influence on the management of a patient. The goal of this chapter is to increase awareness of the impact that negative judgmental attitudes and opinions have on the care of the emergency patient, discuss the ethical considerations involved and propose strategies for minimizing this negative impact.

The difficult patient

The difficult patient has been defined as one who interferes with a physician's ability to establish a normal patient–physician relationship.[4] It is during encounters with difficult patients that we often expe-rience a host of negative emotional reactions. Examples include disgust for a patient's physical appearance (such as patients with maggots in their wounds), intoxicated patients, violent patients, demanding patients, non-English speaking patients (requiring repeated use of translator phones), non-compliant patients, and patients with chronic complaints. We thrive on difficult diagnostic and therapeutic challenges, but we dread the challenge of the difficult patient encounter. However, we cannot escape from this encounter. All emergency physicians have patients who they find difficult. It is important to keep in mind that it is not just the patient that determines a difficult encounter. The interplay of patient characteristics, the physician's skills and the ED environment all combine to create a difficult encounter.[5] Of these three components, the physician is the variable that we can most easily manipulate to successfully manage these patients.

Physician factors

Emergency physicians are skilled at rapidly forming an opinion based on appearances of a patient. The skill that makes us astute clinicians is the very same skill that creates personal bias and prejudice. Especially in inner-city university hospitals, few patients we care for have cultural or social behaviors that seem normal to us. The more we judge our patients, the less we want to be their physicians.[1] Our preconceived stereotypes for difficult patients can lead to misperceptions, misdiagnosis and maltreatment when caring for a patient. Negative thoughts about a patient can lead to negative actions and compromised patient care. Good interpersonal skills are an essential component to the successful patient–physician relationship. Its importance in recent years has made the teaching of professionalism a required core competency in EM residency programs.[6]

Specific ethical considerations

Much emphasis in recent years has also been placed on EM physician oaths and physician code of ethics. First adopted in 1997 and then updated in 2008, the American College of Emergency Physicians published a policy statement on the code of ethics for emergency physicians and stated "emergency physicians shall embrace patient welfare as their primary professional responsibility".[7] Allowing judgmental attitudes and opinions to interfere with this basic professional obligation is an issue that each of us experience at one point of time or another in the care of the emergency patient. This code of ethics asks that we respond "promptly and expertly, without prejudice or partiality, to the need for emergency medical care." A similar code of honor was adopted by the Society of Academic Emergency Medicine.[8] This virtue-based code of conduct included statements of being "committed to serve humanity", "keeping patient welfare my first consideration," being "considerate . . . and just in all my dealing with patients", to "maintain the utmost respect for human dignity" and "advance the ideals of the profession." One aspect of this academic code specific to teachers of EM is the vow for mentorship "nurturing and encouraging the . . . moral virtues of the profession in students of every kind through my words and deeds." The principles of respect for persons, beneficence, non-maleficence, and justice which apply to the patient–physician relationship are concepts that have direct implications on this topic. Morally valuable attitudes known as virtues are important to our practice and the concepts of justice, impartiality, and compassion have particular relevance in minimizing the impact of judgmental attitudes and opinions. Emergency physicians serve the principle of beneficence by acting in the best interests of the patient. Each decision a physician makes about a patient should uphold this fundamental duty to benefit the patient. Making judgments about a patient is part of the practice of EM, and it is part of the process in making a diagnosis for the patient and determining correct management. Making negative judgments about a patient comes with this practice, but it is incumbent upon us to recognize when this occurs so that we can prevent their influence on patient care.

The corresponding duty of non-maleficence and promise to "do no harm" has a higher degree of implication. Judgmental attitudes and opinions are made on every patient we see, and we have an obligation to make sure that any negative attitudes we have do not inflict harm on the care of the patient. Negative attitudes are harmful in themselves when they influence learners such as resident physicians. Many would argue that a higher ethical standard exists in academic environments where the beliefs of the attending often become the beliefs of the resident. Most importantly, when negative attitudes do occur,

their impact on patient care needs to be eliminated, or at the very least, minimized.

Justice or fairness refers to providing care for patients regardless of certain characteristics such as race, gender, or other factors that are not relevant to the appropriate care of a patient. Emergency physicians have a responsibility to provide equal care in similar situations. An example of equal care would be providing consistency in the care to a Caucasian person with chronic pain as you do to an African American person with chronic pain. Many studies find that race and socioeconomic barriers may affect the quality of care received. In one qualitative study of sickle cell disease, patients report being "neglected, stigmatized and experiencing mistrust" from healthcare providers.[9] Another study finds that disparities exist in EDs with inferior analgesic management in African Americans and Hispanics as compared with Caucasians.[10] Stereotyping has been shown to influence physician attitudes about minorities.[11] Since many of these negative stereotypes are subconscious, we need to be prudent in examining and being consistent in our practices.

Justice is classically known as one of the main principles in bioethical theory. In EM justice is also regarded as one of the timeless virtues.[12] Emergency physicians should have the "disposition to give each person what is due to him or her." Justice guarantees a basic level of care to all patients. We should treat all patients with the highest standards of care and equally.

Another timeless virtue of EM is impartiality whereby "unconditional positive regard" is given to every emergency patient. Emergency physicians must treat patients in an unprejudiced way, and be tolerant of cultural differences. We must recognize the worth of every individual and value each person as one who deserves our best effort every time. In other words, we must live by the golden rule of "do unto others as you would want them to do unto you."

A final virtue that is important is that of compassion. Patients in the ED need to feel cared for in order for them to have trust. Harm can come to patients when physicians lack compassion. Consistent high levels of compassion need to be present in all encounters.

Potential solutions

Evidence shows that physicians are guilty of having preconceived stereotypes that can lead to disparities in healthcare.[11] In addition, certain patient encounters elicit strong negative emotions in us. The combination of these two issues leads to the ethical dilemma of letting negative judgmental attitudes affect patient care. The first step in tackling this difficult problem is recognizing that we are influenced by stereotypes and controlling our reactions to patients. Knowledge of those patients and situations that trigger hostile reactions before you enter the patient room is ideal. This early recognition allows the clinician the chance to mitigate the effect of his or her emotions, and to use prior wisdom and experience to approach the patient in a manner that leads to a satisfactory encounter. When difficult patients are anticipated, keeping a healthy emotional distance is critical. It is important to be engaged with the patient, and to feel compassion for the patient to ensure that the patient receives appropriate care, and to make sure no serious medical issue exists. We should give the patient the benefit of the doubt and trust that patients are being honest unless we know otherwise with certainty. If we constantly feel mistrust, we will undertreat patients, and this can lead to failure of the physician to provide appropriate care. By maintaining a healthy distance, when patients respond with hostile emotions, we will avoid reacting with hostility, and avoid the human tendency for countertransference. One way to deal with a negative tirade from the patient is to avoid speaking, and to just listen to the patient. With time, the majority of patients will eventually have nothing left to say. Allowing the patient to vent and acknowledging their frustrations can be therapeutic for the patient. When listening does not work, remove yourself from the patient's presence for a period of time. This gives everyone a chance to reframe their attitudes and expectations. Let the patient know that you will return. When you return, it is important to set limits on what the patient can expect, and to be up front about any specific impasses you have in mind.[13] The key is in the art of presentation and at all times, showing the patient you care about his or her well-being. "I will get your pain under control in the ED, but you will need to get prescriptions from your primary care doctor who is monitoring you, and who can best keep you safe from overdosing or becoming addicted to narcotic medication." Another method for success is incorporating teamwork. Make sure every individual involved in the clinical care of the patient is on board with the plan. The nurse, the resident, and the attending need to present with a united front and maintain compassion and consistency of care. If even just one of the caregivers involved reacts in a hostile manner, the ability to achieve a successful patient encounter will be less likely. Finally, accept that some patients will not be happy with the outcome. The ED is often a thankless environment, and our professional satisfaction should not entirely depend on how patients feel about us. Take solace, for example, in the knowledge that you provided the patient with best care possible.

Conclusion

Judgmental attitudes and opinions are made on every EM patient. Negative judgments of patients can have negative consequences on patient care. One of the greatest challenges of EM is maintaining our humanity when caring for the difficult patient, so that we provide each patient with the highest quality care. Emergency physicians operate under the mission to save lives, mitigate disease, and relieve pain and suffering. We need to remember these ideals as we practice EM and train the future generations of emergency physicians.

Section IV: Recommendations

• Recognize preconceived stereotypes and negative judgments you make about a patient.
• Acknowledge frustration, and separate yourself from the patient if necessary, in order to regain perspective and mitigate the effect of your emotions.
• Reframe your attitudes and expectations with the principles of beneficence, nonmaleficence, justice, impartiality, and compassion in mind.
• Follow standard of care, protocols, or evidence-based guidelines when they exist. Be consistent.
• Consider using a similar course of action as you used in a similar situation previously, in order to achieve a positive outcome.

References

1. Rosen P. (2009) No opiates for headache. *J Emerg Med.* 36(3), 302–4.
2. Lavoie F. (2010) No opiates for headache—reply. *J Emerg Med.* 38(1), 61.

3. Rosen P. (2010) Reply to letter to the editor on the management of headaches without opiates. *J Emerg Med*. 38(1), 61–2.

4. Simon J, Dwyer J, Goldfrank L. (1999) The difficult patient. *Emerg Med Clin North Am*. 17(2), 353–70.

5. Adams J, Murray III R. (1998) The general approach to the difficult patient. *Emerg Med Clin North Am*. 16(4), 689–700.

6. Larkin G, Binder L, Houry D, et al. (2002) Defining and evaluating professionalism: a core competency for graduate emergency medicine education. *Acad Emerg Med*. 9(11), 1249–56.

7. American College of Emergency Physicians. (2008) Code of ethics for emergency physicians. *Ann Emerg Med*. 52, 581–90.

8. Iserson K. (1999) Principles of biomedical ethics. *Emerg Med Clin North Am*. 17(2), 283–306.

9. Maxwell K, Streetly A, Bevan D. (1999) Experiences of hospital care and treatment seeking for pain in sickle cell disease: qualitative study. *BMJ*. 318, 1585–90.

10. Pletcher M, Kertesz S, Kohn M, et al. (2008) Trends in opioid prescribing by race/ethnicity for patients seeking care in US emergency departments. *J Am Med Assoc*. 299, 70–8.

11. Van Ryn M, Burke J. (2000) The effect of patient race and socioeconomic status on physicians' perceptions of patients. *Soc Sci Med*. 50, 813–28.

12. Larkin G, Iserson K, Kassuto Z, et al. (2009) Virtue in emergency medicine. *Acad Emerg Med*. 16, 51–5.

13. Harrison DW, Vissers RJ. (2002) The difficult patient. In: Marx J, Hockberger R, Walls R. (eds) *Rosen's Emergency Medicine: Concepts and Clinical Practice*, 5th ed. St. Louis, MO: Mosby, pp. 2604–13.

6

Using physicians as agents of the state

Jeremy R. Simon

Assistant Professor of Clinical Medicine and Scholar-in-Residence, Center for Bioethics, Columbia University, New York, NY, USA

Section I: Case presentation

The local police brought two prisoners to the emergency department (ED). They had noticed a car driving erratically, and, as they pulled it over, they noticed the passenger appeared to swallow several golf-ball sized white objects. After stopping the car, the driver, who appeared to be intoxicated, refused a breathalyzer test. Furthermore, he appeared so intoxicated that the police did not feel comfortable taking him to the station house. Instead, they brought him to the ED for medical evaluation. They asked that in addition to treating the driver, that also a blood alcohol level be obtained, so that they could know if he really had been driving while intoxicated. They also expressed their belief that the white objects they saw the passenger swallow were drugs, and asked for an imaging study to identify the drug bags, as well as for the gastrointestinal tract to be emptied in order to use the effluent for drug evidence.

Just as the police finished their story, the emergency medical services bring in a patient on a back board. It appeared that while trying to stop the car of the apparently intoxicated driver, the police struck a civilian car. The driver, who was not wearing a seatbelt, struck the steering wheel. After a thorough examination, you discover only point tenderness over the lower left anterior ribs, approximately the seventh rib. Although you do not ordinarily order X-ray studies to confirm the presence of rib fractures, when the physical examination is consistent with isolated rib fractures, you wonder if you should obtain an imaging study since there ultimately may be a lawsuit against the police.

Section II: Discussion

Dr. Peter Rosen: This is a much more common problem than is thought to be true. The appropriate response to this situation is somewhat dependent on where you work. For example, this occurred relatively frequently in Denver where there existed an advantage for the emergency physician, namely the hospital had a police ward. As a result, the police could arrest a patient, the emergency physician could then admit the patient to the police ward, where they could receive whatever medical screening and testing the police felt was legally necessary without emergency physician participation in actions potentially defined as not in the best interest of the patient.

At one point, however, I cared for a patient who had a gunshot wound to the leg from whom the police requested that I retrieve the bullet in the leg so that it could be used as evidence. The patient had allegedly killed a 7–11 clerk and a police officer. I explained to

Ethical Problems in Emergency Medicine: A Discussion-Based Review, First Edition. John Jesus, Shamai A. Grossman, Arthur R. Derse, James G. Adams, Richard Wolfe, and Peter Rosen.
© 2012 John Wiley & Sons, Ltd. Published 2012 by John Wiley & Sons, Ltd.

the police that the bullet in his leg was no longer a bullet, but had shattered into multiple fragments and could not represent useful evidence. The police were angry that I had refused their request, and went to a local judge who ordered that I retrieve the bullet fragments despite my earlier protests. I responded to the order by saying that if the judge wanted the fragments out then he should take them out because I wasn't going to. Finally, the district attorney agreed with my assessment. The only reason for their removal at that point was if there had been any medical indications for their removal, of which there were none. If the district attorney hadn't offered this help, however, I was actually prepared to go to jail rather than perform an operation I didn't think was indicated. One fascinating aspect of our particular case is the notion of changing our medical practice in order to accommodate potential litigation.

Dr. James Adams: This case outlines important questions for the specialty. At the heart of our profession we are the agents of the patient. In very important ways we're also responsible professionals for society. When the police make a request, we would like to cooperate as we all recognize that public safety is important. If, however, their request requires us to overrule the ethics of the profession, there must exist law that directs us to do so. For example, there are state laws that direct us to report suspicions of abuse, penetrating stab wounds, and gunshot wounds. In the state of Illinois, they can use any blood alcohol test that we may have done medically for state evidence. These are just a few examples of state or federal laws that require us to provide law enforcement with evidentiary information. The state cannot run over our professional ethics without the backing of legislation.

Dr. Jeremy Simon: Emergency physicians do have to know the law within their state, though I acknowledge that the laws are not exactly the same in all 50 states. Despite the variability, the law often does address the tension we're discussing between patient and public interests. Usually our primary role is to maintain the patient's health and life. As medical professionals, however, it is also often our role to provide society and our patients with medical information. At times we order diagnostic tests and imaging not because we will act upon the information, but because it provides a diagnosis that can reduce patient anxiety

and increase patients' piece of mind. It's perfectly reasonable to perform tests for this purpose.

Dr. Shamai Grossman: I'm bothered by the notion of performing diagnostic studies, such as X-ray studies or CT [computed tomography] scans, when these studies are not medically indicated. As a purist, my goal is to take the best possible care of my patients. Exposing a patient to the radiation of a CT scan when it's not indicated is truly not within the spectrum of appropriate medical care. To the extent possible, I believe these sorts of studies should not be performed in the ED, but rather should be referred to outpatient facilities that offer MRI [magnetic resonance imaging] and CT scans.

Dr. John Jesus: When I think about police officers attempting to have me perform tests on their behalf that cannot be construed as in the interests of my patients, I get very irritated. That said, I acknowledge that the government still limits the scope of my practice. In some way, I'm still "an agent of the state." For instance, I can't legally prescribe narcotic medications for recreational use. The practice of abortions has been limited by the state. I know that psychiatrists in some areas are not allowed to forcibly give condemned prisoners medications in order to make them competent in court. My interpretation of those laws is that they were designed to keep the public and the patients safe. The use of police officers to gather forensic evidence may speak to public beneficence, but doesn't speak to patient beneficence. Without that factor included in the ethical analysis I don't think it's appropriate.

Furthermore, emergency medicine is not forensic medicine. It makes little sense to try to gather evidence in the ED where we are not trained to document well how each piece of evidence is collected, who handles it, who has access to the evidence, etc. I would assume that evidence collected in the ED is much more easily contested in court than if that evidence was collected by forensic specialists.

PR: The issues may be as difficult to address when there exists clear medical benefit to the patient. For example, the body-packer in our case would likely receive a lethal dose of the drug he ingested if one of the balloons were to rupture. There are times when there is medical benefit to comply with police requests, not because you want to help the police particularly, but because you want to help the patient. Examples like this one highlight the tension between patient and police interests when treating patients who have allegedly broken the law.

Our case also compels us to explore the question of whether we have a duty to help patients obtain information that might be in their future legal and financial interests. In my opinion, the answer depends on what test is being asked for and on the particular medical situation. For example, I don't think there is much radiation risk from a chest X-ray study, and therefore I wouldn't have an objection to ordering a film that I don't think a patient necessarily needs. Recent literature suggests that a CT scan, however, carries with it a significant amount of radiation exposure and risk for future complications. As a result, I would be unwilling to order a CT scan unless there was a medical indication to order one. Even though the physician in our case suspects the patient may sue the police, a chest X-ray study in the setting of blunt trauma is medically indicated, and would not represent a study for the sole purpose of gathering information the patient might use in court. When I try to analyze my ethical position of a certain situation, I start with the question, "Is there a medical to do what the patient is asking me to do," as opposed to simply assisting in a potential lawsuit, for example.

The other option emergency physicians have if they feel uncomfortable with ordering unnecessary imaging requests, is to point out that what the patient wants is evidence that will work for his or her behalf. The physician can state a willingness to document in the medical record clinical evidence of a newly fractured rib, and is prepared to testify in court if necessary. What the physician is not prepared to do, is to order a procedure which is not medically indicated. Thus the physician can demonstrate a cognizance the patient's needs, and is willing to work within the physician's set of professional values to help the patient, even if it means some sacrifice of time and effort.

The last issue I would like to address is the tension between societal and patient interests. In other words, what are our ethical obligations when we encounter information that leads us to believe a patient has become a danger to our society; does it matter if the patient doesn't want us to report the information? I once had a patient who was an airline pilot who presented with his first seizure. His first words to me were, "I don't want you to report this to anybody because it'll mean my job and my career." In California, a physician can state simply that there's a law that mandates that I report your seizure activity to the motor vehicle bureau. That isn't true, however, for most conditions that place the public at risk to an even greater degree than epilepsy. Given this consideration, how should emergency physicians approach the patient who for example, you discover has AIDS, and doesn't want to report it to anybody for fear of losing insurance coverage, suffering the social stigma attached to the diagnosis, or losing a spouse upon the disclosure of the information?

JA: These are great points to discuss, because we do have a responsibility to society. Even when we overrule our obligations to the patient because of a higher social obligation, we must do so carefully and thoughtfully. The Tarasoff case and precedence has dictated that physicians have a duty to warn third parties whom any physician feels are in immediate danger due to potential actions of a patient. The more difficult issue, however, is when a patient has the "potential" to become a danger to society, such as the previously described patient airline pilot with a seizure disorder. A very stressful experience within my own practice involved a patient with HIV [human immunodeficiency virus infection], who continued to have intercourse with his wife who did not know the patient's HIV positive status. This revelation was pretty shocking. I called the person's primary doctor who said, "Yes I know. I've encouraged that patient to tell his spouse, but I'm not going to tell the spouse myself." I felt a great deal of conflict at this point, and sought out legal guidance to help me navigate my duty of confidentiality, and my obligation to warn a third party whose life and health I felt were in danger. Ultimately, the lawyer said that in this particular state, the duty of confidentiality held more weight, and that I shouldn't reveal the patient's HIV status to the patient's wife.

PR: I wrote an editorial about the Tarasoff case, and argued that it was an example of bad medicine rather than an example of why a law stipulating a physician's duty to warn was needed.[1] The psychiatrist who heard the homicidal threats of the patient didn't need to warn the fiancé, instead he should have ordered a mental health hold on the patient, involuntarily committing him to a mental facility. Before we worry about the ethical dilemmas, let's define the medical issues and ensure appropriate medical care.

SG: Sometimes we are forced to use our clinical judgment when our obligations to society and our patients conflict. Ideally physicians could work within the confines of their abilities and local and legal regulations in place. At times this position requires appropriate medical care or legal representation, at other times it may mean going against our own laws. That should be the exception, and far from standard practice. If physicians are able to take a broader perspective, they are often able to solve problems without putting both personal values and clinical judgment at risk.

PR: Addressing my societal obligations when interacting with my patient who was an airline pilot was harder. I was able to convince him, however, that what he was asking for was time to come to terms with what he knew he had to do. I helped him understand by speaking with his wife on the phone, and asking her to come to the ED. I sat them both down for about an hour, explaining the ramifications of his disease and what it meant to have a seizure. After discussing the issue with his wife, he agreed that the last thing he would want to do is fly a 747 into the ground, because he had a seizure and kill 350 people on board. The interaction took a lot more time than I like to spend on individual patients, but I don't think we have any choice but to try to do the right thing even if it's the most difficult one.

There is definitely a competition between our patient responsibilities and societal responsibilities. Who among us would fail to report smallpox or anthrax or some other really highly infectious disease that might be a sign of a bioterrorist attack as well as a threat to thousands, if not millions, of lives, and yet the far more common scenario is one in which a patient may pose a danger to a small number of people, and the resultant conflict of duties a physician will feel is a reality of our profession

JS: Emergency medicine has overlapped with the field of forensic medicine for some time. In fact, a residency program in Louisville included a forensic emergency

medicine fellowship at one point. Furthermore, we perform forensic medicine every time we perform an examination with a sexual assault kit that portends no medical benefit, and serves only to gather evidence.

PR: It is incumbent upon us to have some idea of how to handle evidence we discover and collect in the ED. We don't do a great job of it because we don't do it very often. That said, it isn't all that hard to identify what we've taken from a patient. Not only do we collect evidence with the sexual assault kits, but we also collect foreign bodies, and can carefully document this for the purposes of evidence collection.

PR: We need to remember that any of our charts are able to be subpoenaed, and whether we want to or not, we may end up testifying in court about what we found on that patient as well as what our medical opinions were at the time. I found out the hard way that the better my record looks at the time I make it, the more comfortable I am when I'm called upon to testify in court. I try to make my chart abundantly clear with the details and decision-making I feel are important. If I'm called upon to testify in court, I will not remember my interaction with one particular patient from the thousands with whom I interact on a yearly basis.

SG: Do you perform studies in order to protect yourself from legal repercussions?

JA: To a large degree we do studies when there are medical indications for them, though sometimes those indications are admittedly marginal. Patients sometimes present with an agenda—complaining of back pain and acting out with a little bit of drama because they would like a certain study or medication. My impression of those clinicians who order marginally indicated tests more frequently is that they are striving for certainty. Clinicians order studies with a low likelihood of positive findings for all kinds of reasons. If a person is having legitimate rib pain after blunt trauma, and wishes to have an X-ray study, I think there are many emergency physicians who would consider ordering the test, a rational and an ethically appropriate choice. Really good clinical documentation is far better than anything else clinicians can do to protect themselves from legal repercussions. It is important to describe a clear story in a chart, and we don't have to push our ethics to justify it.

JS: It seems to me that the concept of defensive medicine acknowledges that a clinician only performs low yield tests when he believes there actually is something wrong with the patient. To the extent that a physician believes it's necessary for self-protection, it's necessary to protect the patient. I almost don't see it as an ethical issue, so much as an inability to assess the risk to which a patient is exposed.

PR: The issue for me has become more and more simplified as I have acquired more experience with malpractice cases. Trying to out-guess a plaintiff's attorney based upon a prediction of an interpretation of the evidence is impossible. Therefore, I don't order tests to protect myself because I don't know what to order. My best protection is making sure, to the extent possible, that the patient has a good outcome. If I can't ensure a good outcome, then I try my best to facilitate a safe outcome. For example, I am a firm believer in intercostal nerve blocks for rib fractures. I perform them frequently, and I've never caused a pneumothorax. For years, however, I obtained post-procedure chest X-ray studies looking for complications. I finally realized that the act of ordering a chest X-ray study that I didn't think was indicated, I was doing simply as an act of defensive medicine. I've since stopped ordering the chest X-ray study as it prolongs the patient's stay by 1–3 hours, and instead, I document very carefully what the post-procedure condition of the patient is, including the vital signs and including the chest physical examination.

What I've learned over the years is that since I cannot guess for what I will be accused and sued, why bother trying. The problem with defensive medicine is that we often choose the wrong test, and we interpret it haphazardly due to our preconceived low likelihood of positive results. We are much more likely to miss subtle, small findings that simply make more trouble for ourselves.

SG: You articulated exactly what I believe is the correct approach. Ultimately, our goal is to take appropriate care of the patient. Your best protection from legal action is to provide appropriate care of a patient.

PR: Nothing a physician does, however, will perfectly protect against lawsuits. Though you can be sued at any time for any reason and lose, you can look at yourself in the mirror each morning with self-respect, and feel good about your efforts and decisions. Just take care of the patient, and most ethical problems will take care of themselves.

Section III: Review of the literature

On occasion, emergency physicians are called upon by law enforcement officials to assist in gathering evidence of a crime from a patient in the ED. Often, the patient in question is the victim of the crime, as when emergency physicians collect specimens using a sexual assault kit. Such cases pose few ethical dilemmas for the emergency physician, as the evidence collection is generally in the patient's interest, and takes place with the patient's consent. Sometimes, however, the patient is the suspected perpetrator, and evidence collected by the emergency physician may be used to work to the patient's detriment. In that case, the physician's civic duty and perhaps legal obligation to assist law enforcement will come into direct conflict with the obligation to act in the patient's best interest, and, most significantly, with the obligation to protect confidentiality. This gives rise to an ethical dilemma with serious potential consequences for both the patient and the physician.

Principles and background

Because the dilemmas discussed in this chapter revolve around the conflict between ethics and law, we must be familiar with the relevant principles from each area before we can understand the proper course of action.

Ethics

The ethical principles involved in these cases are the physician's duties to act in the patient's best interests and to protect patient confidentiality.

Acting in a patient's best interests Physicians have an indisputable responsibility to act in the best interests of their patients.[2] In general, this means that in deciding how to act with respect to a patient, a physician must make decisions based on what will benefit the patient, and not in the interests of any other party, be that the patient's family, the physician, the physician's employer, or society at large.

The need to adhere to this standard should be clear. Without the assumption that physicians act in the best interest of their patients, people would not, and could not, trust doctors. They might avoid doctors altogether out of fear of how physicians might exploit their vulnerable position. This would be a great loss to society, and it is for this reason that, in general, society accepts and even mandates that the physician focus on the patient's interests.[3,4] The price paid when the interests of an individual patient diverge from those of society at large is small relative to the benefit of the presence of an effective trustworthy profession. Though wide ranging, this duty is not absolute. In some cases, such as public health emergencies, it has been determined that the cost of ignoring society's interests in favor of the patient's is too high, and doctors may be required to report their patients to enable a quarantine, even if the patient's interests would best be served by being treated at home with full freedom.

Protecting patient confidentiality The obligation to keep confidential all aspects of the doctor–patient relationship has been recognized at least since the Hippocratic Oath was composed. ("What I may see or hear in the course of the treatment . . . which on no account one must spread abroad, I will keep to myself, holding such things shameful to be spoken about.")[5] More recently, it is affirmed in a policy statement by the American College of Emergency Physicians (ACEP), and it was incorporated into several codes of medical ethics and conduct in the interval.[6-8]

This duty can be grounded in the value it has for fostering a strong doctor–patient relationship, and the effective practice of medicine. Unless patients feel free to speak openly with their doctors, physicians may not have access to all of the information needed for proper management.[7] To assure that no breach in the trust between patient and doctor occurs, patient confidentiality is protected by law as well as ethics, most notably by The Health Insurance Portability and Accountability Act of 1996 (HIPAA), but also by many state statutes protecting such information from legal scrutiny.[9]

Law
The legal background to these situations is found in both state legislation and case law (i.e., court decisions). Furthermore, HIPAA, a federal law, addresses these circumstances as well.

Legislation A sample of legislation relevant to our topic concerns obtaining alcohol levels from drivers suspected of driving while intoxicated. For example, New York State Vehicle and Traffic law states that:

> Any person who operates a motor vehicle in this state shall be deemed to have given consent to a chemical test of one or more of the following: breath, blood, urine, or saliva, for the purpose of determining the alcoholic or drug content of the blood provided that such test is administered by, or at the direction of a police officer with respect to a chemical test of breath, urine or saliva, or, with respect to a chemical test of blood, at the direction of a police officer.[10]

However, if such a person "refuses to submit to such chemical test or any portion thereof, unless a court order has been granted . . . , the test shall not be given".[11] Most other states have similar laws, although the scope of the driver's right to refuse, and the penalties for doing so, vary widely.[12]

Case law Much of the law on this topic, including some related to intoxicated drivers, has been established through court cases. When a lower court decision is appealed, the decision of the higher, appellate, court not only affect the case that was appealed, but becomes binding in future cases in the courts jurisdiction. Thus, determinations by appellate courts can have the force of law. In several criminal cases, the US Supreme Court, whose jurisdiction extends to all federal courts and whose decisions are considered even by state courts, has rules on the admissibility of evidence obtained by a physician without the patient's consent. These cases, therefore, speak directly to the question at hand. The most relevant of these are *Rochin* v. *California*, *Breithaupt* v. *Abram*, *Schmerber* v. *California*, and *Winston* v. *Lee*.

In *Rochin*,[13] after seeing a suspect swallow capsules believed to contain morphine, the police brought their prisoner to the hospital, and directed that the capsules be retrieved for evidence. As a result of this request, doctors in the ED inserted an orogastric tube into the patient and administered an emetic, thereby retrieving the capsules. The Supreme Court overturned Rochin's conviction, saying that forced "pumping" of a prisoner's stomach "shocks the conscience," and, therefore, violated Rochin's right to due process.

In *Breithaupt*,[14] hospital personnel drew an alcohol level from an unconscious prisoner suspected of driving while intoxicated. The driver was subsequently convicted based partly on the results of this blood test. The Supreme Court upheld the conviction, finding that blood tests are not objectionable in the way identified in *Rochin*, and that, therefore, there was no violation of due process.

In *Schmerber*,[15] the Supreme Court extended its ruling in *Breithaupt*, upholding the conviction of a driver whose blood was drawn in the ED over his objection. That is, the driver was not merely unable to consent, as in *Breithaupt*, but actively objected to the procedure. The question was whether taking blood without a search warrant constituted an unreasonable search and seizure. Because of the minimal invasion involved in a blood draw, and because of the legitimate concern that the alcohol would be metabolized and the evidence lost, the Court held that a search warrant was not needed in this case.

The Supreme Court showed the limits of its expansive ruling in *Schmerber*, however, in *Winston*.[16] In *Winston*, a shop owner and a thief exchanged gunfire. The thief was struck in the chest by a bullet that lodged approximately 2.5 cm (1 inch) below the skin in muscle. The prosecutors filed a motion to compel the suspect, Rudolph Lee, to undergo surgery under general anesthesia to retrieve the bullet. This surgery was not medically indicated, but would have allowed the state to prove that the bullet came from the store owner's gun, thus strengthening the case against Lee. The Supreme Court held that compelling such surgery was such a substantial intrusion that it would violate Lee's right to "be secure in his person," and would constitute an unreasonable search, even with a warrant.

HIPPA HIPPA generally serves to limit the information physicians are allowed to release regarding their patients. It also sets out circumstances in which it is permissible to release otherwise protected information (though in and of itself, HIPPA never *requires* the release of such information). In particular, HIPPA allows hospitals to release protected information specifically demanded by a court subpoena. Furthermore, official requests from other government agencies for HIPPA-protected information may be met if the request is relevant, specific, and cannot be met with redacted information. Hospitals may also supply limited information to law enforcement to aid in identifying and locating a crime suspect, and under certain circumstances, a victim of a crime.[17]

These cases all involve responding to official requests. HIPPA also allows hospitals to contact agencies with information in some cases. HIPPA permits hospitals to make reports, such as gunshot injuries, which are required by law. It also allows hospitals to report criminal activity taking place on its premises, and to release relevant information to law enforcement.[17]

A note on the relationship between law and ethics
The reader interested in the ethics approach to requests from law enforcement may wonder why such emphasis is placed here on the law. Ethics, after all, pertains to what one ought to do as a matter of right and wrong, whereas law pertains to what we ought to do to avoid legal sanctions. Although the demands of ethics and law **might** align in any given case, there is no guarantee that they will. One might therefore think that while understanding one's legal obligations is indeed important, a discussion of law has no place in a chapter on ethics, which should provide guidance of a different sort.

There are several reasons it is necessary to discuss legal matters here. First, as a practical matter, when deciding how to act, it behooves us to be aware of the law and consider it along the side of ethics considerations, because violating the law often has serious consequences. Second, as citizens, we have an independent ethical duty to follow the law. We *may* decide that certain obligations to our patients outweigh this obligation to society, but this decision can only be made if we understand both sets of obligations. Finally, societal values both establish and limit some of our ethical obligations. As we saw above, both the duty to act in the patient's best interest and the duty to protect patient confidences are at least partly based on the value these principles have to society. Consequently, to some extent, societal value judgments at least partially determine the strength and extent of these ethical obligations. These judgments are often expressed in law. Sometimes, these judgments are made explicit, as in *Tarasoff* v. *Regents of University of California*,[18] which mandates the violation of patient confidentiality in certain cases through a duty to warn the potential victim when a patient poses an imminent danger to another person.

Other limitations society places on the value of these principles may only be implicit, and only an understanding of the relevant law will allow these values to be ascertained. For example, in one of the cases discussed above, *Breithaupt*, throughout the court's discussion of the potential reasons to suppress the blood test obtained without the patient's consent that the court considered, breach of confidentiality was never raised. This indicates that the court did not feel that in such a case patient, confidentiality should be maintained, thus creating a clear, albeit implicit, limitation on confidentiality. Indeed, our professional standards themselves explicitly incorporate legal-based limitations on the ethical duty to respect patient confidentiality. The ACEP policy on patient confidentiality recognizes confidentiality as an important but not absolute duty, with the qualifying factors largely related to legal obligations and societal consensus.[6] Ethics thus incorporates law.

Applications

It is important to be aware of local laws as well as hospital policies regarding law enforcement requests for information regarding patients. These laws and policies vary from state to state and from hospital to hospital, and all discussions below must be understood in this light. As general guidelines, however, the ACEP policy on "Law Enforcement Information Gathering in the Emergency Department" lays out two negative principles which can guide all such interactions. First, law enforcement requests should never be allowed to interfere with patient care. Second, unless it is legally required, patient information should never be released without the patient's (or surrogate's) permission.[19]

In addition, even if one concludes that it is appropriate to share information or evidence with law enforcement, information should never be released without the guidance of the hospital's legal department if at all possible. This will assure that no inappropriate information is released, and that anything that is released is released in the proper manner (e.g., in response to a search warrant).

Alcohol testing

A relatively common situation is for police to request that an alcohol level be drawn on a patient suspected of driving drunk. If the patient is conscious, one should not draw the specimen without the patient's consent. The patient may well consent, however, as refusal to consent to such a test under these circumstances will result in the patient's license being suspended in all 50 US states.[20] In this case, if one is already drawing blood, it is reasonable to draw the specimen even if it does not serve a clinical goal, as it will minimize the number of needle sticks the patient undergoes. However, it is not generally the physician's responsibility to draw this specimen, and this task can be passed on to law enforcement as well.

If the patient is not conscious, one may rely on the fact that in all 50 states the law specifies that by operating a motor vehicle one has implicitly consented to undergoing alcohol testing.[20] Although this implicit consent can be overridden by a conscious patient, it can be relied on for an unconscious patient. Again, however, the collection of evidence can be left to law enforcement.

Drugs and other evidence

Body-stuffing and body-packing are common means of hiding drugs.[21] When law enforcement agents suspect that a patient has ingested packages of drugs, or concealed them elsewhere in the body (rectum, vagina), the suspect may be brought to the ED with a request that the drugs be retrieved and turned over to law enforcement. Under such circumstances, only medical considerations should guide action. It is not the physician's place to perform cavity searches that serve no medical purpose. Sometimes, however, especially when there is a concern for ingested drugs, imaging studies to find the drugs and removal of the drugs (through whole-bowel irrigation or surgery) may be clinically indicated.[21] In this case, treatment of the ingestion should be executed like any other clinical plan. Once the drugs have been passed or retrieved, one has an obligation to dispose of them in a legal manner, which should be coordinated with the hospital's legal and security departments. Note that while one should turn over the drugs, this does not necessarily mean that their source may be identified. Although the police may be present when the drugs are recovered, if they are not, the physician may be asked to testify as to where the drugs were found. This information may fall under the proper domain of physician–patient confidentiality, though physicians refusing to testify should be aware that they may be charged with obstruction of justice.

With other potential pieces of evidence removed from the body of a patient, such as a bullet (as well as drugs retrieved in the operating room), there are two potential courses of action. As with all other surgical specimens, these items can be sent to pathology. Certainly, if there is any question that pathological examination of the specimen will help the patient, this is what should be done. Once in pathology, the specimens will be the hospital's responsibility. Hospitals generally have no clear obligation to proactively turn over or report such contraband to the police, though they may choose to do so. If contraband is turned over to the police, it should certainly be done without identifying the source patient. If, however, a physician is concerned that the hospital will inappropriately identify the patient to law enforcement, it would be ethical, and quite possibly legal, to destroy the specimens. Before doing so, one should be aware of both local laws and hospital policies, which may bear on the issue.

Mandatory reports

Most US states (and several Canadian provinces) have laws mandating the reporting of certain injuries and events such as gunshot wounds, stab wounds, serious burns, and animal bites.[22,23] As these reports generally serve legitimate public safety and public health purposes, it is generally appropriate to make these reports. Should a physician feel that a report serves no legitimate public purpose, it would be ethically reasonable to not make the report. The physician should be aware, however, that failure to make these reports is sometimes a criminal offense, that could result in time in jail.[24,25]

Sexual assault kits

A final case of some relevance to this discussion is the collection of evidence in cases of suspected sexual assault. Although most of the evidence collected is not relevant to clinical care, emergency physicians are often asked to collect evidence using "rape kits." Although these forensic examinations may seem to be beyond the practice of emergency physicians, when necessary, as when no other professional is available to collect the evidence, the emergency physician should assist in gathering this evidence if at all possible. The patient presents as the victim of a sexual assault, and the successful prosecution of the assailant may be important in the patient's recovery. It is, there-fore, reasonably part of the emergency physician's care of the victim. Furthermore, the emergency physician is usually the first healthcare provider the victim encounters, and, as evidence degrades over time, the emergency physician may be the only person with the opportunity to collect satisfactory evidence. These same considerations make it appropriate to examine even unconscious victims (if it is not expected that they will soon become alert), to collect suitable forensic evidence under the presumption that they will want to assist in the prosecution of their assailant. The evidence, however, should be stored securely, and not released to the police until the patient is alert and gives consent.

Section IV: Recommendations

- Be aware of all local laws, hospital regulations and professional policies bearing on interactions with law enforcement.
- Collecting blood from a patient who is a criminal suspect for use by law enforcement may be appropriate if the patient desires it, but can in general be left to law enforcement personnel.
- Drugs and other contraband that are recovered while treating a patient must be disposed of in a legal manner, which may require law enforcement involvement. In general, however, the identity of the patient who was the source of the contraband should not be revealed.
- Complying with local mandatory reporting laws is generally appropriate.
- When in doubt regarding the appropriateness of collecting evidence from a suspect or releasing information to law enforcement, it is best to contact hospital administration if possible.
- Emergency physicians should facilitate the collection of evidence from rape victims, and sometimes collect it themselves.

References

1. Rosen P, O'Connor M. (1986) The practice of medicine v. the practice of law. *J Emerg Med.* 4, 67–8.
2. Beauchamp TL, Childress JF. (2008) *Principles of Biomedical Ethics*, 6th ed. New York, NY: Oxford University Press.

3. Brody H. (1997) The physician-patient relationship. In: Veatch RM. (ed.) *Medical Ethics*, 2nd ed. London: Jones and Bartlett.

4. Geiderman JM, Moskop JC, Derse AR. (2006) Privacy and confidentiality in emergency medicine: obligations and challenges. *Emerg Med Clin North Am*. 24, 633–56.

5. Reich WT. (1995) Oath of Hippocrates. In: Reich WT (ed.) *Encyclopedia of Bioethics*, vol. V. New York, NY: Macmillan, p. 2632.

6. Patient Confidentiality. Available at: www.acep.org/Content.aspx?id=29600&terms=patient%20confidentiality. Accessed July 1, 2010.

7. Larkin GL, Moskop J, Sanders A, et al. (1994) The emergency physician and patient confidentiality: a review. *Ann Emerg Med*. 24, 1161–7.

8. Moskop JC, Marco CA, Larkin GL, et al. (2005) From Hippocrates to HIPPA: privacy and confidentiality in emergency medicine—part I: conceptual, moral, and legal foundations. *Ann Emerg Med*. 45, 53–9.

9. Alexander LC. (1993) Should Alabama adopt a physician-patient evidence privilege? *Ala L Rev*. 45, 261–74.

10. N.Y. Veh. & Traf. Law § 1194 (2.) (a).

11. N.Y. Veh. & Traf. Law § 1194 (2.) (b)(1).

12. Black KP. (2007) Undue protection versus undue punishment: examining the drinking and driving problem across the united states. *Suffolk Univ L Rev*. 40, 463–84.

13. Rochin *v.* California, 72 S. Ct. 205 (1952).

14. Breithaupt *v.* Abram, 77 S. Ct. 408 (1957).

15. Schmerber *v.* California, 86 S. Ct. 1826 (1966).

16. Winston *v.* Lee, 105 S. Ct. 1611 (1985).

17. American Hospital Association. (n.d.) *Guidelines for Releasing Patient Information*. Available at: www.aha.org/aha/content/2005/pdf/guidelinesreleasinginfo.pdf. Accessed June 25, 2010.

18. Tarasoff *v.* Regents of University of California. 17 Cal. 3d 425, 131 Cal. Rptr 14, 551 P. 2d 334 (1976).

19. *Law Enforcement Information Gathering in the Emergency Department*. Available at: www.acep.org/Content.aspx?id=29538&terms=law%20enforcement%20information%20gathering. Accessed July 8, 2010.

20. Beauchamp RB. (1987) "Shed thou no blood": the forcible removal of blood samples from drunk driving suspects. *So Cal L Rev*. 60, 1115–41.

21. Flomenbaum NE, Goldfrank LR, Hoffman RS, et al. (eds.) (2006) *Goldfrank's Toxicological Emergencies*, 8th ed. New York, NY: McGraw-Hill.

22. Hyman A, Schillinger D, Lo B. (1995) Laws mandating reporting of domestic violence: Do they promote well-being? *JAMA*. 273, 1781–4.

23. Massinon S. (2010) Hospitals to report gun, stab wounds: new rules require ER staff to notify police. *Calgary Herald*. April 2, B2.

24. N.Y. Penal Law § 265.25.

25. N.Y. Penal Law § 70.15.

SECTION TWO
End-of-life decisions

7

Family-witnessed resuscitation in the emergency department: making sense of ethical and practical considerations in an emotional debate

Kirsten G. Engel,[1] Arthur R. Derse[2]

[1]*Assistant Professor, Department of Emergency Medicine, Feinberg School of Medicine, Northwestern University, Chicago, IL, USA*
[2]*Director, Center for Bioethics and Medical Humanities and Julia and David Uihlein Professor of Medical Humanities, and Professor of Bioethics and Emergency Medicine, Institute for Health and Society, Medical College of Wisconsin, Milwaukee, WI, USA*

Section I: Case presentation

A 59-year-old man has a high speed collision while riding his motorcycle. A friend who was driving a motorcycle behind him calls the patient's son while the emergency medical technicians arrive and begin resuscitation efforts. The patient is brought to the emergency department (ED) intubated, with ongoing cardiopulmonary resuscitation (CPR). He has decreased breath sounds on the right with evidence of significant chest, facial, and right lower extremity trauma. A junior resident is preparing to place a chest tube when the care team is notified that the patient's son and wife have arrived and are demanding to be present in the resuscitation room. The senior trauma resident raises concerns about the family being present during an invasive procedure and in the setting of the significant blood and facial deformity. "The family will get upset if they see all this blood and gore. Plus, I'm teaching the junior resident to place this chest tube. We can't have family in here while we do that!"

Section II: Discussion

Dr. Peter Rosen: Let's start then by separating two issues. The first is the ethics of training younger physicians, and the second involves the ethical challenges involved in allowing family members to witness resuscitations.

Dr. Kirsten Engel: For the general uncomplicated medical resuscitation during which there are few to no invasive procedures, I believe we are approaching widespread acceptance of family presence. The two remaining frontiers in family-witnessed resuscitations, beyond expanding its practice across the United States, are family presence during trauma related resuscitation, and the teaching of junior residents. There is not a great deal of evidence to help guide our efforts through these issues, and that data which do exist generally come from medical resuscitation research.

PR: If we allow family observers to be present during resuscitations are we breaking any legal rules about

Ethical Problems in Emergency Medicine: A Discussion-Based Review, First Edition. John Jesus, Shamai A. Grossman, Arthur R. Derse, James G. Adams, Richard Wolfe, and Peter Rosen.
© 2012 John Wiley & Sons, Ltd. Published 2012 by John Wiley & Sons, Ltd.

patient privacy? Even though we have only referenced situations in which family members are present during resuscitations, there are many instances of patients sharing information with the physician that they wouldn't have shared with their family. Shouldn't we assume that there are a significant portion of patients who would not want their own families to witness their resuscitation if they were given the choice? Doesn't the burden of proof lie with those who would want to limit the rights and privacy of others to say that the overall benefits outweigh the possible burdens? I don't believe the patient–doctor relationship is at all enhanced by having families present, and I wonder if we assault our patients' legal right to privacy when we allow families to be present during medical and traumatic resuscitations.

Dr. Arthur Derse: The presence of family members in a resuscitation, no matter the severity of the injuries, can change the dynamic between the doctor and the patient. In that situation, physicians are not only attending to the patient, but the physician must also be cognizant of family reactions to what they witness. To the extent that their presence alters or changes a physician's effectiveness, the patient may not receive the best medical care. There is an issue, as well, of patient privacy. HIPPA (the Health Insurance Portability and Accountability Act of 1996) regulations allow you to reveal personal health information to family members when the patient is unconscious, *and* a physician can reasonably conclude that the patient would want the information communicated if that patient had been able to make independent decisions. Allowing family members to be present during resuscitations might fall under the same principle. The heightened scrutiny that would occur should something go wrong would leave one at a higher legal risk. It is difficult to know how relatives will interpret common interventions, but some may think that routinely performed interventions caused the bad outcome by virtue of the temporal relationship of the procedure to the patient's morbidity or mortality, even if the two events are in actual fact, unrelated.

PR: The data on the utility of family presence during a resuscitation from what I have read, is all wish-fulfillment fantasy, without compelling evidence that it does anything to improve the quality of care for the patient. What I would be more concerned about as a departmental chairman, is how I would control an institution that wants to increase "patient satisfaction" by having families view resuscitations without a favorable risk–benefit ratio.

Dr. Richard Wolfe: I am chairman of my department, and though my institution hasn't presented me with this particular issue, this is the way I might handle it. I would make the argument that having untrained observers will at best add nothing to the patient's care, and would probably act as a distraction. The point I've pressed when this has come up in the past is analogous to the following: just as you wouldn't want passengers in the cockpit of a crashing plane, you don't want a lot of other people who are not medical professionals in the room during a resuscitation; you want the providers focused solely on their job of saving the patient's life. If we wish to enable family presence during resuscitations, we need to determine how it would work from a process standpoint. Do you offer it to all family members? Do you insist that everybody be accompanied by an escort? Should there be a screening process to identify family members more vulnerable to the psychological stress of watching family members die? It seems to me that those people most qualified to make these judgments are the very same people who should be running the resuscitation.

PR: The issue of family presence during resuscitations is not unique to the United States. I've read a number of articles recently based out of Jerusalem that discuss the current tensions in Israel that appear to mirror our own. Dr. Grossman, I wonder if you see any particular value in allowing family members into the trauma bay that I may be missing.

Dr. Shamai Grossman: I agree that there is little value to family presence appreciated by the physician. I do, however, believe that there may be some value ascertained by a patient's family through mere exposure to the intricacy of a resuscitation. That doesn't require that a family member stay in the resuscitation room for 30 minutes watching each procedure done. In fact, looking in on a resuscitation for 30 seconds is more than adequate for any family member to be convinced of the authenticity and of the values with which we approach resuscitations. A few moments like these allow brief intervals of exposure, would allow family members to appreciate what we are trying to do, and reassure them that their family member is in the best of hands.

PR: I'm aware of at least one lawsuit in which a mother was allowed to view the laceration repair of her son, passed out, and struck her head. She sued the doctor for the concussion that she claimed ensued. Isn't there some legal risk we expose ourselves to when exposing family members to psychologically stressful situations?

AD: You don't necessarily bear the responsibility for that patient's relative passing out. It would, however, be preferable to have someone devoted to both preparing a family member before you approach the resuscitation bay, and to have someone talk that person through the resuscitation or any particular procedure. This staff person could also ensure that the family member is seated, and doesn't get hurt if there is a syncopal event.

PR: Furthermore, how are medical professionals, during times of crisis, supposed to ensure that people are who they say they are? I've been involved with a family in which three different women claimed to be the patient's wife. It turned out that they all had been his wife at one time or another, but there was no way the medical team could sort out the facts of the situation at the time. It would seem to me that the risks of the visitation far outweigh the benefits.

AD: Most of the time a physician can reasonably rely on the fact that a person presenting him or herself as a family member is a relative. There is, of course, the possibility of asking for identification, but in a case where you're caring for a critical patient and someone ushers in a family member, you may sit them down and tell them about the situation using a concept called **reasonable reliance** (what a prudent person would believe and act upon if told something by another) to at least justify the disclosure of information.

At our adult university hospital, we do allow family members into our resuscitation bays. Moreover, the feedback from family members has been fairly positive. There is benefit for some family members who can be with their loved ones before death is pronounced. To the physicians, it has been only a minor distraction, and while most physicians would prefer to be able to do their work without having this extra factor, we haven't had a lot of resistance from our emergency physicians or trauma surgeons. In fact, we've also employed chaplains and social workers to accompany family members during procedures, so that we can obviate the issues in placing the responsibility of caring for them upon the resuscitation leader to describe what is happening.

PR: I personally find it difficult to have strangers watching complex medical procedures. Even people who should know something about medicine are frequently confused as to what is happening, and misinterpret voice inflections and subtle interactions between team members. It may be helpful to the grieving process to the family of the dying patient, but I don't see that it enhances the quality of the care. I personally am strongly opposed to it.

SG: In truth, I have found myself distracted when family is present. I find myself obliged to explain each detail of the resuscitation to the family rather than focusing on the patient.

PR: Let's move on to medical education as there are two issues I would like us to address: the first is being supervised while performing procedures important to the patient's care, and the second is the performance of procedures on the nearly dead with marginal to no benefit to the patient. If there is a normal interaction between teacher and student during the performance of various procedures, will witnesses conclude the performance is inept?

Dr. John Jesus: I recently read a piece in the *New England Journal of Medicine* by Truog, who favors futile resuscitation of children who can no longer suffer, in order to address the psychological needs of particular families who believe in fighting illness to the very end.[1] He quoted Thomas Mann when he wrote, "a man dying is more the survivors' affair than his own," which is an idea that continues to resonate with me. With regard to people in cardiac arrest, an optimistic survival rate is on the order of 5–10%, which also suggests that resuscitation efforts may actually benefit families more than they have the potential to benefit the patients themselves.

I think we assume too much if we believe that families routinely scrutinize every action we make while trying to resuscitate a patient, especially if they are witnessing their family members in the dying process. It is far more likely that they will remember that they were given the option to be with their family member during the last moments of life, than they will remember if the airway was secured before a chest tube was placed. In regards to education, I remember feeling mildly self-conscious early in my residency when performing procedures on patients with family members present or on conscious patients. We all must learn how to perform a lumbar puncture or other procedure on an awake patient. The mild amount of stress involved is a natural variable in the educational process, and one to which most every emergency physician grows accustomed. Now that I am more comfortable with the process, talking patients and their families through procedures has become second nature.

RW: There are true resuscitations, in which there exists the sincere expectation that our efforts are increasing the chances of a patient's survival, and then there are death rituals, which involves the resuscitation of patients whom you know have very little to no chance of survival. When I have been in the latter position, I have brought family members into the room for the purposes described. In this situation, I agree with focusing the priority of the medical team on the family's grieving process. During resuscitation with a viable patient, the focus must remain solely upon the patient. For example, if you find yourself managing a patient in respiratory failure with a difficult airway, there are frequently a number of intubation attempts, with actual disagreement between professionals, a process that can sometimes be less than calm and diplomatic. Having family in the room might well exaggerate the difficulties being experienced during similar situations. I have no issue with family involvement during the death ritual, but I fail to see why we would want to embrace the risk involved with a patient who is potentially viable.

PR: I still maintain that there is a difference between the needs of a patient during a time-sensitive, life-saving resuscitation, and the needs of grieving family members that are not as time sensitive, and may be addressed after the resuscitation attempt. There has been a lot of study about grief alleviation, and I haven't seen any evidence that says the process is ameliorated by allowing family members to witness the death pronouncement. Furthermore, one of the major forces pushing emergency physicians to allow more people into the resuscitation bay is that which is sensationalized on televised sitcoms, public performance. Publicity is not part of our jobs in the ED, and it should not be part of the medical discipline.

AD: Medical practice in academic centers serves two purposes: to treat patients **and** to educate the next generation of emergency physicians. Teaching procedures in front of family members may heighten the possibility of distrust and risk. If we are to teach junior residents, it would be best to do it in a situation where family was not present. We expect trainees to make mistakes. Within this context, there exists the possibility for misinterpretation on the part of the family at a critical time of need for their loved one.

JJ: The benefit of being present during a trauma resuscitation does not stem from the observation of procedures, but rather from the concept that family members might have the opportunity to witness the suffering of their loved ones, and spend time with them during the last moments of his or her life. Furthermore, the love and sorrow that impregnates the air when families are present for the death of their family member, brings a certain dignity to the resuscitation, which is often far removed from the patient's humanity. In regard to trauma resuscitations, we generally have more time than we do with patients in cardiac arrest. We should be able to reach a compromise, therefore, between performing invasive procedures without the presence of family members, and addressing the grieving needs of the family by allowing them in the room as soon those procedures have been performed. A nurse, social worker, or chaplain should accompany any family member, in order to explain the interventions and terminology being displayed and performed. Finally, the number of family members probably shouldn't exceed two, in order to limit the crush of people that commonly attend major resuscitations.

SG: If having an inexperienced person perform a procedure is a detriment to a dying patient, then it may be ethically or morally unjustifiable to allow the junior resident the opportunity to perform the procedure.

PR: How then do we train the next generation of emergency physicians? I think there is ample evidence that the experienced operator does a better job, and generally has better outcomes than an inexperienced operator. There is plenty of evidence from the surgical literature proving this point. But how will you ever become an experienced operator if you never have the opportunity to perform any of these procedures? Having to do your first life-saving procedure on a patient who needs you to save his or her life is not as good if you can acquire that experience on someone who is already dead. When I first became a physician, patients presented to academic centers voluntarily, knowing that they would be cared for by physicians in training. They found this desirable because they were assured that they would receive better care than at a community hospital where there were fewer physicians or no trainees. It seems to me that we have lost that attitude in our society, and I fear that the potential miscommunication and distrust that may arise from including families in the resuscitation bay may only further enable a loss of respect for academic tertiary care centers.

KE: My anecdotal experience performing procedures with families present is similar to John's experience, in that family members rarely notice the details of a particular procedure. At our institution, we currently perform invasive procedures first, and then invite the family into the resuscitation bay. At this point, I don't have enough evidence to argue that we should change medical culture to include families throughout the resuscitation. I also believe that we may be inflating the physical risk we impose on family members by allowing them to witness a resuscitation. There is no evidence with which I am familiar that shows that patients' family members will reliably pass out in rooms. For example, in the 9 years of studies that have been done at Ford Hospital in Michigan, not a single family member passed out, had any physical difficulty in witnessing the resuscitation, or behaved in such a way as to disrupt the efforts of the clinical team. In fact, as a fellow there, I was made to sign an agreement to permit family members to be present during resuscitations. A cultural shift is occurring, and it is going to take time and further engagement of the medical community about the issues involved and the importance for the family grieving process before we will be able to move forward.

AD: Our ED has changed its practice, and it's not going back, because families really appreciate it, and that was the driving factor at my institution.

Section III: Review of the literature

ED studies, conducted in the 1980s, of people who had experienced the sudden death of a loved one find that their most frequent criticisms centered on frustra-tions with inadequate information or updates during resuscitation.[2] This prompted early interest in the practice of family-witnessed resuscitation. In addition, they noticed that families of critically ill or dying patients often complained about feeling helpless, uninformed, and uninvolved. These findings, along with requests by some family members to be present during resuscitation procedures, called into question the standard practice of excluding families from the resuscitation room.[3]

In two pioneering studies, at Foote Hospital in Jackson, Michigan, and at Parkland Hospital in Dallas, Texas, relatives were allowed to witness resuscitation events while accompanied by a facilitator.[4,5] Participants reported that the opportunity to be present during the event helped to relieve their own anxiety, by reducing feelings of helplessness and the "agony of waiting".[4] Relatives also indicated that this experience eased their subsequent grief and bereavement process. The Parkland study participants expressed that family-witnessed resuscitation facilitated their understanding of the critical nature of their loved one's illness, and also enabled them to appreciate the significant efforts made by providers to ensure that the patient received the best possible care.[4] In the Foote study, 76% of family members surveyed said that they thought the experience facilitated their adjustment to the patient's death, and 94% stated that they would choose to be present again if given the opportunity.[5] Other studies demonstrate similar positive responses to family-witnessed resuscitation by participating families.[6] Enrollment in one randomized controlled trial was suspended early because the ED staff became convinced of the benefit of family-witnessed resuscitation for family members.[7]

In some ways, it may seem surprising that family members would desire to be present during the critical and desperate moments of medical care for their loved ones. However, the potential benefit of this experience is better understood when one considers the deep desire that family members have to help and support their loved ones when faced with grave circumstances. At the moment that life-threatening illness or injury strikes, family members are left feeling helpless by a process they do not understand and are unable to control. Family-witnessed resuscitation is empowering because it engages family members, brings them closer to their loved one, and allows them to witness the significant efforts that are directed at helping their loved one. A young woman, Sarah Adams, whose brother was critically injured during an equestrian accident in 1994, poignantly expressed these feelings,

> the overwhelming desire is to stay close to the injured person. This overrode any fears that I experienced.

In the commentary that follows Sarah Adams personal account, Dr. Roger Higgs indicates that family-witnessed resuscitation may help to reduce shock and disbelief following sudden death and, in turn, offset guilt that can inhibit normal bereavement.[8]

Due to the severity of the illness or injury requiring resuscitation and the small number of survivors, it is difficult to directly assess patients' perspectives regarding family-witnessed resuscitation. In one survey, general ED patients were presented with a hypothetical scenario of critical resuscitation, and asked for their preferences with respect to family-witnessed resuscitation; 72% of patients indicate that they would want to have a family member in the room while they received care.[9] Additional insight into the patient perspective was obtained in follow-up work at Parkland Hospital. In this study, patients provided direct feedback after undergoing either cardiac resuscitation or invasive procedures with family present. Although only a small number (n = 9) of patients were interviewed, the responses identified some consistent and interesting elements. Patients indicate that the presence of family members was comforting to them, and also felt that this opportunity helped to humanize their care by reminding ED staff of their personal connections within a family.[10] These findings are supported by patients' individuals stories and experiences shared in powerful anecdotes, one of which comes from a patient who survived cardiac resuscitation at Wooster Community Hospital in Ohio, which adopted a program for family-witnessed resuscitation in 1994. This 60-year-old man stated that he was:

> very much aware of his wife's presence, which was enough of an encouragement for him to continue his fight for survival.[6]

Despite the evidence that family-witnessed resuscitation provides a benefit for family members (and, perhaps, some patients as well), it is not surprising that there remains marked uncertainty and variability in provider attitudes and clinical practice. Family-witnessed resuscitation evokes strong emotional responses because it raises valid concerns regarding its potential for undesirable ramifications. In particular, emergency medicine providers are worried that relatives will get in the way of medical staff or otherwise interfere with resuscitation attempts.[6,11-14] They also fear that watching a resuscitation attempt will be excessively stressful and upsetting to family members,[12-14] possibly leading to posttraumatic stress disorder or other psychological damage.[11,15] Some providers have expressed concern that the presence of relatives might intimidate the medical team[12] or increase their stress levels, causing them to lose their concentration and objectivity and thereby impeding their performance.[11,13,14] While some physicians worry that observation might reveal inadequacy in the medical care provided, others are concerned that relatives without medical training will misunderstand the actions of the team.[11,12] In addition, many medical professionals worry that family presence programs will lead to an increase in malpractice litigation.[4,6,11,12]

In the initial Foote study,[5] as well as a follow-up review of their continued family-witnessed resuscitation program, anticipated problems failed to occur. Over the 9 years reviewed, there were no situations in which a family member interfered with a resuscitation attempt, and participants demonstrated no signs of emotional trauma as a result of family-witnessed resuscitation, but instead, consistently responded positively to this experience.[16] Similarly, the Parkland study finds that family members do not cause any disruptions during CPR or any invasive procedures; 97% of the healthcare providers surveyed said that family member behavior during visitation is appropriate. Furthermore, family members surveyed 2 months after witnessing resuscitation do not report any psychological trauma resulting from their participation.[4] These findings have been substantiated by additional studies that find no negative sequelae for family members who witness resuscitation events compared with controls.[7,17] On the provider side, a study of 114 ED personnel at a hospital in the United Kingdom concludes that the presence of relatives at a resuscitation attempt does not affect self-reported stress symptoms.[18] Several recent studies have considered the impact of family-witnessed resuscitation on disruptions and delays in care as well as physician performance of critical actions and provide growing evidence to suggest that it does not significantly effect patient care.[19-21] In one of these studies, the authors simulated a cardiac arrest event with and without family present, and measured time intervals to critical actions (chest compressions, defibrillation, and pronouncement of death). For these simulated events, family witnesses were either quiet (no overt grief reaction) or overtly grieving (crying, trying to hug a patient, or asking numerous questions of physicians). This interesting study finds no difference between the groups without a family witness and those with either type of family witness, with the exception of time to first defibrillation for the group with an overtly grieving family. Qualitative responses from providers following their participation in these simulation events emphasize the importance of screening mechanisms to ensure that family witnesses are emotionally stable, and that they receive the support they need during the resuscitation event.[20]

Very little work has been done to directly consider the differences between trauma and medical resuscitations with respect the impact on the witnessing family members and providers. It is reasonable to consider that traumatic injuries, frequently associated with deformity and bleeding, and trauma-related procedures (e.g. chest tubes, thoracotomy) may be more difficult for family members to observe. Although some of the research in this area has included both medical and traumatic resuscitations, and demonstrated positive experiences for family members without evidence of negative sequelae other studies have focused solely on medical patients to avoid the complexities introduced in the setting of trauma.[5,7,17] A recent study specifically evaluated the impact of family-witnessed resuscitation for family members of trauma victims who were subsequently admitted to critical care, and finds that there are no differences in outcomes (including measures of coping, communication and wellbeing) between those who witnessed and those who did not witness the resuscitation of their loved one.[22] Of note, this study did not consider family members of patients who died as a result of their trauma. In the future, more rigorous investigation is needed to directly explore the differences between medical and trauma resuscitations, and how they should have an impact upon policies for family-witnessed resuscitation in clinical practice.

The integration of resident teaching and family-witnessed resuscitation has been identified as a significant concern for providers at academic hospitals.[23] Although some of the research in this area has been conducted at teaching hospitals,[4] it is difficult to assess the interplay between teaching and family-witnessed resuscitation. Future studies may consider simulation as a means for both investigation and training in this area. Although there are gaps in our existing research on family-witnessed resuscitation, there is growing evidence to indicate that provider experience, education and training have a significant impact on attitudes towards it.[23-25] The role of experience in influencing provider views of family-witnessed resuscitation is most poignantly conveyed in a letter to the *Journal of Trauma* by Dr. James Barone, in which he explains how allowing the family of a 9-year old girl in to see her while resuscitation activities were in progress changed his opinion of family presence:

I had previously opposed any intrusion into the sacred domain of the trauma resuscitation room by patients' families. I now realize that under the proper circumstances . . . the presence of the family may actually be a good thing for everyone, including the caregivers.[26]

The importance of experience and education in shaping the attitudes of medical professionals towards family-witnessed resuscitation is further substantiated by studies that demonstrate a gradient of support for this practice corresponding with staff experience. The Parkland study finds that only 19% of residents support the family presence program, compared with 79% of attendings.[4] Another study at a London hospital finds that young physician respondents are less likely to favor family presence than nurses or more senior physicians.[12] This phenomenon is likely due to younger physicians having less confidence in their resuscitation skills, and emphasizes the critical need for staff education, training, and preparation prior to implementation of a program for family-witnessed resuscitation.

Ethical analysis

The question of whether to allow family members to witness attempts to resuscitate may not seem at first to be an ethical issue at all, but merely a practical one.

Beneficence, the duty to act for the patient's benefit, and non-maleficence, the duty not to harm, both would support acting to maximize the likelihood of success in resuscitation by minimizing any extraneous activities or distractions that might interfere with resuscitation.[27,28] Autonomy, the principle that patients may choose to accept or decline treatment, mandates that physicians respect the medical choices of the patient who has decision-making capacity.[29] Generally, this mandate would not extend to family members' desire to be with patients at this crucial time, though a physician should accommodate the patient's preference, if known, as to whether family or loved ones witness these activities, as long as this activity does not harm the patient.

Although the doctor–patient relationship is generally recognized legally as a one-to-one relationship (the physician's duty is to the patient), the doctor–patient relationship and its corresponding responsibilities have more recently widened at times to include duties to third parties including family members.[30,31] As well, when the patient wishes the emergency physician to include family in communication and discussion about the patient's acute medical problem, emergency physicians usually do so. Additionally, both the concern for the wellbeing of family members and the wish not to be a burden to family members have been recognized to be significant concerns for patients.[32,33] Thus, with no evidence of harm to the patient from the practice, and benefits to the family, there are good ethical reasons emergency physicians should consider accommodating family presence, and with increased family satisfaction and no evidence of increased malpractice litigation, there are also good practical reasons to do so. Nonetheless, individual emergency physicians should weigh all the factors carefully in any given situation when making this decision.

Conclusion

The debate over family-witnessed resuscitation represents an important crossroads in the evolution of our specialty. As emergency medicine providers we are deeply committed to providing the best possible care to our patients. On a daily basis, we are faced with serious illness and injury, and must make rapid decisions with significant and, potentially life-saving, consequences for our patients. Our dedication to this important responsibility makes it difficult to consider anything that might distract us from critical tasks. In this way, family-witnessed resuscitation challenges us at a vulnerable core by seeming to threaten our primary commitment to our patients with the introduction of family members during times of intense focus and effort. Moreover, family-witnessed resuscitation frequently confronts us in our most difficult moments as physicians—times when we feel least successful and most distressed because our efforts to save our patient are desperate or failing. Thus, it is clear that the adoption of this new and controversial practice is anything but straightforward.

Research demonstrating the benefit and safety of this practice is critically important as a means of defining policies and strategies in clinical practice. However, research alone will not resolve this controversy because the emotional responses to this change in practice are so intense. As this debate evolves, it is important that we do not dismiss the important issues facing us as providers, but rather embrace them and discuss them openly. Reservations and fears are understandable and represent laudable reflections of a deep commitment to patient care. They should form the basis for education and training that facilitate skill development and enable providers to move past their concerns with confidence and security. With this approach, it will be possible for us to enter a new frontier of care that integrates the needs of our patients with their closest loved ones, while ensuring the best outcome for all.

Section IV: Recommendations

• Promote a candid discussion of family-witnessed resuscitation at your institution and in your department.
• Assess the support mechanisms for families (e.g., social work, nursing) during critical resuscitation events in your department.
• When faced with the critical resuscitation of a patient, consider offering families the option to be present during the resuscitation event.
• In the event that a family is given the opportunity to be present in the resuscitation room, ensure that all members of the team are aware of decision and that adequate support is provided for the family (e.g., social work, nursing) during the events.

References

1. Truog RD. (2010) Is it always wrong to perform futile CPR? *N Engl J Med.* 362(6), 477–9.
2. Parrish GA, Holdren KS, Skiendzielewski JJ, et al. (1987) Emergency department experience with sudden death: a survey of survivors. *Ann Emerg Med.* 16, 792–6.
3. Post H. (1989) Letting the family in during a code. *Nursing.* 19, 43–6.
4. Meyers TA, Eichhorn DJ, Guzzetta CE, et al. (2000) Family presence during invasive procedures and resuscitation. *Am J Nurs.* 100, 32–42.
5. Doyle CJ, Post H, Burney RE, et al. (1987) Family participation during resuscitation: an option. *Ann Emerg Med.* 16, s673–5.
6. Belanger MA, Reed S. (1997) A rural community hospital's experience with family-witnessed resuscitation. *J Emerg Nurs.* 23, 238–9.
7. Robinson SM, Mackenzie-Ross S, Campbell Hewson GL, et al. (1998) Psychological effect of witnessed resuscitation on bereaved relatives. *Lancet.* 352, 614–7.
8. Adams S, Whitlock M, Higgs R, et al. (1994) Should relatives be allowed to watch resuscitation? *BMJ.* 308, 1687–92.
9. Benjamin M, Holger J, Carr M. (2004) Personal preferences regarding family member presence during resuscitation. *Acad Emerg Med.* 11, 750–3.
10. Eichhorn DJ, Meyers TA, Guzzetta CE, et al. (2001) Family presence during invasive procedures and resuscitation: hearing the voice of the patient. *Am J Nurs.* 101, 48–55.
11. Helmer SD, Smith RS, Dort JM, et al. (2000) Family presence during trauma resuscitation: a survey of AAST and ENA members. *J Trauma.* 48, 1015–22; discussion 1023–4.
12. Mitchell MH, Lynch MB. (1997) Should relatives be allowed in the resuscitation room? *J Accid Emerg Med.* 14, 366–9; discussion 370.
13. McClenathan BM, Torrington KG, Uyehara CF. (2002) Family member presence during cardiopulmonary resuscitation: a survey of US and international critical care professionals. *Chest.* 122, 2204–11.
14. Pafford MB. (2002) Should family members be present during CPR? *J Ark Med Soc.* 98, 304–6.
15. Osuagwu C. (1991) ED codes: keep the family out [comment]. *J Emerg Nurs.* 17, 363.
16. Hanson C, Strawser D. (1992) Family presence during cardiopulmonary resuscitation: Foote Hospital emergency department's nine-year perspective. *J Emerg Nurs.* 18, 104–6.
17. Compton S, Levy P, Griffin M, et al. (2011) Family-witnessed resuscitation: bereavement outcomes in an urban environment. *J Palliat Med.* 14(6), 715–21.
18. Boyd R, White S. (2000) Does witnessed cardiopulmonary resuscitation alter perceived stress in accident and emergency staff? *Eur J Emerg Med.* 7, 51–3.
19. Sacchetti A, Paston C, Carraccio C. (2005) Family members do not disrupt care when present during invasive procedures. *Acad Emerg Med.* 12(5), 477–9.
20. Fernandez R, Compton S, Jones KA, et al. (2009) The presence of a family witness impacts physician performance during simulated medical codes. *Crit Care Med.* 37(6), 1956–60.
21. Dudley NC, Hansen KW, Furnival RA, et al. (2009) The effect of family presence on the efficiency of pediatric trauma resuscitations. *Ann Emerg Med.* 53(6), 777–84.
22. Leske JS, Brasel K. (2010) Effects of family-witnessed resuscitation after trauma prior to hospitalization. *J Trauma Nurs.* 17(1), 11–8.
23. Engel KG, Barnosky AR, Berry-Bovia M, et al. (2007) Provider experience and attitudes toward family presence during resuscitation procedures. *J Palliat Med.* 10(5), 1007–9.
24. Bassler PC. (1999) The impact of education on nurses' beliefs regarding family presence in a resuscitation room. *J Nurses Staff Dev.* 15(3), 126–31.
25. Feagan LM, Fisher NJ. (2011) The impact of education on provider attitudes toward family-witnessed resuscitation. *J Emerg Nurs.* 37(3), 231–9.
26. Barone JE. (2001) Family presence during trauma resuscitation [comment]. *J Trauma.* 50, 386.
27. Beauchamp TL, Childress JF. (2009) Respect for autonomy. In: *Principles of Biomedical Ethics.* New York, NY: Oxford University Press, pp. 99–148.
28. Beauchamp TL, Childress JF. (2009) Beneficience. In: *Principles of Biomedical Ethics.* New York, NY: Oxford University Press, pp. 197–239.
29. Beauchamp TL, Childress JF. (2009) Nonmaleficence. In: *Principles of Biomedical Ethics.* New York, NY: Oxford University Press, pp. 149–96.
30. Junkerman C, Derse A, Schiedermayer D. The physician's professional responsibilities. In: *Practical Ethics for Students, Interns and Residents: A Short Reference Manual*, 3rd ed. Hagerstown, MD: University Publishing Group, pp. 78–80.
31. Schuster *v.* Altenberg, 144 Wis. 2d 223, 424 N.W.2d 159 (1988).
32. Berger JT. (2009) Patients' concerns for family burden: A noncomforming preference in standards for surrogate decision making. *J Clin Ethics.* 20(2), 158–61.
33. Derse AR. (2009) When I lay my burden down: Commentary on Berger. *J Clin Ethics.* 20(2), 172–4.

8

Palliative care in the emergency department

Tammie E. Quest,[1] *Paul DeSandre*[2]

[1]*Interim Director, Emory Palliative Care Center, Chief, Section of Palliative Medicine, Atlanta VAMC, Fellowship Director, Hospice and Palliative Medicine, Division of Geriatrics and Gerontology, Associate Professor, Department of Emergency Medicine, Director, EPEC-EM, Atlanta, GA, USA*

[2]*Assistant Chief, Section of Palliative Medicine, Atlanta VA Medical Center, and Associate Program Director, Fellowship in Hospice and Palliative Medicine, and Assistant Professor, Emergency Medicine and Hospice and Palliative Medicine, Emory University, Atlanta, GA, USA*

Section I: Case presentation

An 82-year-old woman with advanced dementia presents with shortness of breath shortly after routine percutaneous endoscopic gastrostomy (PEG) tube feedings at home. She has become bed bound, and has lost the ability to speak over the last several months. This is her fourth emergency department (ED) visit in the last year for pneumonia and a urinary tract infection. Her daughter, the primary caregiver who has a documented Durable Power of Attorney for Health Care, is at the bedside and is frustrated that her mother is not getting better. On examination, the patient is lethargic with clinical symptoms of pneumonia, but appears to be protecting her airway. She appears to be in pain during the examination with grimacing and moaning. She is noted to have a stage II decubitus ulcer and contractures of all extremities. There is leakage around the PEG tube site with skin breakdown. Her vital signs are temperature 39.2 °C, blood pressure 82/50 mmHg, heart rate 120 beats/minute, respiratory rate 24 breaths/minute, oxygen saturation 93% on supplemental high flow oxygen. The emergency clinician and her daughter establish the goals of care as comfort. The patient is found to have a right lower lobe pneumonia on the portable chest radiograph. Peripheral intravenous access cannot be obtained.

Section II: Discussion

Dr. Peter Rosen: We have many patients who, on initial assessment, appear not to belong in the ED. In this case, for example, the daughter likely has unrealistic expectations for her mother's outcomes, and has not accepted the reality that medical care cannot improve her mother's quality of life. What do we need to consider in deciding what to do for this patient?

Dr. Shamai Grossman: Because emergency physicians do not have an established relationship with the patient, it is difficult to fully understand what the patient's quality of life actually is, and furthermore, what quality of life the patient considers sufficient to justify the medical interventions we have to offer and their sequelae. In many cases, patients with similar states of health will have several admissions, with only transient improvements. This cycle is frustrating for everyone involved. We must explain to patients and their families that despite our interventions, patients in this cycle will have a similar outcome. We should then attempt to understand what the patient would have wanted if she were able to communicate to us, or what the family understands of what the patient would have wanted. Unfortunately, the time constraints of the ED often make such a conversation impractical.

Ethical Problems in Emergency Medicine: A Discussion-Based Review, First Edition. John Jesus, Shamai A. Grossman, Arthur R. Derse, James G. Adams, Richard Wolfe, and Peter Rosen.

Ideally, the primary care physician should have this conversation before a patient has lost her faculties, and is able to participate in the conversation. Ultimately, our obligation is to do what is best for the patient. In a critical scenario, this means stabilizing the patient, and moving them somewhere conducive to a conversation about what long-term plans are appropriate.

PR: Physicians are not likely to agree on what constitutes the best care for this patient. Many would focus on the fact that they don't know the patient, haven't already participated in discussions about goals of care and quality of life, and would simply conclude that it would be best not to become involved with those issues. They might admit the patient to the intensive care unit (ICU), and allow the inpatient team to tease apart the patient's true goals of care.

Dr. Arthur Derse: If a power of attorney has been activated in the past, then the daughter does have the authority to express her mother's wishes and make decisions she feels are in the best interest of her mother. Emergency physicians should become more comfortable speaking with family members about the trajectory of a patients' illness, even if they don't know the patient well. To talk about prognosis, quality of life, and goals of care with the family is important and legitimate. They have the legal authority to speak for their loved ones, and you can help them better understand the situation and reach an informed decision.

Dr. John Jesus: In addition, we must consider the importance of stewardship of ED resources and protecting the interests of other patients in the department as we address the acute needs of the patient in our case. Ideally, we ought to clarify with the family and patient the trajectory of their condition and their goals. If there are other unstable patients in the department, taking the time to discuss these issues with the family would be inappropriate. In this setting, I would arrange an interaction between the family and the physician who is in the best position to have an in-depth conversation about goals of care and code status. In terms of what should be done clinically, I think in many cases, treating the patient's acute care need is consistent with reducing their suffering. Even in the setting of a poor long-term prognosis, as in this case, I might treat the pneumonia, not

necessarily in the interest of extending the patient's life, but as a means of reducing her suffering to the extent of my abilities.

PR: The question I would ask is, "Why does this patient need to be admitted at all?" I would rather place the patient in an observation unit, and then have a longer discussion with the daughter and the primary care physician about either arranging hospice care or allowing her to die at home. It has become a custom to not allow patients to die at home or in the nursing home. This is something we must address if we hope to control our shortage of inpatient beds and healthcare costs.

Dr. Tammie Quest: The World Health Organization defines palliative care as the physical, spiritual, psychological, and social care of a patient and family from the diagnosis of a life-threatening illness to cure, or death and bereavement. Comfort measures are those aspects of care directed at the physical, spiritual, psychological, and social suffering of both the patient and the family. These are not categorically different from the care that we provide in the ED every day, and I don't view any of these measures as inappropriate as long as they relieve distress.

SG: Would that include intubation?

TQ: Yes, it could include intubation, though some evidence suggests that in most patients at the end of life, intubation or invasive respiratory management often fails to relieve the distress associated with dyspnea. These considerations should be focused less on how invasive a procedure is, and more on the evidence that it might palliate a particular symptom.

PR: We are not necessarily accurate at determining who is and who isn't having pain, and in fact, the patient in the case presented is not in a condition to perceive her own comfort. I think palliative care is a useful concept for patients who have cognizance. When patients are aware that they have an incurable disease, it makes sense to try to maximize their quality of life until their death. I would distinguish this concept from that of comfort care, which is often more concerned with the comfort of the family and the physician than that of the patient.

TQ: Palliative care can apply to patients with curable illness. The emphasis is on life-threatening illnesses, but these may be curable illnesses. For example, there are many palliative care interventions that apply to a patient awaiting a transplant who will be virtually cured of their illness posttransplantation.

PR: If you say that palliative care applies to curable illnesses, then it's not clear to me how it differs from what we do for every patient. I don't believe palliative care includes curable care, at least in the way it is commonly understood. In thinking about comfort care, ethical problems arise for physicians in considering specific measures namely food, water, antibiotics, and analgesia. What circumstances justify withholding any of these?

TQ: The decision to give or withhold an intervention is based on the goals of care and how that intervention relates to their goals. In this case, my suspicion is that food and water would increase her risk for respiratory distress, and thus these would not be comfort care measures. Antibiotics might prolong life, which would also prolong the dying process and thus appear to work against the goals of care. There are circumstances, however, in which the family may accept that the patient is dying, but want the patient to live long enough for another loved one to arrive and say goodbye. Evaluation of what interventions are in line with the goals of care can be complex and based on motivations that conflict with one another. There are also alternative, non-invasive interventions to palliate symptoms such as low-dose opioids for dyspnea and subcutaneous administration of medications and fluids instead of intubation and central venous catheterization, respectively.

SG: One needs to make an assumption in that case that the patient would have preferred prolonged suffering to allow a family member to say good bye to her. If not, I believe it would be unethical to place the family's needs above the needs of the patient.

PR: If I was truly convinced that this patient was having pain, the only comfort care I would consider is pain relief. I don't know how long it will take her to die. I don't believe the hospital has anything to offer her that couldn't be provided in hospice care or at home.

SG: If the patient's family desired further curative treatment rather than comfort care, I would treat the patient as I would any other. Though her prognosis is poor overall, sepsis is potentially treatable with antibiotics, fluids, pressors, and whatever other support that doesn't exceed what the family deems appropriate. Such an intervention may allow the patient to get over this immediate illness, and the subsequent process of dying from her underlying illness could take years. It is possible that during the time the patient is DNR/DNI [do not resuscitate/do not intubate] she could survive recurrent small diseases without draining significant resources and avoid critical care.

PR: In this case, we cannot do anything to enhance the comfort of this patient's life, because I don't think she is capable of perceiving whether she is comfortable or not. She moans and appears to be in pain, but can't communicate what is bothering her, and we therefore can't tell if she actually has discomfort. The fact that she has developed a potentially curable disease that could end her apparent suffering is a blessing in my mind, not a curse. I do not believe this patient fits into the mission of medicine, because she does not have a curable disease, she does not have a disease that we can make bearable while she lives with it, and she does not have a life that we can make comfortable. Our major task is therefore to allow her to die, and do so in a way that will not tax the resources of the hospital. This is an important concern, because in my view it is this kind of situation that can reduce the availability of beds for patients that have curable disease. In addition, this situation is one that creates enormous financial burdens on our healthcare system with very little impact to show for it. While I can understand the perception that life is a wonderful thing and we should appreciate and maintain it, there is nothing left to appreciate about this woman's life.

JJ: I would like to reassert a point you made earlier that it is very difficult to assess whether or not the patient is having pain. My inclination, therefore, is to be conservative, and attempt to reduce whatever suffering she may be having, rather than assume that she is not suffering. That said, I do recognize the importance of stewardship of hospital resources, and agree that the patient does not necessarily require an admission. Instead, I would be inclined to treat her with antibiotics and attempt to place her at home under hospice care.

PR: One of the reasons you frequently encounter families who want all possible interventions performed to prolong the life of their loved ones, is that they bear no risk for the burden of the patient's care. It is natural to say, "Do everything" when you are not confronted with the costs, financial and otherwise. At some point, we have to define the utility of the care we are asked to provide.

SG: Israel has a socialized medicine system, and spends approximately 7% of the gross national product on healthcare. That's roughly half as much as we spend in the United States, and they have a higher life expectancy. It is the standard practice to give patients full care at the end of life unless the family or the patient express wishes to the contrary. Though it is clear that end-of-life care does introduce financial burdens, it alone does not explain the high cost of healthcare in this country. The case of Israel demonstrates that one can have aggressive end-of-life care and low healthcare costs. This is because their universal healthcare system is substantially cheaper overall, and there are many potential methods of lowering costs other than terminating healthcare in the elderly that they have been loathe to implement in Israel. Quality of life cannot be the sole determinant of who lives and who dies.

PR: Our hardest task here is to define what constitutes futile treatment, and better evaluate what treatments offer utility under different circumstances.

TQ: This is a major goal of palliative care specialists. On a basic level, it is the goals of care that define whether an intervention is useful or not. In considering specific interventions, there are many studies in palliative medicine that will assess an intervention's effectiveness in palliating a symptom to provide evidence-based guidance for clinicians. Another important consideration is the patient's palliative prognostic score. In this case, the patient's score is quite low, suggesting the patient would not survive long even if her sepsis were effectively treated. In general, physicians are poor at predicting prognosis, and are not typically equipped with objective evidence when making such estimates. A physician's ability to make evidence-based evaluations of utility serves not only the interests of the patient and her family, but also other patients in the department insofar as such determinations are important to stewardship of ED resources.

PR: These are difficult problems, and this has been a wonderful discussion. The most important consideration that we have repeatedly discussed is the importance of communication with families, and the demonstration that their goal, as representatives of the patient, and our goal, as their clinical team, is the same: patient comfort. Once they understand that some interventions serve only to extend their loved one's suffering, they tend to be much happier about the decision to avoid futile treatments. We need to change our attitudes regarding what we should do for patients whose lives we can't improve.

Section III: Review of the literature

Palliative care is the physical, spiritual, psychological, and social care provided to patients and families from diagnosis to death or cure of a life-threatening illness.[1] The focus is on the relief of suffering, and is best provided as an interdisciplinary approach. It is appropriate at any stage of illness and is appropriate in any setting. The palliative approach accepts death as a normal process. Bereavement care is also an important aspect of palliative care. Practical elements of palliative care include pain and symptom management, advance care planning, communication about goals of care, truth-telling, social support, spiritual support, psychological support and risk/burden assessment of treatments. Palliative care, practically speaking, amounts to "good interdisciplinary care." Palliative care and life-prolonging care can coexist. For example, a patient may have terminal lung cancer, but while functional, would accept antibiotics for a hospital-acquired pneumonia or even an aggressive attempt at reversal of sepsis during neutropenia while receiving palliative chemotherapy. However, when life-prolonging care is no longer possible or not indicated based on the therapy's inability to achieve identified goals of care, palliative care may be the entire focus. In the United States, when an illness reaches a prognosis of 6 months or less if the disease runs its usual course, patients are considered eligible for hospice care[2] (Figure 8.1). Applications of palliative care in the emergency setting continue to be defined.[3–6]

Setting the scene

Seriously ill older adults have significant palliative care needs.[7] Emergency clinicians are uncomfortable

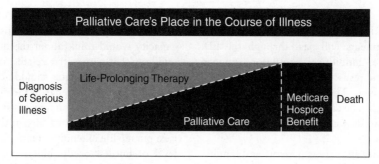

Fig. 8.1 Palliative care's place in the course of illness.

with the details of palliative care, and have limited knowledge of palliative and end-of-life care. Thematically, emergency clinicians equate palliative care with end-of-life care; may disagree about the feasibility and desirability of providing palliative care in the ED; care for families of patients distressed by end-of-life symptoms and a palliative approach; may experience a lack of communication between outpatient and ED providers leading to undesirable outcomes (e.g., resuscitation of patients with a DNR order); commonly experience conflict around withholding life-prolonging treatment (e.g., between patient's family and written advance directives); and feel their training in pain management is inadequate.[8] All of these factors make the ability to care for a patient with a life-threatening illness difficult. However, the emergency clinician will continue to face these cases with increasing frequency. An attempt to start understanding the issue with respect to trajectories of life, goals of care/quality of life, pain management, prognosis, and the bias of emergency care, may assist in providing competent and compassionate quality care.

Trajectories of end of life encountered in the ED
End of life can be considered a phase, not an event. Global trajectories experienced at the end of life have been described.[9] The ability to identify where a patient is on the trajectory of end of life, particularly in the ED where longitudinal care is not the construct, can be of particular importance. With advancements in medicine, patients are living longer with serious, life-threatening, and terminal illnesses, with heart failure and malignancy being notable examples. With the introduction of the left ventricular assist device and biventricular pacing, patients with severe, advanced heart disease may live years longer than even 5 years ago. The common denominator for all, however, is death.

Due to symptom burden, caregiver breakdown or need for primary disease management, patients with advanced illness often present to the ED for care, some in the end-of-life phase. The emergency clinician first evaluates the clinical scenario based on identification and reversibility of a life threat with nearly simultaneous attention to the relief of suffering and risk/burden assessment. There is often an assumption that presentation to the ED means that reversals of life threats are desired. This may not be true. Seven trajectories specific to ED presentations at or near the end of life have begun to emerge: dead on arrival; prehospital resuscitation with subsequent ED death; prehospital resuscitation with survival until admission; terminally ill and comes to the ED; frail and hovering near death; alive and interactive on arrival, but arrests in the ED; and potentially preventable death by omission or commission.[10] Another framework of end of life in the ED is the spectacular or subtacular trajectory. The **spectacular** death yields a public display of the end of life in the ED, involving additional nurses, physicians, technicians, and often a variety of specialties within the hospital; **subtacular** dying occurs in patients who present to the ED for symptom management as their underlying condition deteriorates or they experience a periodic crisis.[11]

Risk–burden–benefit assessment
While the majority of adult patients in America state that they would prefer to die at home, most will not. Approximately 70% of all deaths occur in a nursing home, long-term care facility, or acute care hospital.[12]

83

Of those who die in acute care hospitals, it is estimated that approximately 20% will die in the ICU.[13] Many of these patients will pass through the ED. They will receive antibiotics, ventilator support, blood products, and resuscitation, to name just a few possible interventions. They often are admitted to critical care settings. The critical question is often not what we are able to do for a patients, but what is in their best interests.

We must recognize and advise patients and families when it appears that interventions are delaying the death process, and are distracting clinicians from a potentially more important goal of relieving patients' suffering. The patient discussed in our case met the criteria of frail and hovering near death. The patient had not previously been deemed terminally ill, but may meet those criteria objectively. The patient's family and perhaps her primary care physician, however, may see her as merely frail, even though on presentation she hovers near death.

Recent studies suggest that in patients with advanced dementia, treatment of infection may extend life, but does not enhance comfort.[14] The role of the emergency clinician is to recognize the trajectory of illness on which the patient presents, considering the global illness process, and then guide patients and families with advice regarding the likelihood of treatments and therapies to achieve the patient's goals of care. If no goals have been defined, it is the ethical and legal responsibility of the emergency clinician to inform patients and their surrogates the risks, benefits, and alternatives of a given treatment. For some clinicians, death is a very uncomfortable alternative. The palliative approach makes peace with death as a normal and natural process. The choice is not whether one will die, but how and when it will happen. Most patients and their surrogates have not considered the end of life in the intensive care setting or nursing home as the likely site of their end-of-life process, and do not realize there is another choice.

Quality of life, goals of care, and prognostication
How one defines quality of life is highly personal. When weighing options for medical interventions, patients and their surrogates are often faced with the determination of the quality of life that they are experiencing, or that which is believed to be medically anticipated—is it "worth it?" What may be good quality of life to one person may not be to another.

A surrogate is asked to perform a substituted judgment of what the patient, who has lost decision-making capacity would think about the quality of their life, and how that perspective relates to available medical interventions. Surrogates should not utilize their own feelings about the patient's or their own quality of life. The emergency clinician may assist patients and families by assessing goals of care in three broad categories: pursue life extending interventions no matter the level of burden or disability; pursue life extending interventions that may be minimally or moderately burdensome, but could ensure some defined quality of life; and do not pursue life extending interventions, only pursue measures that would be directed at symptom relief and allow death to occur naturally. In practice, patients and surrogates might choose a blend of the three—they might want comfort measures as well as the pursuit of life extending therapies. For those patients and surrogates who do not fit squarely in one category, it may be helpful to define the minimally acceptable outcome of an intervention, beyond which if attempted and unsuccessful, interventions should stop. In all cases, the clinician must be able to discuss with the patient and surrogate what the minimally acceptable outcome, often described in terms of functional status, that one would be hoping to achieve. Some questions that begin to assess the patient's perspective on quality of life might include: What are you expecting to happen with your illness? At the end of your life, whenever that is, what will you find important for yourself or for your loved one?

For most patients and their surrogates, the answer would change based on the prognosis. Emergency physicians may be uncomfortable with the prognosis, feeling that other providers might be more skilled at prognostication. While this may be true with respect to specific illnesses, the true art of prognostication combines not just one disease entity or episode of illness, but incorporates a multifactorial approach. The emergency physician ideally should be comfortable with basic tenets of prognostication. There are several scores and scales that can allow the emergency physician to estimate prognosis from a disease-specific as well as global sense.[15–20]

Pain management
More than 50% of patients at the end of life will die in pain.[21] Emergency physicians have identified lack of knowledge with respect to pain management to be

a significant barrier to the provision of optimal palliative care in the ED.[5] In particular, older adults appear to be less likely to receive analgesics.[22] Skill and comfort with pain management at end of life is a deficit in many specialties of medicine, but in the ED, there are particular barriers that exist that include assessment, lack of knowledge, lack of longitudinal relationship with the patient and environmental factors.

Bias toward life-saving interventions

Once a **subtacular** dying trajectory is identified in the ED, it has been observed that these patients may become lower priority, in particular, after a DNR order has been written or decisions to withhold or withdraw treatments have been made.[11] The emergency physician must strive not only to identify the trajectory and proceed appropriately, but make sure those patients on less **spectacular** trajectories are still adequately attended. The emergency physician can be skillful in discussing the risks, benefits, and alternatives to invasive interventions in a non-biased and informative matter. Advising patients and families on interventions that consider not just the extension of life, but the likely functional outcome of the proposed interventions, would be most beneficial. Cardiopulmonary resuscitation can reliably be presented as a therapy that universally has a low probability of restoring life outside the hospital.[23–25] In some conditions, antibiotics should be described as a therapy that may deliver more days of life, but not more comfort or quality.[14]

Future directions and potential solutions

Current training and practice do not yet sufficiently equip emergency physicians to meet the expected challenges of patients presenting to the ED with palliative care needs. Acknowledging these challenges, in 2006 the American Board of Emergency Medicine became one of 10 sponsoring boards for the newest subspecialty of the American Board of Medical Specialties: Hospice and Palliative Medicine (HPM). As the fifth recognized subspecialty of Emergency Medicine (EM), the door is now open for EM specialists to receive formal training and board certification in HPM. One of the goals for fellowship training in HPM is to foster education and practice improvement within the specialty. The number of EM specialists

now board certified in HPM is rising, and palliative care curriculums are already being developed in some EM residency training programs.

To address the broader group of clinicians interfacing with patients suffering from advanced progressive illness, practice guidelines were released in 2007 to provide information to guide future training and practice development.[2] In addition to these general guidelines, several resources exist to build curricula for training and provide guidelines for improving practice in the ED. One excellent teaching tool for general training in principles of palliative care in the ED the Education in Palliative and "End-of-Life Care-EM" (EPEC-EM). It is an important vehicle for professional practice development for the full range of professionals functioning in EDs. This curriculum is open to physicians, nurses, social workers, psychologists, and chaplains interested in bringing structured principles of palliative care practice into the ED. The program has been in place since 2007, and remains one of the most influential educational tools in emergency medicine exploring teaching and training methods to integrate palliative care practices in the ED.

To provide tools for practice improvement in the ED, the Center for the Advancement of Palliative Care (CAPC) is sponsoring an effort targeted to professionals in emergency medicine. It is intended as a comprehensive source of information and resources to foster optimal care of patients with advanced illness who present to the ED. The project, Improving Palliative Care in Emergency Medicine (IPAL-EM), intends to become the primary repository for education, assessment, and intervention tools for practice improvements in the ED. Administrators, clinicians, and HPM specialists will all likely benefit from content in their efforts to improve the care of patients presenting to the ED with advanced progressive illness.

A majority of hospitals now have access to palliative care services in some form. Some institutions have access to HPM specialists at all times; most institutions have at least phone access during off-hours. Depending on current availability, EDs can begin to foster improved access to these specialists to help in difficult situations arising in the ED, much like other consultation services. Formal training in EM residency training programs in basic principles of palliative care, targeted training related to the ED interface in HPM fellowship programs, the EPEC-EM program, and the IPAL-EM resource project are the beginnings of an effort to change the culture of care for an increasingly large population of vulnerable patients. Effective training and practice development to improve the care of these patients can allow rapid and reliable interventions with intended and beneficial outcomes.

Conclusion

The primary goal of emergency clinicians is to prioritize and physiologically stabilize the patients with the greatest life threats, provide curative therapies and interventions when possible, alleviate suffering and pain, and communicate effectively. These are shared goals with palliative care. In the United States, the median age of death is 77.7 years. It is estimated that the proportion of people over 85 years of age will double to 10 million by 2030, and nearly one quarter of patients over the age of 85 will likely continue to experience dementia.[26] Excluding infants under 1 year, patients over the age of 75 represent the age group with the highest rate of ED use.[27] The elderly are only a portion of patients with advanced progressive illnesses who are becoming an increasingly large and important segment of the ED population. The majority of patients who die in the United States experience an anticipated or **subtacular** death that is the result of advancing progressive illness, and they are likely to require emergency care along their trajectory with increasing frequency as the illness progresses.[26] The current training, practice, and comfort of emergency physicians is not yet sufficient to meet these needs. Specific barriers to providing intended and beneficial interventions illustrate both a need and an opportunity for improvements in education and practice development. With new opportunities available for formal training, teaching curricula, and practice development tools, emergency clinicians will be better equipped to address the care of these patients in the future.

Section IV: Recommendations

• Awareness of the known trajectories of illness and dying enables the emergency physician to contextualize the presenting condition of the patient, and provides an opportunity for assessing options for medically reasonable intervention.

• The risks, benefits, and burdens of all treatment options should be well understood in terms of outcomes in order to provide accurate information to the patient or surrogate. It is only with a clear understanding of expected outcomes that a true presentation of options can guide informed consent.

• Interventions must be guided from the patient's perspective. This information may come directly from the patient, either verbally or through a previously completed advance directive, or from an established surrogate. Understanding the outcome goals of the patient and the likely prognosis, reasonable recommendations and goals for intervention can be quickly established.

• Improving pain management skills in the ED would enhance both physician and patient comfort. Either through formal training or continuing education, the confidence and ability to provide adequate pain and symptom relief encourages reasonable alternatives to potentially non-beneficial therapies.

• Recognizing the bias in emergency care for life-prolonging therapies can redirect the emergency physician to question whether the available options for intervention are best aligned with the patient's perspective and realistic goals.

References

1. World Health Organization. (2011) *National Cancer Control Programmes: Policies and Managerial Guidelines.* Geneva: World Health Organization. Available at: www.who.int/cancer/palliative/definition/en/. Accessed 2 December 2011.
2. Betty F, Stephen RC, Anne C, et al. (2007) The national agenda for quality palliative care: the national consensus project and the national quality forum. *J Pain Symptom Manage.* 33, 737–44.
3. Lamba S, Quest TE. (2011) Hospice care and the emergency department: rules, regulations, and referrals. *Ann Emerg Med.* 57, 282–90.
4. Quest TE, Marco CA, Derse AR. (2009) Hospice and palliative medicine: new subspecialty, new opportunities. *Ann Emerg Med.* 54, 94–102.
5. Alexander KS, Jonathan F, Mara AS, et al. (2009) Am I doing the right thing? provider perspectives on improving palliative care in the emergency department. *Ann Emerg Med.* 54, 86–93.e81.
6. Waugh DG. (2010) Palliative care project in the emergency department. *J Palliat Med.* 13, 936.

7. Grudzen CR, Richardson LD, Morrison M, et al. (2010) Palliative care needs of seriously ill, older adults presenting to the emergency department. *Acad Emerg Med.* 17, 1253–7.

8. Smith AK, Schonberg MA, Fisher J, et al. (2010) Emergency department experiences of acutely symptomatic patients with terminal illness and their family caregivers. *J Pain Symptom Manage.* 39, 972–81.

9. Lunney JR, Lynn J, Foley DJ, et al. (2003) Patterns of functional decline at the end of life. *JAMA.* 289, 2387–92.

10. Chan GK. (2011) Trajectories of approaching death in the emergency department: clinician narratives of patient transitions to the end of life. *J Pain Symptom Manage.* May 28 [Epub ahead of print].

11. Bailey C, Murphy R, Porock D. (2010) Trajectories of end-of-life care in the emergency department. *Ann Emerg Med.* 57, 362–9.

12. Centers for Disease Control and Prevention/National Center for Health Statistics. (2008). Mortality statistics: worktable 309: deaths by place of death, age, race, and sex: United States.

13. Angus DC, Barnato AE, Linde-Zwirble WT, et al. (2004) Use of intensive care at the end of life in the United States: an epidemiologic study. *Crit Care Med.* 32, 638–43.

14. Givens JL, Jones RN, Shaffer ML, et al. (2010) Survival and comfort after treatment of pneumonia in advanced dementia. *Arch Intern Med.* 170, 1102–7.

15. Anderson F, Downing GM, Hill J, et al. (1996) Palliative Performance Scale (PPS): a new tool. *J Palliat Care.* 12, 5–11.

16. Mitchell SL, Miller SC, Teno JM, et al. (2010) Prediction of 6-month survival of nursing home residents with advanced dementia using ADEPT vs hospice eligibility guidelines. *JAMA.* 304, 1929–35.

17. Lau F, Maida V, Downing M, et al. (2009) Use of the Palliative Performance Scale (PPS) for end-of-life prognostication in a palliative medicine consultation service. *J Pain Symptom Manage.* 37, 965–72.

18. Tassinari D, Montanari L, Maltoni M, et al. (2008) The Palliative Prognostic Score and survival in patients with advanced solid tumors receiving chemotherapy. *Support Care Cancer.* 16, 359–70.

19. Wilner LS, Arnold RM. (2006) The Palliative Prognostic Score #62. *J Palliat Med.* 9, 993.

20. Glare P, Eychmueller S, Virik K. (2003) The use of the Palliative Prognostic Score in patients with diagnoses other than cancer. *J Pain Symptom Manage.* 26, 883–5.

21. Investigators SP, Connors AF, Dawson NV, et al. (1995) A controlled trial to improve care for seriously ill hospitalized patients. *JAMA.* 274, 1591–8.

22. Hwang U, Richardson LD, Harris B, et al. (2010) The quality of emergency department pain care for older adult patients. *J Am Geriatr Soc.* 58, 2122–8.

23. Miller W, Levy P, Lamba S, et al. (2010) Descriptive analysis of the in-hospital course of patients who initially survive out-of-hospital cardiac arrest but die in-hospital. *J Palliat Med.* 13, 19–22.

24. Sasson C, Rogers MAM, Dahl J, et al. (2010) Predictors of survival from out-of-hospital cardiac arrest. *Circ Cardiovasc Qual Outcomes.* 3, 63–81.

25. Meaney PA, Nadkarni VM, Kern KB, et al. (2010) Rhythms and outcomes of adult in-hospital cardiac arrest. *Crit Care Med.* 38, 101–8.

26. Heron M, Hoyert D, Murphy S, et al. (2009) Deaths: final data for 2006. *Natl Vital Stat Rep.* 57, 1–135.

27. Niska R, Bhuiya F, Xu J. (2010) National Hospital Ambulatory Medical Care Survey: 2007 emergency department summary. *Natl Health Stat Report.* 26, 1–31.

Web resources

Education in Palliative and End of Life Care—Emergency Medicine. Available at: www.epec.net.

Improving Palliative Care—Emergency Medicine. Available at: www.capc.org.

Refusal of life-saving therapy

Catherine A. Marco,[1] Arthur R. Derse[2]

[1]*Professor, Department of Emergency Medicine, University of Toledo College of Medicine, Toledo, OH, USA*

[2]*Director, Center for Bioethics and Medical Humanities and Julia and David Uihlein Professor of Medical Humanities, and Professor of Bioethics and Emergency Medicine, Institute for Health and Society, Medical College of Wisconsin, Milwaukee, WI, USA*

Section I: Case presentation

A 72-year-old man presented with complaints of shortness of breath and chest pain. The patient had a history of end-stage chronic obstructive pulmonary disease (COPD), and cardiomyopathy with an ejection fraction of 15%. He had a recent prolonged intensive care unit (ICU) stay for sepsis and congestive heart failure (CHF), with difficulty in being weaned from the ventilator. At baseline, the patient was bedridden, and cared for at home by his elderly wife. On physical examination, the vital signs were as following: blood pressure 88/52 mmHg, heart rate 86 beats per minute, respiratory rate 42 breaths per minute, and temperature 36.7 °C. Oxygen saturation on a non-rebreather mask was 80%. The chest X-ray study showed extensive CHF. The patient requested: "Please make me comfortable, but I don't want to be on a ventilator. I'd rather die."

Section II: Discussion

Dr. Peter Rosen: What's your feeling about people who demand comfort care, and have an oxygen saturation of 80%?

Dr. Shamai Grossman: This depends on the individual patient. A patient who normally lives and functions with an oxygen saturation of 80% is more able to make realistic personal decisions than someone who's suddenly develops the same level of hypoxia. Because this patient is in respiratory distress **and** is severely hypoxic, I'm very concerned this patient lacks adequate decision-making capacity.

PR: We know that patients with chronic COPD are chronically hypoxic. In fact, their hypoxic state may be their only drive to keep breathing. We can't use numbers to make judgments about whether or not a patient has capacity to make decisions. The real problem in the emergency department (ED) is deciding when to make judgments about capacity during tenuous situations, and when to provide a decisive intervention in the E.D. that will allow for a more informed decision about ongoing care by the inpatient clinical team. In the process of waiting, however, you may have to do something the patient doesn't want you to do. As the patient's treating physician did you know anything about his past medical history? Perhaps there was further information that might have helped to guide our decision?

Dr. Catherine Marco: We eventually did receive more information. At the time the patient presented, however, that's all the information we had available. Later we discovered that he had had several admissions for worsening congestive heart failure.

Dr. Arthur Derse: This case involves a very definitive statement from the patient, but lacks a long description of the kinds of interventions he wants. The patient simply states, "Please make me comfortable, but I don't want to be on a ventilator I'd rather die," which seems fairly straightforward and definitive. One of the burdens that emergency physicians bear is that they have the responsibility for making quick bedside determinations of decisional capacity—sometimes for extremely important, life-sustaining medical treatment. The traditional approach would be to push forward and treat the patient, refusing to acknowledge the refusal. Over the past 30 years there has been a sea of change toward the recognition that patients have the right to refuse even life-sustaining medical treatment.

Although the patient has the right to refuse life-saving treatment, there first must be proof of decision-making capacity. Rather than focusing on baseline vital signs and oxygen saturation, the treating physician needs to determine the patient's capacity to make decisions. The key to this analysis is to assess the patient's ability to understand pertinent information, compare it against his or her values, and balance the risks and benefits of treatment and treatment refusal with the ability to make a consistent choice.

Dr. John Jesus: What role do other people, such as the patient's family, have in making this decision?

AD: In the American legal system, the decision is made by the individual. But the doctor–patient relationship involves two people; and we know that people often make decisions within a community, or within a relationship. Family and children all may have different things to say, which may change an individual's mind. Initially, a patient may wish to refuse life-sustaining medical treatment. After speaking with the family, listening and considering their concerns, however, the patient may change the decision. Once you choose to make a decision regarding a patient's decision-making capacity, you are then obliged to explain to the spouse and family your assessment of whether or not the patient is capable of making a decision at that time.

JJ: Would you criticize a physician who intubated this patient?

AD: I'm very sympathetic to any physician in this situation. It is very difficult to make a quick assess-ment of capacity when the patient has strong opinions about intubation, but is too hypoxic to understand and make appropriate treatment decisions. Even if you intubate the patient and begin artificial ventilation, the medical team may withdraw ventilation once the patient's preferences are better understood. The ability to forego and the ability to withdraw life-sustaining medical treatment are seen as legally and ethically equivalent, even though they may not **feel** equivalent.

SG: I would argue that not all ethical belief systems or even legal systems would agree that the ability to forego and the ability to withdraw life-sustaining medical treatment are equivalent. In Judaism, this clearly is not the case. Similarly, in Israeli law, provisions for withdrawal of care, particularly of ventilation are very limited, and only very recent legislation allows the possibility of withdrawal of a ventilator when the machine either must be turned off for cleaning, or when a built-in pause in ventilation takes effect.

AD: Many clinicians have initiated an intervention to see whether or not it held any utility knowing that if it did not, they would have the ability to withdraw it. If clinicians do not maintain the ability to withdraw therapy, I believe some physicians would tend to err on the side of never starting therapy.

PR: Even if they are morally and ethically equivalent, functionally it's much harder to withdraw care once it's started than it is to not start it. Once the patient is placed on a ventilator it becomes much harder to say, "Well he didn't want us to do this so we're going to stop."

AD: In this case, we should use temporizing measures first that do not involve intubation. If, however, you need to intubate the patient to prevent a cardiopulmonary arrest, and you don't have the time to assess the patient's decision-making capacity, then you might consider saying to the patient: "Unfortunately, I don't have enough information to allow you to make the decision to refuse intubation. We need to temporarily begin pulmonary resuscitation. Just because we've decided to intubate you, doesn't mean we won't be able to stop. I understand how you feel, but we need more time and the opportunity to gather more information." In retrospect, I would not fault an emergency physician for intubating this patient. If the patient has a DNR/DNI [do not resuscitate/do not intubate] order or a prehospital POLST [Physician's Order for Life-Sustaining Treatment] document we would know much more about the end-of-life preferences. These documents are created by a physician when the patient has decision-making capacity, and is able to communicate end-of-life preferences. With these documents in hand, we can feel more comfortable doing exactly what the patient asks of us.

PR: A common problem in ethical debates is the failure to resolve medical decisions before considering the ethical nuance of a situation. The only patient I would automatically intubate for congestive failure is the patient who is in pump failure. Many patients who are volume overloaded, however, never need to be intubated with modern management of CHF. Perhaps we're making an ethical problem where one need not exist. Could you comment on the appropriate medical management of this patient?

SG: First-line therapy for this patient would not be intubation, but it would certainly be in the back of our minds. First-line therapy would be non-invasive ventilation such as bilevel or continuous airway pressure ventilation (BiPAP or CPAP), the use of nitroglycerin or some other afterload-reducing agent, and perhaps a diuretic as well. The fact the patient has a systolic blood pressure of 88 mmHg, however, necessitates cautious use of these medications. Renal dose dopamine might be useful here in both elevating blood pressure and enhancing diuresis. You may end up getting stuck between a rock and a hard place; unless you see a good response to non-invasive therapy, you may need to intubate this patient as you have nothing else left to offer.

I would also add that it's very hard to make a decision that is irreversible. If I decide that I'm going to avoid intubating a patient in extremis, who may not be making a well considered choice, there's no going back to make a different decision once the patient expires. Intubating this patient may be the right thing to do regardless of what the patient's stated wishes are. If we intubate this patient, I don't believe we're acting against the patient's wishes per se. Rather, I simply think he may be in the wrong place to make that decision.

JJ: Capacity needs to be thought of as a concept that is dynamic. In a certain unique presentation, someone may have capacity in one hour, but not in the next. For example, there are numerous conditions classically referenced that variably impair capacity—transient ischemic attacks (TIA), transient global amnesia, epilepsy, delirium, and perhaps in this case: hypoxia. Here, we could try non-invasive measures such as CPAP, and then reevaluate the person's capacity once, and if, the hypoxia resolves.

PR: In addition, the presentation of our thought processes can make a difference as well. The patient's decision may depend on how you answer that patient when he says, "I don't want to be on a ventilator." You could say, "I can accept your desire but I don't have any other way to save your life." He then may acquiesce with this change in perspective and say, "Oh, okay, that's a different story." There is another salient concept to consider in this situation. When I was a young physician, I had a great deal of trouble accepting the older patient's refusal of life-saving interventions. It didn't fit with my vision of what life was all about. As I got older, I began to find it more acceptable to allow patients to die—not from a desire to avoid helping them, but from an acceptance that patients have different attitudes towards what quality of life they believe is acceptable. The problem we face in the ED is that we often don't know the patient attempting to refuse further care. You don't really know what the quality-of-life issues are, or what he or she truly wants. I believe that there are times when I might be willing to accept that patient's decision. Without knowing more about the patient or his family or his circumstances, however, I would have a hard time doing so in our case. As a young physician, do you have difficulty accepting patients' refusal of life-saving therapy?

JJ: In the materials we study and the classes we attend, attention is almost entirely focused on how to reverse life-threatening conditions. I don't believe medical students are given enough training or guidance on how to navigate the medical management and ethical nuance of situations like the case we are discussing. It is for these reasons difficult for me to accept refusal of life-saving interventions.

I would also note that it is difficult to deny an older patient what may be perceived as the respect to make his or her own choice. If a physician has made the decision to administer an intervention against the will of the patient, he should also realize that even though we are precluding the patient from making a decision regarding one particular intervention, the physician can still include the patient in the conversation about other interventions. You can explain why you are making a decision, and at least attempt to obtain agreement. If you intend to go ahead with the intervention regardless of the response, keeping the patient included in your thought process helps address the perception of degrading or disrespecting the patient—a perspective that may help younger physicians who want to act with respect toward their elder patients. Furthermore, even if the patient doesn't have capacity to make a decision about intubation, he may well have the capacity to make lesser decisions about sedation, or other possible interventions.

PR: In this ED environment, sometimes we don't have the luxury of waiting to see if something will work. It may well be that the most appropriate management of this particular patient at the time he arrives to your ED is to intubate him, get him up to the ICU, and get him out of the ED.

AD: This is a point that the ethics literature infrequently recognizes. The doctor–patient relationship is seen as a 1:1 ratio, when your responsibility actually includes all other patients in the ED.

PR: What if the wife had come in with the patient and said, "Don't listen to the old fool, he's always that way, just take care of him?"

CM: I would have wanted to discuss her comment in more detail with her. I'd want to ask if his current mental status is at his baseline mental status. I would want to know more history regarding his preferences for end-of-life care during less stressful times in his life.

PR: Let's say the wife comes in with the patient and says, "I don't want you to intubate him," and the patient changes his mind and says, "Well, that's what she wants, but I actually don't want to die just now."

AD: This situation does occur, and represents a significant challenge for involved clinicians. We have sometimes been derided by ethicists for only questioning a patient's decision-making capacity when he or she disagrees with us. Although the truth of the matter is that we don't recommend interventions that we don't believe are in the patient's best interests; the burden of proof increases when patients attempt to

make decisions that are contrary to decisions we believe are in their best interests. Though you haven't done an analysis of the decisional capacity of the patient in this scenario, the default understanding is that patients may always change their minds regarding their end-of-life preferences. As a result, it is fairly straightforward when a patient states, "I revoke the DNR order, I no longer want to be DNR." There are times, however, when we ask leading questions—"Do you want us to help you?" The answer to this question will invariably be "Yes," though the patient may actually choose comfort care measures without intubation if presented with the choice.

PR The only grounds on which a relative can legally refuse life-sustaining care for a patient is if that person is a court-appointed guardian for the patient who lacks decision-making capacity.

AD: Somebody who holds the power of attorney for healthcare has the same ability to accept or refuse life-sustaining medical treatment. The power of attorney for healthcare can be revoked, but it must be done orally with witnesses, or in writing, or the patient must tear up the document. Interestingly, in some [US] states, patients don't have to have decision-making capacity to be able to revoke such a document.

JJ: If the physician doesn't feel that the healthcare proxy or the power of attorney is acting in the best interests of the patient, however, the physician still has the right to ignore bad advice.

AD: Generally, one would need a legal procedure to be able to replace that person as guardian or as power of attorney for healthcare. For this purpose, you would need strong evidence as to why you think they're not acting in the patient's best interests.

PR: I can remember a case in which the patient had three daughters and two sons, each one of whom had a different idea about what should happen to the father, and they didn't want to listen to the wife because she was a step-mother. What would you do if there is more than one family member and they're not in accord?

SG: I've been in this situation myself a number of times. If there's a healthcare proxy, it becomes a little easier. You can say, "Well, who's your healthcare proxy? Who is legally appointed as the decision-making person?" If there isn't a healthcare proxy, then to some extent you must ignore what the family says and make the decision yourself. You have to say, "I can only act in the patient's best interests." To the degree possible, you should find a way to communicate your decision in a way that is acceptable to the family. Though this can prove even more difficult than the clinical challenges of the situation, it remains a part of our clinical responsibilities.

PR: Tell us what you did for this patient.

CM: I am a very firm proponent for following patients' wishes. It was my judgment that the patient truly did not want to be on a ventilator, even though there were some potential threats to his decision-making capacity. We treated the patient with non-invasive ventilatory support, and he survived without the need for intubation. Even if he had succumbed, however, I would have felt good about the decision I had made.

AD: Once the patient survives this particular episode, someone should ensure that his end-of-life preferences are well documented to avoid future confusion. DNR and POLST documents can facilitate this process.

PR: I don't think you need to feel apologetic about accepting the patient's wishes. As an older physician, I have no problem accepting a patient's wishes when he has decision-making capacity, even when they are in direct opposition to my own view of what is good for the patient.

Section III: Review of the literature

Informed consent and informed refusal of care are basic medical rights of patients, and are important aspects of emergency medical care. Emergency physicians should use the appropriate processes for informed consent and refusal of care to assure that patients have the opportunity to be informed about proposed medical treatment and procedures. Many potential barriers to the informed consent process exist in emergency medicine, including impaired decisional capacity, language barriers, illiteracy, insufficient time, problems with communication, and differences in values, among others. Because many ED patients are vulnerable due to a variety of factors, particular attention should be paid to ensure appropriate decisional capacity of patients, adequate delivery of information, and to the extent possible, an understanding by the patient of the proposed intervention and its risks and benefits.[1]

The doctrine of informed consent includes several essential elements, including disclosure of information to the patient prior to consent, and voluntariness on the part of the patient to consent. Similarly, informed refusal of care requires a similar standard of disclosure of information and voluntary decision-making by the patient. This fundamental principle is based on the concept that healthcare providers have training and experience to diagnose and treat medical conditions, but the patient is best prepared to make his or her own medical decisions, based on the patient's value system and goals of treatment.[2] The right to refuse medical care has been established by the justice system, both in state courts based in the law of battery, and by the US Supreme Court, based on the liberty interest of the 14th Amendment of the Constitution.[3,4]

Informed consent for emergency medical interventions

Informed consent and informed refusal of care are important components of patient autonomy, or self-determination, in medical decision-making.[5-10] Although many routine ED procedures, such as intravenous lines and blood drawing, may be appropriately performed after general consent to treatment, invasive emergency procedures may require additional disclosure of information regarding the procedure, its purpose, risks, benefits, and alternatives to the proposed procedure or intervention.[11-13] Exceptions to requirements of informed consent exist when emergency treatment must be initiated for patients with life-threatening conditions who cannot consent, when there is a duty to treat according to public health or legal requirements, and in circumstances in which patients waive their right to consent. The American College of Emergency Physicians (ACEP) has summarized these issues in its code of ethics: "Emergency physicians shall communicate truthfully with patients and secure their informed consent for treatment, unless the urgency of the patient's conditions demands an immediate response."[14]

Some states have enacted informed consent statutes that require patients diagnosed with a terminal condition to be informed (or informed when the physician is asked) that the patient may choose to forego curative treatment and be treated with palliative measures.[15,16]

Informed refusal of medical care

Just as all patients with appropriate decisional capacity have the right to participate in the informed consent process, patients also have the right to refuse medical care. Patients may elect to refuse all treatments, refuse hospital admission, or refuse certain specific tests or therapies. Informed refusal, like informed consent, is a **process**, not merely a signature on a form. Some erroneously believe that merely documenting a patient leaving against medical advice (AMA), using an "AMA form," is sufficient to meet legal and ethical standards. Importantly, the process of refusal of care, including a patient leaving AMA, should include determination of decisional capacity, and when practical, delivery of relevant information, including risks of refusing treatment, alternative treatments, and documentation of these elements. When a patient refuses medical treatment, care should specifically be taken to ensure that the patient understands the consequences, and that the physician expresses a willingness to treat the patient, including providing reasonable alternative treatments, as well as providing appropriate follow-up recommendations.

Special challenges near the end of life

Near the end of life, special circumstances pose unique challenges when patients wish to refuse life-saving medical interventions. Numerous threats to decisional capacity may exist, including hypoxia, medications, central nervous system lesions, metabolic and electrolyte disturbances, infection, hypotension, hypovolemia, and others. Decisions regarding life-saving medical interventions by definition carry greater significance than other medical decisions, and as such, require intense scrutiny to ensure that the patient's goals of medical treatment are adhered to. Refusal of life-sustaining medical treatment presents emergency physicians with the responsibility of determining whether the patient has the capacity to refuse treatment, and whether the patient's refusal is informed.[17]

For many patients, the ED may not be the ideal location for end-of-life care. Many barriers exist in the ED that may interfere with a peaceful and dignified end-of-life experience for families and patients, including high noise levels, distractions, lack of privacy, uncomfortable settings, and the unfamiliar environment. Ideally, patients near the end of life should have previously completed advance care planning with their primary care physician, including advance directives, family education, and planning for a peaceful death in the environment preferred by the patient, often in the home or hospice environment. However, patients with terminal conditions frequently are transported to EDs for symptom management, or perhaps because of anxiety or lack of education about other alternatives. A variety of terminal conditions are frequently encountered in emergency medicine include malignancy, neurologic disease, and cardiorespiratory diseases.[15] Independent predictors of decisions to forego life sustaining treatment include: age, underlying disease, living in an institution, preexisting cognitive impairment, admission for medical reasons, and acute cardiac failure, acute central neurologic illness, or sepsis.[18] Quality improvement goals directed toward improved end-of-life care can be effective in improving satisfaction of patients and families.[19]

Communication with the primary care provider and appropriate consultants is useful in end-of-life decision-making. Patients with improved continuity of care by primary care physicians may have reduced utilization of EDs.[20] Patients and families should be educated to anticipate the expected course of events, including symptoms and management, and appropriate actions, to ensure the desired setting at the end of life.

Many patients refuse medical interventions because of fear of the loss of dignity near the end of life. Communication with patients and families about goals, expectations, personal preferences, and the development of a long-term plan to help meet individualized goals can improve a patient's sense of dignity and control at the end of life. When possible, privacy may improve the sense of dignity and peace with family.

Accurate information is important to help patients develop realistic goals and expectations.[21] In many cases, the communication, care, and counseling provided for survivors (family, friends, and others) of victims of cardiac arrest will have more impact than the actual resuscitative efforts.[22] The approach of the physician to the patient has an impact on refusal of life-saving medical interventions.[23]

The assessment of decisional capacity

Decisional capacity is the ability of the patient to make a decision regarding medical treatment.[24] Decisional capacity is affected by cognitive and affective functions, including attention, intellect, memory, judgment, insight, language, emotion, and calculation. Appropriate decisional capacity for medical decision-making includes the following elements:

- The ability to receive information
- The ability to process and understand information
- The ability to deliberate
- The ability to make and articulate a choice.

Decisional capacity should be carefully assessed in patients who may wish to refuse life-saving medical interventions, because of the likelihood of threats to capacity, as well as the magnitude of the consequences of the decision.[25] Impaired decisional capacity may result from disruption of any of the essential elements: the ability to receive, process, and understand information, the ability to deliberate, or the ability to communicate a decision. Numerous conditions and circumstances near the end of life may impair decisional capacity, including dementia physical communication impairments, severe pain, organic disease states and other conditions.[25–31] Reversible etiologies of impaired capacity should be addressed, if possible, to improve the patient's capacity. Even in cases of some impairment of decisional capacity, some patients may demonstrate sufficient understanding of the decision at hand to make an appropriate informed choice for a particular decision.

Disclosure of information

When patients wish to refuse life-saving medical interventions, appropriate disclosure of information is of crucial importance. The information to be disclosed includes the nature of the proposed intervention, benefits, risks, alternatives, including no treatment. The necessary amount and detail delivered as part of the informed refusal of care process varies according to the nature and urgency of the clinical condition. Sufficient information should be presented to allow the patient to weigh the risks and benefits.

At times, patients or families may express concern regarding insurance payment for medical care, when certain interventions have been refused or if the patient signs out against medical advice. Patients may be appropriately reassured that insurance companies do not deny payment based on these circumstances.[32]

Documentation of informed refusal of care

Informed refusal of care is a process, not merely a signature on a form. The process includes necessary elements, including the discussion between the physician and patient, delivery of material information, including a description of the intervention, risks, benefits, and alternatives, and the patient's agreement to, or refusal of, the proposed intervention. The documentation does **not** comprise informed consent and is not a substitute for the discussion between physician and patient. Documentation may serve to provide evidence of the patient's agreement that the informed consent process did take place and that the patient voluntarily agrees or disagrees with the intervention. Appropriate documentation should include confirmation of the informed discussion, information disclosed, patient's decisional capacity, and the patient's consent or lack of consent to the intervention.

Conclusion

Informed consent and informed refusal of care are basic rights of patients, and are important aspects of emergency medical care. Discharge against medical advice remains a complex, unavoidable, and challenging situation for emergency physicians. In all cases, decisional capacity should be evaluated, and if the patient is deemed to have decisional capacity, the physician should communicate with the patient regarding the proposed interventions, risks, benefits, and alternatives, and the patient's goals and values. When a patient refuses medical treatment, care should specifically be taken to ensure that the patient understands the consequences, and that the physician expresses a willingness to treat the patient, including providing reasonable alternative treatments, as well as providing appropriate follow-up recommendations. The voluntary decision of the patient regarding medical care and important aspects of the discussion should be documented in the medical record.

Section IV: Recommendations

- Assess decisional capacity for all patients who wish to refuse life-saving medical interventions.
- Correct reversible threats to decisional capacity.
- Inform the patient of the risks and benefits, alternatives, and expected outcomes of the proposed life-saving medical intervention.
- Assure that the patient is making a voluntary, autonomous decision.
- For patients who possess appropriate decisional capacity, who have been adequately informed, respect and carry out their wishes to refuse life-saving medical intervention.
- Document the informed refusal of care process in the medical record.
- Provide appropriate medical care, comfort care, psychosocial and spiritual support, and ongoing communication with the patient and family.
- Recall that no matter what the circumstance, a physician's obligation is to attempt to do what is best for the patient.

References

1. Simon JR. (2007) Refusal of care: the physician-patient relationship and decisionmaking capacity. *Ann Emerg Med.* 50, 456–61.
2. Junkerman C, Derse A, Schiedermayer D. Informed consent. In: *Practical Ethics for Students, Interns and Residents: A Short Reference Manual*, 3rd ed. Hagerstown, MD: University Publishing Group, pp. 17–19.
3. Wons *v.* Public Health Trust of Dade County, 500 So. 2d 679 (Fla. App. 3 Dist. 1987).
4. Cruzan *v.* Director of Missouri Department of Health, 497 U.S. 261, 110 S. Ct. 2841, 111 L. Ed. 2d 224 (1990).
5. Prentice ED. (1999) Informed consent: the most important protector. *Acad Emerg Med.* 6, 774–5.
6. Moskop JC. (1999) Informed consent in the emergency department. *Emerg Med Clin North Am.* 17, 327–40.
7. Hansson MO. (1998) Balancing the quality of consent. *J Med Ethics.* 24, 182–7.
8. Young WF Jr. (1997) Informed consent. *Ann Emerg Med.* 30, 350–1.
9. Etchells E, Sharpe G, Walsh P, et al. (1996) Bioethics for clinicians: consent. *CMAJ* 155, 177–80.
10. Faden RR, Beauchamp TL, King NMP. (1998) *A History and Theory of Informed Consent.* New York, NY: Oxford University Press.
11. Braddock CH, Edwards KA, Hasenberg NM, et al. (1999) Informed decision making in outpatient practice: time to get back to basics. *JAMA.* 282, 2313–20.
12. Meisel A, Kuczewski M. (1996) Legal and ethical myths about informed consent. *Arch Intern Med.* 156, 2521–6.
13. Tardy B, Venet C, Zeni F, et al. (2002) Death of terminally ill patients on a stretcher in emergency department: a French specialty? *Intensive Care Med.* 28, 1625–8.
14. ACEP Board of Directors. (revised 2011). *Code of Ethics for Emergency Physicians.* Available at: www.acep.org/Content.aspx?id=29144. Accessed December 20, 2011.
15. New York Palliative Care Information Act. N.Y.S. Public Health Law Sec. 2997-C (2010).
16. California Right to Know End-of-Life Options Law, California Statutes, Chapter 683 (2008).
17. Derse AR. (2005) What part of "no" don't you understand? Patient refusal of recommended treatment in the emergency department. *Mt Sinai J Med.* 72, 221–7.
18. Reignier J, Dumont R, Katsahian S, et al. (2008) Patient-related factors and circumstances surrounding decisions to forego life-sustaining treatment, including intensive care unit admission refusal. *Crit Care Med.* 36, 2076–83.
19. Lynn J, Nolan K, Kabcenell A, et al. (2002) Reforming care for persons near the end of life: promise of quality improvement. *Ann Intern Med.* 137, 117–22.
20. Burge F, Lawson B, Johnston G. (2003) Family physician continuity of care and emergency department use in end-of-life cancer care. *Med Care.* 41, 992–1001.
21. Fallowfield LF, Jenkins VA, Beveridge HA. (2002) Truth may hurt but deceit hurts more: communication in palliative care. *Palliat Med.* 16, 297–303.
22. Marco CA. (2005) Ethical issues of resuscitation: an American perspective. *Postgrad Med.* 81, 608–12.
23. Garland A, Connors AF. (2007) Physicians' influence over decisions to forego life support. *J Palliat Med.* 10, 1298–305.
24. Junkerman C, Derse A, Schiedermayer D. The physician's professional responsibilities. In: *Practical Ethics for Students, Interns and Residents: A Short Reference Manual*, 3rd ed. Hagerstown, MD: University Publishing Group, pp. 20–3.
25. Larkin GL, Marco CA, Abbott JT. (2001) Emergency determination of decision making capacity (DMC): Balancing autonomy and beneficence in the emergency department. *Acad Emerg Med.* 8, 282–4.
26. Rockwood K, Stadnyk J. (1994) The prevalence of dementia in the elderly: a review. *Can J Psychiatry.* 39, 253–7.
27. Fellows LK. (1998) Competency and consent in dementia. *J Am Geriatr Soc.* 46, 922–6.

28. Derogatis L, Morrow G, Fetting J, et al. (1983) The prevalence of psychiatric disorders among cancer patients. *JAMA.* 249, 751–75.

29. Marson DC, Ingram KK, Cody HA, et al. (1995) Assessing the competency of patients with Alzheimer's disease under different legal standards. *Arch Neurol.* 52, 949–54.

30. Dresser R, Whitehouse PJ. (1994) The incompetent patient on the slippery slope. *Hastings Cent Rep.* 24, 6–12.

31. Freer J. (1993) Decision making in an incapacitated patient. *J Clin Ethics.* 4, 55–8.

32. Wigder HN, Propp DA, Leslie K, et al. (2010) Insurance companies refusing payment for patients who leave the emergency department against medical device is a myth. *Ann Emerg Med.* 55, 393.

10

Revisiting comfort-directed therapies: death and dying in the emergency department, including withholding and withdrawal of life-sustaining treatment

Raquel M. Schears,[1] Terri A. Schmidt[2]

[1]*Associate Professor of Emergency Medicine, Department of Emergency Medicine, Mayo Clinic, Mayo Graduate School of Medicine, Rochester, MN, USA*
[2]*Professor of Emergency Medicine, Department of Emergency Medicine, Health and Science University, Portland, OR, USA*

Section I: Case presentation

A 28-year-old man with incurable glioblastoma multiforme, diagnosed 3 years ago after he presented with a headache and seizures is brought into to the emergency department (ED) by his sister for worsening lethargy and confusion, after vomiting all of his medications. For a week he has been escalating the opiates and steroids prescribed for the headaches. During the past month, he has been increasingly depressed, fatigued and short of breath. He has not had any seizures recently or fever, neck pain, or rash. He is emaciated and curled up in a fetal position on the hospital gurney. He looks pale against the sheets, and is markedly dehydrated. He moans when moved, and mumbles "headache" repeatedly when touched. He keeps his eyes tightly closed. Vital signs reflect tachycardia, tachypnea and hypotension, but the patient is afebrile and saturating 94% on room air. He has a couple of well-healed scars, overlying the right cranium and upper abdomen. The sister relates his medications, and past medical history, which includes a partial hepatectomy for her (she pulls up the corner of her jersey to showcase her matching right midriff). "Tylenol overdose 10 years ago" she says, and gives his arm a playful squeeze. The palliative chemotherapy he has endured in the last year is summed by the sister as: "he is DNR [do not resuscitate], but without plans to go gently." She reiterates that if his heart stops beating, he doesn't want a breathing tube, but will take "anything else" that may help him prolong his life.

Section II: Discussion

Socratic maxim:

> "Primum non tacere."
> (First, do not be silent.)

Dr. Peter Rosen: I'm constantly surprised at how little guidance patients with incurable diseases are given by their treating physicians. One problem we have in trying to deliver ethically appropriate care in the ED to patients like these is our attempts to navigate the medical wish fulfillment fantasies of the families involved.

Ethical Problems in Emergency Medicine: A Discussion-Based Review, First Edition. John Jesus, Shamai A. Grossman, Arthur R. Derse, James G. Adams, Richard Wolfe, and Peter Rosen.

Dr. James Adams: This presentation is common. The first step in resolving this issue is to assess what the family already knows. I have been impressed with how little education patients with terminal illnesses are given. Many patients have no idea that their death is near or imminent. I recently took care of a young woman, with widely metastatic breast cancer. For weeks, she hadn't gotten out of bed. It doesn't take a lot of medical knowledge to come to the understanding that she wasn't doing well, and that she would soon die. The family, however, had no idea that her death was quickly approaching. I was shocked at how poorly they understood the situation.

Dr. Terri Schmidt: At the same time, we all know that what physicians tell their patients, and what the patients hear and understand, is often not the same. When I see patients for the first time who are rapidly approaching the end of their lives, I frequently ask the patient or family, "What do you understand about your disease, and what do you expect to happen from here?" Even when I have spoken to the treating physician who believes the patient knows the prognosis, I am often quite amazed at the patient's or family's lack of insight.

PR: Is there an ethical mandate to admit to the hospital patients who harbor false beliefs about the efficacy of care? Can we reach a point when a prudent and caring physician can say truthfully to a family: "There is nothing we can offer your family member that cannot be as well accomplished at home. I'm more than willing to help you with home health nurses, or to help place this patient in a hospice, but I don't have the luxury of admitting to a hospital bed a patient for whom there is no useful treatment."

JA: There is no obligation to provide treatment that is not going to be effective or palliative in the setting of a hospital when the treatment may be administered elsewhere. It is a challenge to avoid choosing the path of least resistance when presented with a patient in this situation, which is to say, "This is a complex situation. There are a number of people who have to be involved in the discussion, and it will take time and resources away from my very busy ED. I want this person admitted." Emergency physicians have a professional obligation, however, to make recommendations based on medical indications, and to communicate honestly, especially information and news

the family doesn't want to hear. In this case, if the patient's family members aren't already aware, they should know that there isn't anything more that can be done to cure their relative. They should then be reassured as to what palliative treatment is available, and then it should be explained that palliative efforts might best be administered in a setting other than the hospital.

PR: When dealing with comfort care for a dying patient, the normal restrictions on how we use pharmacology simply do not apply. We're not giving pain relief in order to euthanize the patient, but we simply shouldn't care if there are complications to the treatments with which we choose to try and make the patient more comfortable; you can ignore the side effects of medications in a way you couldn't under different conditions. This is a distinction that many physicians don't recognize, and about which they are ethically concerned. Do you think that there is a way to overcome this reluctance to treat patients aggressively in the ED, or perhaps this is one of the considerations that pushes many physicians to admit these patients?

Dr. Shamai Grossman: You have described a very fine line we walk in the ED, where giving your patient large doses of narcotics that can cause respiratory compromise is balanced with our attempts to reduce the patient's suffering. When you introduce a deviation from the norm you're always at risk of opening Pandora's box by creating different standards for different patients. It's much more difficult to accomplish the intended goal in the ED, where pressures are greater than they are elsewhere in the hospital to move the patient out of the ED, and where our demands in caring for other patients and time are all severely constrained. It may be more appropriate to create guidelines that allow these patients different dosing schedules for more appropriate analgesia. That said, these efforts ought to be approached with much caution and thoughtful consideration.

PR: When you were caring for this patient, did you have available resources such as social workers who might have helped you with an emergency hospice placement or an observation unit that you might have utilized to begin palliative measures while awaiting hospice placement?

Dr. Raquel Schears: Though we do have an observation unit, end-of-life and palliative care measures are not part of the protocols for that area as they are considered too intensive to manage in an observational setting. We do have 24-hour access to a social worker and a chaplain, both of whom were called [in the present case], but these resources generally don't resolve the medical dilemmas of whether you need to admit such a patient for palliative comfort care to be initiated.

PR: What were the family's expectations? As presented in our case, it doesn't sound like the patient was in a condition to tell you his desires, and his initial end-of-life decisions may have been made in a time when he was more coherent, and had a quality of life that was more worth preserving.

RS: Their goals were to improve his pain, and mitigate some of the symptoms that they had observed over the last couple of weeks. They were very well informed about how long he had to live. Though there had been discussions with their family medicine doctor about palliative care options and hospice, they declined hospice care options in the outpatient setting.

PR: Have you had any experiences getting patients to hospice care facilities? I know it's not that difficult from an inpatient service, but in many communities it is not possible from the ED.

Dr. John Jesus: Though I haven't had the opportunity to send a patient from the ED directly to a hospice center, I have treated many hospice patients who present to the ED seeking symptomatic relief. To the extent possible, we do just that, and discharge the patient back home or back to the hospice. One of the aspects of this case we haven't touched upon yet is whether the patient's sister feels a sense of obligation to prolong the patient's life given the considerable amount of care he took to donate part of his liver to her. It is important to assess the family's and patient's level of insight into the patient's condition, as well as the factors that might influence their decisions. There needs to be some direct questioning about feelings of obligation. This can take a significant amount of time, which is not always practical in the ED, and the patient may need to be admitted for further discussions and deliberation.

RS: The concern about treating pain and causing respiratory depression is overblown and similar to the many years of argument we heard from the surgeons about avoiding analgesics for patients with abdominal pain for fear of masking pathology. The reality is that respiratory arrest from narcotics given to alleviate pain is phenomenally rare, and can be avoided with minimal observation and monitoring.

Dr. Arthur Derse: I agree that respiratory arrest from analgesia is rare in this setting. If it did occur and the patient had a documented preference not to be intubated, would you treat that respiratory depression with an opioid antagonist?

TS: My goal in these situations is to work with the family to best understand the patient's goals of care, and to allow them to recognize that there are times when making the patient more comfortable involves allowing a natural death. It is important for the family and health care professionals to understand that providing adequate pain control is part of treating the patient's symptoms, and it is not the cause of a patient's death, even if it may impact the timing of death. There is some evidence, in fact, that people who are provided good palliative care actually live longer. Our most important palliative care goal is to educate health professionals and families that providing appropriate analgesia does not cause death, rarely leads to respiratory depression, and provides appropriate symptom control.

PR: I agree that it is not that easy to paralyze respiration with analgesic doses of morphine. The fear of doing so, however, is relatively common. This ethical dilemma could often be resolved if we had better education. The solutions to the problems presented in our case are very difficult to address in the ED, and would have been easier had the situation been addressed before the patient had deteriorated. Unlike the physicians who saw this patient before his deterioration, and could have made decisions without the stress of the patient's acuity, emergency physicians are often forced to make difficult choices in less than ideal circumstances.

I once had a patient whose daughter brought him in from home. The patient's spouse, the primary caregiver, had taken the night off from nursing him towards death, but she never explained to the daughter that he was not to be taken to the ED. After the patient lapsed into a coma, the daughter immediately called 911. He had been treated at another hospital, and without any prior records and a family member requesting that we help her father, we intubated him and started the process of admitting him to our ICU [intensive care unit]. The wife appeared suddenly, said that he was a comfort care only patient, and requested that we stop our heroic interventions. We said, "You know, it's too late to tell us this now, where was this information when the patient deteriorated?" I told her that we would sort it out in the hospital since he has already been intubated, and placed on a ventilator.

AD: Is it ever too late? I can think of at least one case in which I extubated a patient in the ED when I later learned of the patient's end-of-life preferences.

PR: It's not impossible to do, I agree. I believe we sometimes act in a cowardly manner when we admit patients prior to withdrawal of care, because it's easier for us to avoid difficult, emotional conversations with families.

JJ: Extubation in the ED can be an ethically appropriate, though logistically difficult intervention. In my experience, this occurs most frequently when a patient has a non-survivable intracranial hemorrhage, and our attending neurosurgeons in conjunction with the family decide to withdraw care or avoid escalating care. Even in this setting, however, the duration of time between extubation and death may be significant. The patient may be there for hours meanwhile, occupying a bed and taking up resources that could potentially be given to other patients with life-threatening but reversible problems. While stewardship of hospital resources is not a reason to treat patients inappropriately, I think withdrawal of intubation should occur only in the very rare circumstance. The difficulty in providing privacy, the nurse to patient ratio, and the situational stress of the ED together produce an environment that is not very conducive to the sensitivity and consideration necessary when withdrawing care.

SG: It is not cowardly to suggest that the ED is not the appropriate place for withdrawal of care. These decisions are not often made in the efficient, expeditious fashion that often constrains all our decisions in the ED. The time devoted to helping a family navigate the difficult decisions inherent in withdrawal of care, is time taken away from the management of other acutely ill patients in the ED. An emergency physi-

cian's threshold for assuming the responsibility of having these conversations will also depend on the state of the ED at any given moment.

PR: You have to accept the reality that death is something that none of us want to facilitate. Particularly in emergency medicine, we look upon it peculiarly as our personal failure. It's shameful that people are no longer allowed to die at home. It's even more shameful that people are not allowed to die in nursing homes. Part of the blame for this change in culture is our own fault, because we abdicate our responsibility for allowing appropriate patients to die in the ED. Instead, we run up huge bills for the act of dying, without clear clinical purpose. This does not represent ethically appropriate care nor good medical practice.

TS: And yet, death does not need to be a failure. In fact, if preventing death was the principal reason most of us went into medicine, we are doomed to fail. Medical care, rather, ought to be about preventing untimely death and ameliorating suffering. Success can and should be defined as making our patients comfortable as they navigate the dying process, and helping their family members accept their death. Most people would prefer to die at home. Encouraging programs like the Physicians Orders for Life Sustaining Treatment (POLST), which helps patients' convey those preferences, is one way to avoid having patients sent to the hospital.

PR: One of the major points of this case is that there comes a time when no matter what the family wants, the physician has to decide whether or not to continue treatment. In San Diego, we attempted to design a policy that placed the final decision about medical futility with the physician. We met with all ethics committees that were part of the University of California communities, and put together a consensus policy to which everyone could agree. The university attorneys, however, refused to endorse the policy, because they felt the final decision should be left to a judge.

The principal reason for creating the policy, however, was because we had bitterly disappointing experiences leaving such decisions to a judge. There was a patient who had been on a ventilator for over two years. The child was brain-dead, and we wanted to remove the child from the ventilator, but the parents refused. The clinicians went to the court, and asked for the authority to remove the patient from the ventilator. In response, the judge asked the physicians what the parents wanted. The answer, of course, was that the patient's parents wanted every possible intervention administered in order to keep the patient's body alive. The judge concluded that the clinicians should keep the patient on the ventilator. Arguing against this conclusion, the clinicians told the judge that the reason he's on a ventilator is because he was beaten into a coma by his parents, and they don't want to be tried for murder. In the end, the judge sided with the parents' wish to keep the patient on a ventilator.

SG: I would add one word of caution. In our assessments of medical futility, we need to take care not to predicate those assessments on what we personally consider an acceptable quality of life and what is not. If we are not careful, we may negate the patient's wishes and the patient's perception of the value of life, even when they have a terminal illness. There are some patients who would decide to pursue maximal care even during the final days of their lives. For example, a patient with metastatic lung cancer may be in favor of intubation if it means that while on the ventilator the patient can be somewhat awake and communicative. If we decide this care is futile based on the decision that the patient would not achieve what we deem an appropriate quality of life to justify the intervention, then we're not treating these patients justly.

PR: We frequently cannot conceive of having an acceptable quality of life if we were to suddenly sustain a major disability. I once had a case where the paramedics found a paraplegic man at the bottom of a flight of stairs, and assumed that he had committed suicide. As a result, they didn't attempt to resuscitate him. In actuality, the patient had a malfunctioning motorized wheelchair that launched him down a flight of stairs. There was a very interesting study done at a rehabilitation hospital in Denver, in which they surveyed their para- and quadriplegic patients when they first had their injury and again a year later. They found that even though they were depressed and often suicidal initially, almost all of them said that after a period of adjustment they were glad to be alive despite their injury.

I'm not trying to suggest that we use our own concepts of what is an acceptable quality of life to justify medical intervention. Rather, I'm referring to situations in which it is clear that further treatment is futile, though the same may not be as obvious to the patient's family members. When patients are able to communicate with the physician, or when family members have the insight and emotional wherewithal to agree with the emergency physician's assessment of futility, there is no conflict. The situation is considerably more difficult when the patient is unable to communicate, and when family members are incapable of understanding the gravity of the situation in which they find their ill family members. In these situations, I would first do my utmost to try to resolve the disagreement by discussing the issues with other attending physicians and utilizing the ethics consult service if it is available. The final decision concerning medical futility, however, ought to rest with the attending physician alone.

JA: There are times when we provide interventions that just prolong a painful dying process and increase the patient's suffering. This is not treatment, it is not care, and it is not warranted. I also believe that we are able to make an assessment of medical futility when we are certain that particular resuscitations or medical interventions will be ineffective. Although there are examples of when emergency physicians should deliver bad news, they can also offer comfort care or advise initiating new treatments based on our scientific evaluation of medical futility. When done properly, that is the most therapeutic and caring thing we can do.

TS: The discussion of futile treatments brings up two important points. First, quality of life is an important consideration, but one that must be interpreted from the patient's point of view, not our own. The second issue concerns how we define futility. We all have heard of the one patient who wakes from a coma after 15 years. Stories like these make it difficult to say that a patient has absolutely no chance of recovery. Should we then define futility as a 1 in a 100 chance, perhaps a 1 in a 1000? And even once we are able to define futility, there will always be families that request a patient be kept alive long enough to have a sister arrive from out of town, in order to say good bye. There are times when we must identify non-beneficial treatment, but we also need to be sure about what our goals are.

PR: The problem is that we can't alter the past. The minute the diagnosis of glioblastoma was confirmed, there should have been a discussion about the natural course of the disease, what the patient should expect, and the role of hospice in the final stages of the disease process.

JA: In our current healthcare landscape, we spend a lot of time struggling over what we're not going to do, and how we should approach the family with these decisions. This approach puts the families in a terrible position, and makes us extremely uncomfortable. We don't spend enough time talking about what we are able to do for the patient who cannot benefit from any curative therapy. If the patient in our case with a glioblastoma developed a creatinine of 5.0, would we suggest dialysis? No, we shouldn't even bring it up. Instead, we should tell the family that the patient's kidneys are failing, and that it is part of the dying process. Rather than focus on why we don't think that dialysis is appropriate, we should focus on the comfort measures we are able to provide. To that end, the priority would be pain control and symptom control.

If we start to change the conversation toward advising patients with what we thought was most appropriate, we would be acting as responsible physicians. This approach provides patients with the options available within the limits of medical science, and allows emergency physicians to feel better about their contributions. Remember, if a medical intervention has no promise of benefit or achieving the goals of the patient or medical team, emergency physicians cannot be accused of withholding an effective therapy when they refuse to administer it.

Section III: Review of the literature

"In the end every ethical rule must be tested against real life stories."
Stephen Gillers (1989). Taking L. A. law more seriously, *Yale Law Journal*. 98: 1607–623.

Calls to emergency medical services (EMS) are often activated for patients near death, and may lead to the ED as the entry point for many adult patients who die in the hospital. As well, the ED portal doubles as the access point used by sick patients whose health spirals chronically downward, with illness trajectories often punctuated by multiple ED visits, and hospital readmission.[1] Dying patients may be brought in by family, or sent in by their primary care physicians, seeking pain relief and other symptom amelioration. Studies show that between one-third to one-half of all patients presenting to the ED report chronic pain of severe intensity (i.e. mean pain scores >8/10 on the visual analog scale), which had not improved on ED discharge in over 30% of cases.[2,3] The progressive trend towards limiting longitudinal or multidisciplinary care for chronic pain may be partially responsible for the increasing number of patients attempting to ameliorate pain via the ED.[4,5] Additionally, many patients may not have other access to healthcare because they lack insurance or because of a shortage of primary care providers.

End-of-life issues arise in the ED when patients with terminal illnesses lose their battle, become wounded, or are disabled by symptoms. Integrating palliative medicine with emergency medicine makes intuitive sense, as all EDs stand at the intersection of life and death. Acute care episodes that involve dying may be part triumph or disaster, but death is always difficult in the emergency setting. Treating symptoms, discussing life-sustaining interventions and considering withholding or withdrawing of non-beneficial treatment with dying patients and their families, are all important parts of a palliative skill set emergency medicine professionals can develop in order to provide expert and compassionate care for patients at the end of their lives.

From an ethical perspective, the principle of beneficence in medicine requires that suffering and pain be treated. This chapter discusses some of the end-of-life issues related to cancer patients who present to the ED. We include a brief review of federal policy protections contributing legal fixes to remediate pain and suffering at the end of life, and also research findings that give some scientific platform to ethical deliberations on treatment aggressiveness and palliative care in terminal cancer patients. Coinciding with the ethical concerns that arise in death and dying episodes specific to emergency physicians, we provide a 10-point checklist (Box 10.1) based on the American College of Emergency Physicians (ACEP) policy to enhance end-of-life care, which fits into a conceptual framework (Figure 10.1) for clinicians to use in an approach to the end of life that emphasizes comfort-directed thera-

Box 10.1 Checklist of ethical issues at the end-of-life

To enhance end-of-life care in the ED emergency physicians should:

- Respect the dying patient's needs for care, comfort and compassion
- Communicate promptly and appropriately with patients and their families about end-of-life care choices, avoiding medical jargon
- Elicit the patient's goal for care before initiating treatment, recognizing that end-of-life care includes a broad range of therapeutic and palliative options
- Respect the wishes of dying patients, including those expressed in advance directives. Assist surrogates to make end-of-life choices for patients who lack decision-making capacity, based on the patient's own preferences, values, and goals
- Encourage the presence of family and friends at the patient's bedside near the end of life, if desired by the patient
- Protect the privacy of patients and families near the end of life
- Promote liaisons with individuals and organizations in order to help patients and families honor cultural and religious end-of-life traditions.
- Develop skill at communicating sensitive information, including poor prognoses and the death of a loved one.
- Comply with institutional policies regarding recovery of organs for transplantations.
- Obtain informed consent from surrogates for postmortem procedures.

Adapted from the ACEP Policy Statement. *Ethical Issues at the End of Life*.[6] Available at: www.acep.org/content.aspx?id=29440/. Accessed June 23, 2011, with permission from American College of Emergency Physicians.

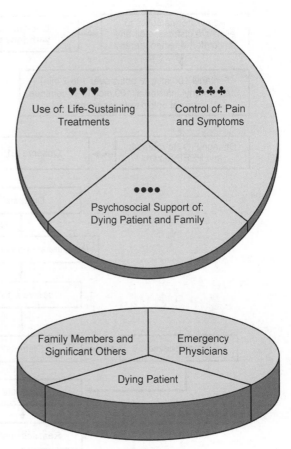

Fig. 10.1 Elements impacting end-of-life decision making and triad of stakeholders: the fragile peace.

pies for patients. A suggested guideline for removing life-sustaining interventions and treating pain in imminently dying patients is also provided (Figure 10.2).

Lastly, we discuss and differentiate the ethical and legal permissibility of withholding and withdrawing life-sustaining treatment and accepted comfort measures including palliative sedation from that of physician-assisted suicide and euthanasia (Table 10.1). This may help readers distinguish some of the relevant ethical and clinical concerns raised by the vignette at the beginning of the chapter.

Pain takes priority

The thought of experiencing a painful death is frightening for many people. At the end of life, patient

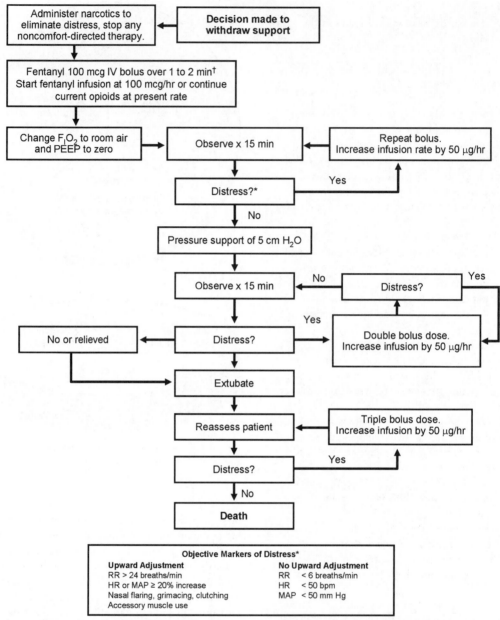

Fig. 10.2 Suggested guidelines for withdrawal of life-sustaining interventions and pain management at end of life. Reprinted from Schears RM. (1999) Emergency physicians' role in end-of-life care. *Emerg Med Clin North Am.* 2(17), 539–59, with permission from Elsevier.

Table 10.1 End-of-life decision making and respective cause of death, intention of intervention, and treatment legality

	Withhold life-sustaining treatment	Withdraw life-sustaining treatment	Palliative sedation and analgesia	Physician-assisted suicide	Euthanasia
Cause of death	Underlying disease	Underlying disease	Underlying disease[a]	Intervention prescribed by physician and used by patient	Intervention used by physician
Intent/goal of intervention	Avoid burdensome intervention	Remove burdensome intervention	Relieve symptoms	Termination of patient's life	Termination of patient's life
Legal?	Yes[b]	Yes[b]	Yes	No[c]	No

[a]Note doctrine of double effect.
[b]A number of states limit the power of surrogate decision makers regarding life-sustaining treatment.
[c]Legal only in Oregon, Washington and Montana.
Reproduced from Olsen ML, Swetz KM, Mueller PS. (2010) Ethical decision making with end-of-life care: palliative sedation and withholding or withdrawing life-sustaining treatments. *Mayo Clin Proc.* 85(10), 949–54. By permission of Mayo Foundation for Medical Education and Research. All rights reserved.

goals may shift to comfort, removal of burdens, and relief of suffering. However, physicians may be uncomfortable providing comfort-directed therapies or removing life-sustaining therapy.

Although most pain is treatable, and patients may benefit from skilled professionals involved in end-of-life care, dual-trained emergency medicine–palliative care specialists and on-site ED consultation for pain management is still rare, and the coincidence of comorbid conditions and terminal cancer is not. Perhaps this disconnection relates to the subjective nature of pain, and how it is expressed in patients with a life-limiting condition, resource limitations, or possibly owing to some lingering concern over the unsettled legal status of the management of pain and other symptoms.

Most barriers to pain management in EOL care are the result of lack of knowledge or longstanding misconceptions, and should not deter providers from following established clinical guidelines (Figure 10.2). Despite the social awareness of healthcare disparities affecting pain control, ethical calls, and recent public policy initiatives including the 2003 National Pain Care Policy Act, and legislative incentives framed upon the appeal of the Decade of Pain Control and Research, estimates indicate more than 70% of ED visits are related to chronic pain or its manifestations.[7] Hospital policy efforts that increasingly frame end-of-life care as a problem of healthcare quality,

may eventually enable committed medical organizations to apply quality improvement strategies institution-wide to consistently inform and educate staff, thereby reducing pain and suffering often mismanaged in the dying process.

Legal fixes = pain remedies for society?

The Emergency Medical Treatment and Labor Act (EMTALA) enacted by US Congress in 1986, recognizes the ethical need to treat pain as a symptom of emergency medical conditions, but stops short of explicitly naming pain as a medical disorder itself. EMTALA requires medical evaluation and stabilizing emergent treatment for anyone presenting to an ED regardless of the ability to pay. Some hospitals left to pick up the costs of required medical treatment have been forced to close their EDs, with well over 20% decline in the number of EDs recorded for the decade ending in 2009.[8] Others have weathered public outcry, and paid federal fines for what amounts to ethical failure to provide emergency care, notwithstanding legal guides encoded for professional behavior.[9,10] Moreover, while pain is the impetus prompting ED visits, it is not viewed uniformly as the justification for such interventions to occur in the ED.

Recent passage in 2010 of the Affordable Care Act (ACA) has also put some hazard lights on the use of EDs in the United States, and includes the possibility that healthcare reform will increase ED waits and crowded conditions, with more patients coming to EDs with end-of-life issues because care is not available elsewhere.[11] (This was the case in Massachusetts, whose model state plan was heavily borrowed from in crafting the national ACA.) In addition, because the final ACA version passed by Congress and signed into law by the President, did not include the provision to authorize funding for advance care planning (blocked by opponents hyping it as a means to deny life-sustaining treatment for vulnerable patients), the new law fails to support patient autonomy and well-being reflected in end-of-life discussions, even as medicine holds patient preferences ethically paramount, clinically relevant, and legally noteworthy. Americans will likely continue to rely on the ED and emergency physicians to do the right thing in matters of life and death, and acute care episodes.

Prolonging life—end-of-life goals

Issues relating to end-of-life cancer care affect a large number of Americans each year, and although cancer diagnoses and deaths have shown some small decrease in the past decade, ED visits for cancer-related emergencies are increasing as a likely result of the expanding therapeutic possibilities for patients with advanced cancer.[12-14] The complexity of emergency care is magnified by the aging of the populace; the growing prevalence of chronic diseases such as cancer; and the widespread availability and use of advanced imaging techniques and other advanced diagnostic modalities and therapy options. Overall, ED visits continue to increase at twice the rate of population growth, reaching 124 million ED visits in 2008, with cancer-related visits up over 20%.[15,16] During the same interval, there has been a revival of interest in the importance of high-quality end-of-life care, including focused efforts to improve three main elements impacting end-of-life decision-making: control of pain and other symptoms, use of life-sustaining interventions, and psychosocial support of those who are dying and their families (Figure 10.1). Each of these three areas may become ethically challenging in emergency settings as medical professionals, dying patients, and their families must interact in goal-directed activities.[17] The decision-makers must negotiate and come to grips with imminent death in the midst of technology.

Many times the financial imperatives of the hospital operations compete with patient safety and quality of care initiatives leading to avoidable suffering and harm. The chaos and limited timeframe for care in the ED makes ethical solutions at the end of life difficult. More often than not, the medical tradition and clinical tendency has been to overdo, in the face of existing human finitude. However, it is possible to provide compassionate, technically skilled care in accordance with patient treatment wishes for patients near the end of life in the ED.

Research studies: got cancer? Fight to the death

Aside from intensive use of chemotherapy, and interventions resulting in ED visits, several other indicators of aggressive patient care in end-of-life treatment have been identified including: hospitalization, readmission, ICU admission, and late and low rates of hospice use. Most of these studies characterizing markers of aggressive care are in population-based cohorts of patients 65 years old on Medicare with advanced solid tumors. These studies rarely include younger adults with terminal malignancy because the proportion of younger patients admitted to hospital is one quarter that of older individuals. As a group, elderly patients account for about 60% of cancer deaths in the United States enrolled by tumor registries participating in the National Cancer Institute's Surveillance, Epidemiology and End Results (SEER) Program.[18] This database captures approximately 97% of incident cases, and covers a representative sample of roughly 14% of the American population linked to Medicare claims data.[19-22] The evidence shows increased ED visits, hospitalizations and ICU admissions near death in terminally ill elders with cancer.[23] Investigators surmise that while comorbidities influence whether chemotherapy is initiated, they do not affect how many cycles of therapy are given, leading to the speculation that aggressive regimens may have resulted in more ED visits or admissions to hospital in the last month of life. Furthermore, despite greater enrollment in hospices, accounting for a decrease in hospital deaths during the 4-year study period, most patients transfer to a hospice very close to the time of death. This last finding suggests that hospices are being used to manage death itself, rather than to palliate cancer symptoms occurring progressively in the dying process, with the typical interval spanning 6 months or more.

There are few randomized controlled trials (RCTs) on the effectiveness of palliative care interventions to improve the care of patients with advanced cancer even though 50% of persons with cancer are not cured of their disease, and may live for years with improved treatment.[24] The National Consensus Project Clinical Practice Guidelines for Quality Palliative Care recommends palliative care referral at the time of a life-threatening diagnosis, and other core elements including a multidimensional assessment to identify, prevent, and alleviate suffering; provide assistance with medical decision-making, and improve effective communication skills; and treatment in selected cases after multidisciplinary team evaluation.[25] However, the evidence supporting these recommendations is limited.[26] One RCT was designed to compare a palliative care intervention concurrent with oncology treatment, as commonly recommended, with usual care in newly diagnosed advanced cancer patients. This investigation does not demonstrate any difference in improvements in symptom intensity scores or reduced days in hospital or ICU or ED visits between the two groups during the 5-year study window ending in 2008.[27] However, a more recent study finds that patients with metastatic non-small-cell lung cancer who receive early palliative care, have significant improvements in the quality of life, receive less aggressive care at the end of life, and have longer survivals.[28]

Other investigators have looked at the intensity and cost of treatment in the last year of life and find extensive regional variations. In 2007, the percentage of deaths in hospital varied by a factor of almost 4 across hospital referral regions, and the average number of hospice days per patient in the last 6 months of life varied by a factor of more than 6. Areas with high in-hospital deaths rate included New York City, with rates over 40%, while rates of death in hospital for Minot (North Dakota), Fort Lauderdale (Florida), and Portland (Oregon) were below 20%. Similarly, the likelihood that a patient spends time in intensive care during his or her final hospital admission varied widely. Almost a third of chronically ill Medicare beneficiaries in New Brunswick (New Jersey), Miami (Florida), and Los Angeles (California) were admitted to intensive care during their final hospital admission, compared with only 4.2% of such

patients in Appleton (Wisconsin), 10.1% in Portland (Oregon), and 11.5% in Madison (Wisconsin).[29] These variations could not be explained by differing patient preferences by region.[30]

Not surprisingly, aging among the US population is one of the causes of the tandem increase in overall ED visits and cancer-related visits. The Centers for Disease Control and Prevention projects that by 2030 the number of Americans aged 65 years and older will have doubled, and represent fully 20% of the population. Looking ahead, to avoid further endangerment of the one right to US healthcare Americans have under EMTALA, healthcare reform advocates and physicians must work to reverse the public expectation that life can be extended indefinitely, and the assumption that if a treatment can be done, it should be done.

With over 139,000 ED deaths per year, down from more than twice that figure in 2000, the continued visible unequal distribution of medical resources may result in secondary effects that fly beneath the radar of societal scrutiny.[16] More insidious is the increasing emphasis of biology on our moral commitments, the need felt to "make live," and avoid death, at any cost, at any age. Physicians often act as if age and disease factors are not transformative, but what hangs in the medical outcome balance, successful versus failure and other likely options can help in framing proposed interventions to counsel patients, and avoid the trap of wishful thinking.

Developing a proactive approach to enhance end-of-life care in the ED may also invoke the novel ethics challenge of the golden rule. ACEP policy gives clear guidance for incorporating respect for patients' autonomous choices, and honoring advance directives (ADs).[6] We add a few twists, including a modern-day checklist (Box 10.1) format, for busy clinicians to help organize compassionate end-of-life responses to prioritize interacting with dying patients and their families, and some coaching interpretation. It is hoped that by demonstrating more respect for the needs of dying patients, the potential tide of ethical conflicts may lessen and the subjective burdens may ease.

Providing end-of-life care—an ethical base

Whether EDs should practically reconsider new aims to deliver sophisticated end-of-life care beyond providing bridging therapeutics for symptoms related to the process of dying, is a matter open to debate. Managing cancer pain, for example, may be impacted adversely by the short time available to evaluate the patient, lack of past history or an ongoing relationship with the patient. Given that emergency physicians typically spend on average 12–15 minutes with urgent (not critically ill) patients, it would be difficult to obtain sufficient past medical history, dig into psychosocial issues, review prescription and non-prescription medication use, and conduct a complete systems review and physical examination to capably render more than stopgap measures to ameliorate severe symptoms.[31] Then add here consideration of the conflicted or questionable DNR status as portrayed in the case scenario. However, we have an obligation to do just that based on respect for patient autonomy and beneficence.

Honoring patient preferences near the end of life

As our opening case highlights, patients with cancer generally do not come into the ED because they "have cancer," they come because the ED is open when they have symptoms such as vomiting and altered mental status for which they are seeking treatment. When a patient arrives in the ED with a serious, life-limiting disease such as cancer, it is important to know and understand the patient's goals of care. Is he or she seeking treatment for the symptom only, seeking life-prolonging treatment or both? For the alert patient with decision-making capacity, we are able to ask the patient. For patients who are unable to speak for themselves, we need to rely on surrogate decision-makers, ADs, and medical orders such as POLST.

An AD is a document completed by a patient when he or she has decision-making capacity that provides direction for the future when the patient no longer is able to express treatment preferences. ADs can take the form of statements about future preferences such as, "If I was permanently unconscious I would not want a breathing tube," or they can be used to designate a healthcare proxy who will be the person making medical decisions on their behalf when the patient is unable to do so. The Patient Self Determination Act of 1991 was designed to encourage completion of ADs, and requires hospitals to offer information about completion of ADs at the time of admission. However, research has found that ADs are ineffective

in consistently relaying patients' wishes, and are often times inaccessible.

The large, multicenter SUPPORT trial concludes that "ADs do not substantially enhance physician–patient communication or decision-making about resuscitation. Increasing the frequency of ADs is unlikely to be a substantial element in improving the care of seriously ill patients."[32] Another study finds that there is no significant difference in the frequency with which mechanical ventilation, inotrope support, cardiopulmonary resuscitation, or renal dialysis is applied in patients with or without an AD.[33] One reason for this may be the misfit between abstract ideals that guide the content of ADs when created and the messy realities that infuse end-of-life situations that develop later. Predicting and outlining directions for all possible scenarios are difficult, thus ADs are rarely sufficiently precise to dictate patient preferences in specific situations as a disease progresses.[34] Furthermore, a 2001 study finds that an AD is lacking in most patients who are transferred from a skilled nursing facility to an ED.[35] Also a retrospective medical record review and qualitative interviews with emergency physicians in a study population of nursing home patients over age 65 transferred to the ED finds that many patients arrive in the ED without their AD, and when it is sent, it might not agree with other information in the record, limiting its use.[36]

The POLST form was developed because of the difficulty in using ADs in a time of crisis. This brightly colored form constitutes a set of medical orders based on the patient's current treatment preferences. In addition to orders either for resuscitation or do not attempt resuscitation (DNAR) when the patient is in cardiopulmonary arrest, the orders allow patients to specify one of three levels of care in other emergency situations: full treatment including mechanical ventilation and ICU, limited interventions including hospital admission and treatment of potentially reversible conditions, but not intubation and ventilation, or comfort measures only. The orders can be modified and changed as the patient's medical condition and preferences for or against certain interventions change.

The POLST program began in Oregon in the 1990s.[37] It has become a national model for portable medical orders, and is now being implemented or used in over 30 states. To validate the form, one study used theoretical scenarios to determine whether or not 19 primary care physicians, 20 emergency physicians, 26 paramedics, and 22 long-term care nurses could correctly interpret the orders. Overall, professionals are able to correctly identify treatments to provide or withhold.[38] Subsequent studies support its effectiveness at honoring patient preferences.[38–43] A group of 180 nursing home patients at one facility that used a POLST form indicating "DNAR and comfort measures only," was prospectively followed for 1 year. During that time, 38 died. For these patients, 100% of the orders regarding cardiopulmonary resuscitation (CPR) were honored.[44] In a recent study across three states where POLST is widely used, finds "POLST orders restricting medical interventions are associated with less use of life-sustaining treatments. Findings suggest that the POLST program offers significant advantages over traditional methods to communicate preferences about life-sustaining treatments."[45]

Preparing for unpreventable death

This process begins with an uncontroversial step: Work at being a better communicator! For example, opening remarks are critical when interacting with patients. The best first question: "How can I help you?" Also consider asking, "What were you hoping we would do when you came to the ED today?" This is more helpful than," What brings you to the ED?" The first questions set the stage for effective information sharing, while the latter fails to adequately communicate the sense of public service and self-effacing tone that regards the welfare of the patient above the doctor's preferences. Further, the second question allows the patient to begin to talk about his or her goals of care. Within the ED context, it is especially important to send the welcome message to a patient facing the end of life, to quickly establish a favorable first impression, and to underpin the implicit prima facie duty of the doctor to take all reasonable measures to deliver safe and effective care related to treatment while honoring preferences for or against specific life-sustaining interventions.

Many physicians are reluctant to discuss ADs, citing lack of time to engage patients meaningfully in end-of-life discussions, even though investigators have demonstrated conversations about ADs only require an average of 5.6 minutes.[46,47] Emergency physicians also find themselves needing to have "The Code Status" conversation. How this conversation is framed is important. Often, the question is asked, "If you were stop breathing or your heart stopped, would you want everything done?" Who is going to say "No" to that question? Emergency professionals need to have a realistic conversation about the likely outcome of intubation or CPR. A better starting point is, "Have you thought about what you do NOT want if your heart stopped or you quit breathing properly?" Then, based on the response and the patient's understanding of his or her current medical condition, it is our obligation to provide an explanation of the likely outcome of these interventions. The patient should be aware that in patients with advanced cancer the chance that they will benefit from CPR and mechanical ventilation is low, and the burdens are high.

Some bioethicists have argued that physicians may be tongue-tied in the presence of a dying patient because they lack a conceptual framework for approaching end-of-life care, similar to how they clinically approach clear disease states such as acute appendicitis or myocardial infarction.[48] This line of reasoning may be less persuasive in ED settings where emergency physicians by necessity are expected to face down the unknown, and be capable of forging ahead to medically manage patients presenting with undifferentiated illness or trauma.

On the other hand, although the dying process and death will confront us all, many people continue to act as if it will not come to **them**, and few of **us** are willing to take responsibility for determining our own fates. Removal of an obstructed appendix, or restoring blood flow to an ailing heart, may seem easy by comparison. To withhold our own preferences when we have the opportunity to provide input into the care we receive in the future is deliberate, albeit uncertain gain.[44] Awareness of this blind spot may prompt doctors to compensate patients for some perceived life shortfall in the moment, by applying life-sustaining technology in preference to admitting the uncertainty of doing nothing or withholding interventions. The medical consequences for patients may emerge through "routine" treatment provided by physicians blinded by their own denial, and possibly powerless to consider withholding or withdrawing what may actually be non-beneficial interventions. While the ED paradigm may make this exchange visible, it is located throughout the medical enterprise, and the social fabric characterized more by the difficulty of saying "no"—even when death is looming large—to life-sustaining, prolonging or extending interventions. The case juxtaposition of having a "DNR [order] but without plans to 'go gently,'" reflects both an awareness and yet confusion in distinguishing the limits of medicine from the limits on life.

Treating pain and suffering

An emergency physician may fear that the use of high-dose opioids will accelerate the dying process. In fact, respiratory depression is rare.[49] Rather, appropriate treatment of pain may allow the patient to relax, be more comfortable and interact more meaningfully with family and friends. Furthermore, the principle of **double effect** has both a legal and an ethical basis. First described by Thomas Aquinas, the principle states that it is ethically justifiable to perform an act for a good reason, such as controlling pain, even if an unintended consequence occurs, such as hastening death. Emergency physicians further worry that they will contribute to addiction when providing large doses of opioids to patients. Again, in the setting of advanced cancer this fear is generally unwarranted.[45] Physical dependence and tolerance can occur, and patients may need escalating doses of opioids both due to progression of disease and because of tolerance. When a patient comes to the ED because of pain, it may be necessary to evaluate the patient for new causes of pain such as new bony metastases, or bowel obstruction, and provide both short- and longer-term pain management. There is no ceiling effect for opioids, and some patients may require very high doses (Figure 10.2). The cross-tolerance to opioids is incomplete, and one strategy to consider when a patient has a high opioid need is to rotate among various alternatives to control symptoms.

Palliative sedation

Palliative sedation refers to the use of medications to induce decreased or absent awareness in patients in order to relieve their otherwise intractable suffering at the end of life. Palliative sedation usually involves continuous sedative administration (i.e., ketamine, benzodiazepines, propofol, or barbiturates) in addition to opioids maintained to avoid triggering narcotic withdrawal (pain) from emerging in the midst of prolonged sedation. Ongoing palliative sedation

can occur at home, in the setting of hospice, or as part of a hospital admission. Although palliative sedation as a strategy for extreme suffering has been granted the legal authority of the US Supreme Court, emergency physicians may be concerned about its application in the ED, for it goes beyond the usual scope of practice. Normally, emergency physicians are comfortable inducing brief episodes of closely monitored conscious sedation for the limited purpose of controlling procedural awareness and pain, such as for fracture realignment or joint reduction. Informed consent for procedural sedation usually includes patient assent for CPR in the event of complications that may arise during treatment. By comparison, candidate selection, medical process variations, and unlimited timeframes of palliative sedation, which routinely includes patient death (although not the goal of therapy), typically occurs off vital sign monitors; and these features may be ethically troubling for physicians, regardless of the informed consent of the suffering patient and family, or formal consultation with the palliative medical service.

Stopping and not starting resuscitation in the ED

Without evidence to the contrary, the automatic response is to provide resuscitation regardless of the patient's underlying medical condition. This is based on the assumption that it is in the best interests of the patient. However, CPR and resuscitation were designed for healthy patients who suffer a sudden cardiac arrest, and are unlikely to be successful in patients with advanced cancer. Most prehospital providers and emergency physicians are willing to honor legally authorized DNAR orders, or valid ADs.[50–52] More difficult for healthcare professionals in the ED is deciding how to proceed once a patient has been intubated and placed on the ventilator. Sometimes, shortly after intubation, information becomes available indicating that an unwanted intervention was facilitated. The response of least resistance is often to rely on the presence of the endotracheal tube to dictate hospital level of care; usually this ensures an ICU admission to in effect "keep the patient alive long enough to make the decision someone else's decision." While this is an understandable and sometimes necessary response in a busy ED, it may not always be the best response. Although certainly emotionally different, there is no ethical distinction between not starting and stopping resuscitation. Withdrawing treatment in the ED can be appropriate to honor patient treatment preferences and avoid ongoing suffering (see Figure 10.2). In reality, withdrawing life support in the ED requires time to prepare the family, along with privacy and compassionate staff who are able to provide support to both the family and the patient.

Assisted suicide and euthanasia

While withholding and withdrawing life support is both ethically and legally justifiable, physician-assisted suicide and euthanasia are illegal in all US states except Oregon, Washington, and Montana (see Table 10.1). These three states allow a physician to write a prescription for a lethal medication that a patient then can self-administer. Due to safeguards in the law (Oregon and Washington) including a 15-day waiting period and evaluation by two separate physicians, emergency physicians are not likely to be involved in decisions about whether or not to write a prescription. However, it is possible that a patient may present to an ED after a failed attempt to hasten death. A survey of Oregon emergency physicians at the time the Death with Dignity Act was enacted finds most respondents (97%) indicate at least one circumstance in which they would sometimes be willing to withhold resuscitation for a patient who was brought to the ED after ingesting medications. The respondents would withhold resuscitation from a patient with an AD (81%), with documentation in writing from the patient's physician (73%), after speaking to the primary physician (64%), if a patient with decision-making capacity verbally confirmed intent (60%), or if the family verbally confirmed intent (52%).[53]

Conclusion

Convention holds that the ED is not well equipped to manage complexities of end-of-life care. However, patients near the end of life often seek care in EDs, and we have an obligation to provide expert and compassionate care to these patients. Emergency physicians are responsible for not only providing immediate treatment, but also for arranging disposition and follow-up care. We need to be able to manage and treat patients' pain and other symptoms, as well as addressing their goals of care.

References

1. Jencks SF, Williams MV, Coleman EA. (2009) Rehospitalizations among patients in the medicare fee-for-service program. *N Engl J Med.* 360, 1418–28.
2. Duchame J, Barber C. (1995) A prospective blinded study on emergency pain assessment therapy. *J Emerg Med.* 3, 571–5.
3. Todd K, Sloan E, Chen C, et al. (2002) Survey of pain etiology, management practices and patient satisfaction in two urban emergency departments. *CJEM.* 4, 252–6.
4. Giordano J, Schatman, ME. (2008) A crisis in pain care—An ethical analysis. Part one: Facts, issues, and problems. *Pain Phys.* 11, 54–62.
5. Schatman ME. (2006) The demise of multidisciplinary pain management clinics? *Pract Pain Manage.* 6, 30–41.
6. American College of Emergency Physicians Policy Statement. *Ethical Issues at the End of Life.* Available at: www.acep.org/content.aspx?id=29440/. Accessed March 28, 2011.
7. Disorbio J, Bruns D, Barolat G. (2006) Assessment and treatment of chronic pain: A physician's guide to a biopsychosocial approach. *Pract Pain Manage.* 6, 11–27.
8. Hsia RY, Kellermann AL, Shen Y. (2011) Factors associated with closures of emergency departments in the United States. *JAMA.* 305, 1978–85.
9. Associated Press. (1998) Boy does after hospital refuses to help: Policy changed when workers do not treat teen who lay bleeding outside. *Milwaukee J Sentinel.* 19 May.
10. SoRelle R. (1998) Teen's death 50 feet from hospital becomes a lesson for emergency medicine. *Emerg Med News.* 9, 12.
11. US Government Printing Office. *Public Law* 111-148/152. Available at: www.gpo.gov/fdsys/pkg/PLAW-111publ148/pdf/PLAW-111publ148.pdf. Accessed January, 5 2011.
12. Hoyert DL, Kochanek KD, Murphy SL. (1999) Deaths: Final data for 1997. *National Vital Statistics Reports: from the Centers for Disease Control and Prevention, National Center for Health Statistics, National Vital Statistics System* 47, 1–104.
13. Bleiberg H. (1998) Continuing the fight against advanced colorectal cancer: New and future treatment options. *Anticancer Drugs.* 9, 18–28.
14. Steward WP, Dunlop DJ. (1998) New drugs in the treatment of non-small cell lung cancer. *Cancer.* 83, 679–89.
15. Institute of Medicine Committee on the Future of Emergency Care in the United States Health System.

Hospital-Based Emergency Care: At the Breaking Point. Washington, DC: National Academies Press, 2006.

16. Nawar EW, Niska RW, Xu J. (2007) National Hospital Ambulatory Medical Survey: 2005 emergency department summary. *Adv Data.* 386, 1–32.

17. Maa J. (2011) The waits that matter. *N Engl J Med.* 364, 2279–81.

18. American Cancer Society. (2000) Cancer statistics 2000. *CA Cancer J Clin.* 50, 7–33.

19. Zippin C, Lum D, Hankey BF. (1995) Completeness of hospital cancer case reporting from the SEER program of the National Institute. *Cancer.* 76, 2343–50.

20. Nattinger AB, McAuliffe TL, Schapira MM. (1997) Generalizability of the surveillance, epidemiology, and end results registry population: Factors relevant to epidemiologic and health care research. *J Clin Epidemiol.* 50, 939–45.

21. Ries LAG, Kosary CL, Hankey BF, et al. (1997) *SEER Cancer Statistics Review, 1973–1994.* NIH Publication No. 97-2789. Bethesda, MD: National Cancer Institute.

22. Potosky AL, Riley GF, Lubitz JD, et al. (1993) Potential for cancer related health services research using a linked medicare-tumor registry database. *Med Care.* 31, 732–48.

23. Earle CC, Neville BA, Landrum MB, et al. (2004) Trends in the aggressiveness of cancer care near the end of life. *J Clin Oncol.* 22, 315–21.

24. American Cancer Society. (2007) *Cancer Facts and Figures 2007.* Atlanta, GA: American Cancer Society.

25. National Consensus Project. (2009) *Clinical Practice Guidelines for Quality Palliative Care,* 2nd ed. Brooklyn, NY: National Consensus Project for Quality Palliative Care.

26. Zimmermann C, Riechelmann R, Krzyzanowska M, et al. (2008) Effectiveness of specialized palliative care: a systematic review. *JAMA.* 299, 1698–709.

27. Bakitas M, Lyons KD, Hegel MT, et al. (2009) Effects of a palliative care intervention on clinical outcomes in patients with advanced cancer: The project ENABLE II randomized controlled trial. *JAMA.* 302, 741–9.

28. Temel JS, Greer JA, Muzikansky A, et al. (2010) Early palliative care for patients with metastatic non-small-cell lung cancer. *N Engl J Med.* 363, 733–42.

29. The Dartmouth Atlas Project. Available at: www.dartmouthatlas.org/downloads/reports/EOLTrend_Report_0411.pdf/. Accessed June 24, 2011.

30. Barnato AE, Herndon MB, Anthony DL, et al. (2007) Are regional variations in end-of-life care intensity explained by patient preferences? A study of the US medicare population. *Med Care.* 45, 386–93.

31. Johnson S. (2005) The social, professional, and legal framework for the problem of pain management in emergency medicine. *J Law Med Ethics.* 33, 741–60.

32. The SUPPORT Principal Investigators. (1995) A controlled trial to improve care for seriously ill hospitalized patient: the study to understand prognoses and preferences for outcomes and risks of treatments (SUPPORT). *JAMA.* 274, 1591–8.

33. Kish-Wallace S, Martin CG, Shaw AD, et al. (2001) Influence of an advance directive on the initiation of life support technology in critical ill cancer patients. *Crit Care Med.* 29, 2294–8.

34. Bomba PA, Vermilyea D. (2006) Integrating POLST into palliative care guidelines: a paradigm shift in advance care planning in oncology. *J Natl Compre Canc Netw.* 4, 819–29.

35. Lahn M, Friedman B, Bijur P, et al. (2001) Advance directives in skilled nursing facility residents transferred to emergency departments. *Acad Emerg Med.* 8, 1158–62.

36. Weinick RM, Wilcox SR, Park ER, et al. (2008) Use of advance directives for nursing home residents in the emergency department. *Am J Hosp Palliat Care.* 25, 179–83.

37. Dunn PM, Schmidt TA, Carley MM, et al. (1996) A method to communicate patient preferences about medically indicated life-sustaining treatment in the out-of-hospital setting. *J Am Geriat Soc.* 44, 785–91.

38. Schmidt TA, Hickman SE, Tolle SW, et al. (2004) The physician orders for life-sustaining treatment program: Oregon emergency medical technicians' practical experiences and attitudes. *J Am Geriatr Soc.* 52, 1430–4.

39. Lee MA, Brummel-Smith K, Meyer J, et al. (2000) Physician orders for life-sustaining treatment (POLST): outcomes in a PACE program. Program of All-Inclusive Care for the Elderly. *J Am Geriatr Soc.* 48, 1219–25.

40. Hickman SE, Hammes BJ, Tolle SW, et al. (2004) A viable alternative to traditional living wills. *Hastings Center Rep.* 34, 4–6.

41. Hickman SE, Nelson CA, Moss AH, et al. (2009) Use of the physician order for life-sustaining treatment (POLST) paradigm program in the hospice setting. *J Palliat Med.* 12, 133–41.

42. Tolle SW, Tilden VP, Nelson CA, et al. (1998) A prospective study of the efficacy of the physician order form for life-sustaining treatment. *J Am Geriatr Soc.* 46, 1097–102.

43. Hickman SE, Nelson CA, Perrin NA, et al. (2010) A comparison of methods to communicate treatment preferences in nursing facilities: traditional practices versus the physician orders for life-sustaining treatment program. *J Am Geriatr Soc.* 58, 1241–8.

44. Go RS, Hammes BA, Lee JA, et al. (2007) Advance directives among health care professionals at a community-based cancer center. *Mayo Clin Proc.* 82, 1487–90.

45. Hojsted J, Sjogren R. (2007) Addiction to opioids in chronic pain patients: A literature review. *Eur J Pain.* 11, 490–518.

46. Morrison RS, Morrison EW, Glickman DF. (1994) Physician reluctance to discuss advance directives. An empiric investigation of potential barriers. *Arch Intern Med.* 154, 2311–8.

47. Tulsky JA, Fischer GS, Rose MR, et al. (1998) Opening the black box: how do physicians communicate about advance directives? *Ann Intern Med.* 129, 441–9.

48. Singer PA, MacDonald N. (1998) Bioethics for clinicians: Quality end-of-life care. *CMAJ.* 159, 159–62.

49. Dahan A. (2007). Respiratory depression with opioids. *J Pain Palliat Care Pharmacother.* 21, 63–6.

50. Schears RM, Marco CA, Iserson KV, et al. (2004) Do not attempt resuscitation (DNAR) in the out-of-hospital setting. *Ann Emerg Med.* 44, 68–70.

51. Marco CA, Schears RM. (2003) Prehospital resuscitation practices: a survey of prehospital providers. *J Emerg Med.* 24, 101–6.

52. Marco CA, Bessman ES, Kelen GD. (2009) Ethical issues of cardiopulmonary resuscitation: comparison of emergency physician practices from 1995 to 2007. *Acad Emerg Med.* 16, 270–3.

53. Schmidt TA, Zechnich AD, Tilden VP, et al. (1996) Oregon emergency physicians' experiences with, attitudes toward, and concerns about physician-assisted suicide. *Acad Emerg Med.* 3, 938–45.

11 Futility in emergency medicine

Arthur R. Derse

Director, Center for Bioethics and Medical Humanities, and Julia and David Uihlein Professor of Medical Humanities, and Professor of Bioethics and Emergency Medicine, Institute for Health and Society, Medical College of Wisconsin, Milwaukee, WI, USA

Section I: Case presentation

An emergency medical technician (EMT) called in to report that they were bringing in a cachectic 82-year-old man with metastatic small cell lung cancer. Vital signs on the EMTs arrival at his home were: 60/40 mmHg, pulse 140 beats per minute, respiratory rate 32 breaths per minute, with an oxygen saturation of 92% on a non-rebreather mask. The patient's physician called the emergency department (ED) as well, before the patient arrived, and told us that the patient had failed chemotherapy, and that she had recommended referral to a hospice, although the referral hadn't yet been made. The patient had been bedbound for 2 months. The physician had also recommended a prehospital do-not-resuscitate (DNR) bracelet, but the patient's wife rejected this suggestion. The patient arrived unresponsive with a thready femoral pulse. He indeed was cachectic and cyanotic. The EMT said the patient's wife and daughter were at the scene, and asked that "everything be done," but they had not yet arrived at the ED. As the patient was placed on an ED stretcher, his cardiac rhythm changed to asystole. He had no pulses and no respiratory efforts.

Section II: Discussion

Dr. Peter Rosen: How can we define medical futility and determine what medical care is appropriate?

Dr. Arthur Derse: One definition of medical futility is an intervention that a physician deems ineffective based upon experience and knowledge of the literature. This definition is one that is ethically defensible. A second definition of futility includes the concept of an intervention that has a vanishingly small chance of meaningful effect, but which would prolong the dying process. Finally, a third definition is an intervention that will prolong someone's life, but would do so in such a way that would either not improve or even threaten the patient's current quality of life. The last two definitions of futility are far more controversial and potentially ethically problematic. In our case, an emergency physician using his knowledge of the literature and experience, along with a good bedside assessment, may reasonably refuse to continue aggressive treatment even if that decision isn't in agreement with the family's wishes.

Dr. Shamai Grossman: Would you ever continue to resuscitate a patient when the medical literature and

Ethical Problems in Emergency Medicine: A Discussion-Based Review, First Edition. John Jesus, Shamai A. Grossman, Arthur R. Derse, James G. Adams, Richard Wolfe, and Peter Rosen.

clinical judgment state that there is no value in the continuation?

AD: Troug of Children's Hospital in Boston argues that futile pediatric resuscitation is not always wrong, and can be performed as an "act of sincere caring and compassion" for those families who identify most with the idea of not "giving up" over and above the concept of dying in peace and comfort.[1] Though there are those families and physicians who believe in this approach, I disagree with Dr. Troug's arguments.

PR: I don't take issue with extending prehospital pediatric resuscitations, in order to better address parental grief in the hospital, even when there is little hope of success. That does not justify, however, initiating ineffective interventions. Part of the problem with medical futility is that while we try to rely upon evidence to define what is and is not effective, we end up with differences of opinion about what it means for an intervention to be futile. We can't prove a treatment to be ineffective 100% of the time, aside from interventions that have never been successfully performed, such as a brain transplant. How do you decide when to ignore family requests for aggressive measures and forego initiating a new procedure or therapy?

Dr. John Moskop: It's not always an easy decision, particularly in the ED. There are cases in which resuscitation is possible, but the patient's underlying disease is such that efforts to prolong life do not necessarily improve or may even threaten the patient's quality of life. The treating physicians might see resuscitation as futile, and yet we know that some believe life is worth prolonging regardless of its quality. If that is the case, decisions about treating the patient become a value conflict. It is not clear who should hold the greatest authority, and there is not a clear opportunity for compromise. Generally, we give the authority to physicians, but where there are potential differences of opinion, we are often inclined to defer to the family's preferences.

PR: We should also consider situations in which there are things we can do to help the patient, but the patient won't give us permission. Is it ever permissible for the doctor to ignore the patient, and move forward with interventions felt to be appropriate?

AD: Although patients don't have the right to demand therapies, they may autonomously refuse interven-

tions, even if they are life-sustaining or life-saving. The only exceptions are if the patient lacks decision-making capacity or authority. Patients who have altered mental status, are minors (not an emancipated or a mature minor), or are under duress are some of the most common exceptions we see in the ED.

PR: In difficult cases, it certainly helps to know the patients and their wishes, since sometimes they can deviate from those of the family who might not even agree amongst themselves as to what should be done. There are situations in which family values should not be given the authority to decide what care is administered. It may be useful to simplify the situation by taking an exaggerated position. For example, a physician would not perform brain transplantation on a patient per family request. In addition, families may be naïve to the fact that prolonging patients' lives may increase their suffering without any clear real benefit. Families generally hope to restore their loved ones to their previous state of health. If they understand the situation more fully, they might well agree that it is preferable to allow the patient to die a natural death. In the case presented, I would have very little problem refusing to resuscitate this patient, feeling that a natural endpoint had been reached.

Dr. John Jesus: Discussions with families along these lines are ethically hazardous, because they often take the form of a physician trying to convince a family of a particular view or cost:benefit ratio. I prefer not to impose my own value system on someone else, and instead try to offer guidance by saying, "These are the set of interventions that we could do that have these possible benefits. If this were my family member, or if this were my sister, this is how I would want them to be treated."

PR: The question here is not whether or not the resuscitation is futile, but rather if it is justifiable, given that prolonging this patient's life may not improve its quality. While I am reluctant to impose my judgments about what constitutes good quality of life, I don't think there is much argument about what the death from metastatic lung cancer is like for the victim. The real question for me in this case is whether it is ethically permissible for a physician to say, "I know what is going to happen to this patient, and I am not going to cause the patient to continue to experience that degree of suffering."

SG: I would approach futility from two perspectives. First, I would consider the futility of healthcare, where we should aim to be objective, though data supporting an objective approach are scarce. In rare situations where we can say that the resuscitation will likely be successful and provide the patient with a non-trivial lifespan, there is objective evidence that it is justified. It is more often the case, however, that the resuscitation might restore spontaneous circulation, only to have the patient arrest again and die within a few days, which would support the conclusion that the situation is futile. I believe this perspective pertains to the case presented. Second, we should consider futility of life, which by nature is subjective, and should depend on the patient's autonomous views of the value of a life of lesser quality.

PR: Do you feel that it is justifiable to extend the patient's life because that is what the family would want?

SG: Yes. If the family wanted me to do everything despite concerns about the patient's quality of life, I would do what I could for the patient.

PR: I'm uncomfortable with the concept that life is a quantitative and not a qualitative event. I'm also uncomfortable with the notion that physicians are merely technicians who offer various procedures off a menu, from which the family is allowed to order. It is the responsibility of the physician to define what is appropriate for end-of-life care. The onset of death is not as troubling as the practice of prolonging life at great cost to the patient in the form of suffering, in addition to the expense to the system or the patient's family. The ability to prolong life does not imply that we should. I personally believe that the medical decisions in this case are simple. I would pronounce the patient dead. I would then sit the family down and explain that we did everything possible. We helped him out of the world with as little suffering as we could, and unfortunately, the disease has ended his life.

AD: I think this case raises the issue of how the concept of futility can be applied ethically and appropriately. I know that many of us are uncomfortable withholding a treatment that has even a miniscule chance of helping, especially given how many families seem to value every minute the patient is alive. Even if the patient himself expressed a desire to live as long as possible, the short-term prolonging of life without

any possible change in the eventual outcome is not a proper goal of medicine, and I see no ethical reason to pursue it.

SG: Cardiopulmonary death is death, and you have no right to pretend that death has not occurred to placate a family regardless of the age of the patient. What if you could resuscitate this patient, and he could open his eyes and see his children, or take a pen in his hand and write his will or open his mouth and say a final prayer? Is this still beyond the goal of medicine? I would say not to do this would degrade my mission as a physician, and might even be considered murder.

PR: Since we have not achieved consensus, perhaps we can start with premises upon which we do agree. Would you agree that the three missions of medicine are to cure disease when possible, to alleviate disease when it is not possible to cure it, and to give comfort regardless of whether the first two goals are achievable? I think that artificially prolonging life without considerations of quality of life doesn't fit within any one of those three missions. Resuscitation is not going to cure disease, it is not going to alleviate disease, and it certainly is not going to give the patient comfort. Those are my ground rules for making decisions, and the family's desires do not overrule them.

SG: All three of these are appropriate missions in medicine. There is, however, subjectivity in defining them. I do not believe that that withholding resuscitation for someone who wants to live longer, even with a poorer quality of life, is failing to give comfort or fulfilling a mission of medicine. It is difficult to know when to stop applying the argument that an intervention extends life only temporarily, as everyone will die at some point. Is 5 days or 5 weeks sufficient time to define life as appropriate for resuscitation? There are democratic countries in western Europe where patients over a certain age are not offered dialysis. Are you really comforting the patient by telling them they could potentially live another 1–5 years, but you can't give them that care because there are others who have more time?

PR: What would you do for this patient?

SG: If the patient will definitely have another arrest in the next 72 hours, I agree the situation is futile. If there is a possibility that this patient will survive for an undefined period of time greater than 72 hours, however, I would attempt to resuscitate the patient. For example, I recently saw a patient with metastatic breast cancer receiving palliative chemotherapy in cardiac arrest. I treated her for hyperkalemia from her tumor lysis syndrome, and she survived her hospital stay. She was able to go home under hospice care and spend time with her family. The patient in our case might not have the same quality of life that he had previously if he were resuscitated, but that doesn't mean the resultant life is not worth preserving.

JJ: I recognize those three missions of medicine, but would argue that the scope of providing comfort may justifiably include not only the patient, but also the patient's family; it is for this reason that we sometimes allow parents to be present during pediatric resuscitations. If we include the family's comfort, then our mission becomes far more complicated when we consider futility.

PR: You could have it both ways. You could wait for the family to arrive, and then explain to the family why the patient's death needs to be pronounced.

JJ: I feel that you either code a patient or you don't, and I think "slow codes" are ethically unjustified. At the very least, the "slow code" is a misrepresentation, and an insincere attempt to make our actions appear to be something they are not.

PD: I've never been a part of a "slow code." I do believe, however, that there are situations in which I would delay the pronouncement of death for the sake of the family, which I do most commonly for pediatric deaths in the field.

PR: If we set out to do everything possible for both the family and the patient, it is important to set limits on what they can ask for, and on the suffering the patient might experience in the course of resuscitation. In addition, at some point we have to face that death is not necessarily a bad end point. I believe that there comes a time in a person's lifecycle when death is not only inevitable and necessary, but desired by the patient.

JJ: Suppose a patient like this man arrives in the ED and is able to communicate personal wishes coherently, and indicates that he is aware that his life is rapidly coming to a close, but when asked if he would want to be resuscitated responds by saying that he

would like to live a little longer, and that we should do what we can to help him. Would that change anyone's mind regarding the appropriateness of resuscitating him?

AD: Though this would change my mind, I wouldn't offer an option that I didn't think was appropriate. I would also be up front in saying that there may be circumstances in which resuscitation would not be successful, and therefore would not be appropriate. Patients have the autonomy to be able to accept or refuse the care we offer them based on our best clinical judgment, but that they can't demand something that we don't think is appropriate.

PR: I believe there are cases when the physician has to say "No" to further resuscitation, not because there is nothing more that we **can** do, but because there is nothing more that we **should** do. The case presented represents such an example in my judgment.

Section III: Review of the literature

Should a physician honor patient or family demands for a treatment that the physician judges to be medically futile? Determining when an intervention in medicine should not be offered on the basis of medical futility is one of the most vexing issues in medical ethics today.[2] Although the issue has long been in the forefront of ethical consideration and debate among intensivists, hospitalists, and neonatologists, it also impinges on emergency medicine. The issue of futility has arisen in medicine because of the development and implementation of interventions such as resuscitation and mechanical ventilation, which were developed to reverse life-threatening medical conditions, such as cardiac dysrhythmia. These interventions, however, are not always effective in reversing these conditions, and they may only prolong the dying process. Physicians may nevertheless feel obligated to provide these interventions because of patient or family request. Because these measures are often initiated in the ED, emergency physicians often make the judgment as to whether to initiate them.

In the case described, the initiation of life-sustaining medical treatment in the form of resuscitation is unlikely to be effective in reversing the patient's cardiopulmonary arrest. The patient's prognosis, having been bed-bound for 2 months with worsening renal failure, is extremely poor. Additionally, even if the patient is resuscitated to the point where pulses return, the likelihood that the patient will survive to discharge from the hospital is minuscule. Nonetheless, family members ask that "everything be done."

Definition of futility

The term "futile" is derived from the ancient Greek word for "leaky," and indeed, in some cases of treatments that seem unable to stave off the inevitable, it may feel to emergency physicians that the boat is sinking and the water is flowing in faster than it can be bailed out. Authors have proffered various definitions of futility in medical treatment, but the meaning and scope of futility remain very controversial issues. Criteria for futility generally can be divided into those that concern the likelihood of effectiveness, including the measure and duration of that success (also known as "quantitative" futility), and those that concern the quality of the patient's life for any duration of effectiveness of the measure (known as "qualitative" futility).

One of the most widely discussed quantitative criteria for futility asserts that a treatment with less than a 1% chance of achieving its goal is futile.[3] However, while a 1% chance that an elderly patient without decision-making capacity with a severe hemorrhagic stroke would be able to be resuscitated from a cardiopulmonary arrest may be an acceptable reason to family members to forego treatment and agree to a DNR order, the same 1% chance that their child might be resuscitated from a drowning may not be an acceptable reason to them. There is no societal consensus as to the percentage of success (other than 0%) at which the physician has no obligation to offer or provide the measure.

However, in thinking about quantitative futility it may helpful to think of two broad categories. The first category is one in which, in the physician's well-grounded judgment, the proposed intervention would not work (or would not achieve the goals expressed by the patient, when the patient had decision-making capacity). If an intervention would not work or would not achieve the goals of the patient, some medical societies' codes of ethics (including that of the American College of Emergency Physicians [ACEP]) recognize that the physician is not obligated to provide the treatment or procedure. The second category is that the intervention may work temporarily, but would only prolong the dying process (e.g., in the example above, the intervention of resuscitation may bring back a pulse and a rhythm, but the patient would not survive to discharge from the hospital, or would not survive to achieve a state that he or she would have wanted to achieve). Some would argue that life prolongation for any period of time has value, and that to forego attempts to prolong life would be making a judgment about the quality of that life, no matter how short. However this situation is categorized (quantitative or qualitative futility), there is less of a consensus in the medical ethical literature about withholding or withdrawing treatment on the basis of the intervention working only for a short time but ultimately failing to result in discharge from the hospital.

Qualitative futility posits that even though the intervention may be successful in its physiological outcome, it is not worth doing because of the cost or the quality of life that the patient would achieve. This is the most controversial category of futility. In the United States, we have nothing close to a consensus on the issue of stopping expensive treatments that prolong a life indefinitely, such as in a persistent vegetative state, except when the patient would not have wanted treatment under these circumstances. Some advocates might argue that resources would be better used for care of patients at the beginning of life, for instance on maternal health for indigent women. The United States, however, has no formal mechanism for allocation of these resources at the bedside, even if these measures result in higher healthcare costs. In contrast, by law or custom in some other countries, physicians commonly withhold or withdraw treatment based on these reasons.

Given these categories, the consensus on futility is strongest in the first (physicians are not obligated to provide interventions that would not work), less strong in the second (would not work for long, and would only prolong the dying process). There is no consensus in the third (not worth it), and there is a general practice of providing interventions that will work without consideration of cost or quality of life.

Professional obligations of emergency physicians

Emergency physicians must decide whether to offer an emergency medical treatment or procedure in a given situation, whether or not a patient accepts that offered treatment is their choice to make [4] However, there is nothing in the emergency physician–patient relationship that requires an emergency physician to provide treatment that in his or her medical opinion would not be medically beneficial to the patient. Simply put, doing everything is not always the right thing to do.

Beneficence is the principle that treatment provided actually benefits the patient.[5] Non-maleficence is the corollary principle that the emergency physician should not harm the patient.[6] Those harms may include pain or prolongation of suffering. If a therapeutic intervention cannot result in benefit, or the harm significantly outweigh the benefit, the emergency physician ought to avoid it, even if requested by the patient or the patient's family.

Professional guidance on futility

The ACEP *Code of Ethics* states that "medically non-beneficial treatment is not morally required."[7] Additionally, the American Medical Association (AMA) code of ethics recommends that all healthcare institutions adopt a policy on medical futility and proposes a "due process" approach, including provision of a second opinion, and an offer of transfer if a willing provider can be found. The AMA opinion concludes that, once the prescribed process is completed, futile interventions need not be offered.[8] However, this approach assumes a patient is in stable condition for such discussions. In the ED, a due process approach may not be practical. Nonetheless, the AMA's code endorses the physician's ability and obligation to determine futility.

The ACEP futility policy states that "physicians are under no ethical obligation to render treatments that they judge have no realistic likelihood of medical benefit to the patient. Emergency physicians' judgments in these matters should be unbiased, and should be based on available scientific evidence, and societal and professional standards . . . [For] patients in cardiac arrest who have no realistic likelihood of survival . . . emergency physicians should consider withholding or discontinuing resuscitative efforts, in both the pre-hospital and hospital settings."[9] The American Heart Association's *Guidelines for Not Starting CPR/Terminating Resuscitative Efforts* is

another example of professional guidance on when resuscitation would be ineffective.[10]

Challenges to the professional consensus concerning ineffectiveness and futility

Despite a general medical consensus that physicians need not offer ineffective treatment, there have been challenges to this consensus. One physician has written that "[I]f family members or legal surrogates for the patient want every possible measure taken to keep the patient alive, professionals should comply with this request."[11] Another physician more recently has stated that "[f]utile CPR has a limited but legitimate place in the practice of medicine." As an example he tells of resuscitative efforts for a 2-year-old boy with a large frontal encephalocele. "At the time we began our resuscitative efforts, I believed that this child was beyond suffering, whereas the psychological needs of his parents were both clinically and ethically significant."[1] This view, that futile treatment (on the basis of ineffectiveness) should nonetheless be done for the benefit of the family, is not required by law, in that there is no obligation to provide ineffective treatment to a patient to satisfy or ameliorate family needs. Additionally, this view does not have a medically supportable stopping point. The question may logically be asked, when are family needs met well enough so that futile treatment may be stopped?

Ethics consultation and futility

In cases where time might allow a bedside consultation in the ED, an opinion by an ethics consultant or ethics team can be of potential benefit, though decisions about effectiveness often must be made rapidly at the bedside in these circumstances, such as in the case that begins this chapter, where an ethics consultation would be impractical. Emergency physicians should be aware that ethics consultations are generally advisory, and the emergency physician still retains the professional authority (and responsibility) for medical decision-making.

Legal considerations

There is no legal obligation to provide ineffective or medically non-beneficial treatment. However, in the

United States there is an obligation under the Emergency Medical Treatment and Active Labor Act (EMTALA) to provide needed emergency treatment, or to stabilize the patient and transfer for treatment of the emergent medical condition.[12] In between those two legal principles lies an area where there is little legal precedent in reported case law. EMTALA would certainly preclude an emergency physician making a unilateral determination to refuse emergency treatment on the basis of the patient's quality of life (the third category), as would current emergency medical treatment standards of care. Sanctions could also include disciplinary actions and criminal charges. However, determination that treatment would be ineffective is a more complex matter.

There are very few reported cases concerning decisions not to provide treatment due to ineffectiveness, and none were found that concerned an emergency physician's bedside decision to do so. However, there are a number of cases concerning withdrawal, or proposed withdrawal, of a ventilator from a hospitalized patient.[13,14] In general, when physicians have gone to court requesting to stop a treatment that was effective in maintaining the patient's physiological functions (e.g. ventilation for a patient in persistent vegetative state), courts have been reluctant to order termination of life support. However, when physicians have made so-called unilateral decisions on futility, they have often won cases litigated after the fact of the patient's death, when the issue has been ineffectiveness.[15]

In the benchmark Baby K case, an appellate court held that physicians could not decide in advance to refuse to intubate a child with anencephaly who was spontaneously breathing as an outpatient, despite the mother's wish to have the child resuscitated when brought to the ED, since respiratory depression, when it would occur, would be an emergency medical condition that could be treated with intubation and ventilation. This case, precedent-setting for the Fourth Federal Circuit Court of Appeals district that includes Virginia, North Carolina and South Carolina, was not about medical ineffectiveness, but concerned a pre-judgment of the child's quality of life, and a blanket a priori refusal to intubate the child presenting with a treatable condition of respiratory failure, such refusal being held to be a violation of the EMTALA requirement to treat or stabilize.[16]

Texas has a unique legislated approach to resolving issues of futility. According to the Texas Advance Directive Act (TADA) "[i]f an attending physician refuses to honor a patient's advance directive or a health care or treatment decision made by or on behalf of a patient, the physician's refusal shall be reviewed by an ethics or medical committee." If the committee agrees with the physician and a 10-day period has elapsed, the physician is free of legal liability. "The attending physician may not be a member of that committee. The patient shall be given life-sustaining treatment during the review."[17] Though nothing in the statute requires physicians to provide ineffective treatment, the statute may add a level of statutory complexity to an ED physician's evaluation of effectiveness, and may actually result in ED physicians erring on the side of what they may judge as highly likely (though not definitely) ineffective treatment to take advantage of the immunity provided by the statute in situations where they would not do so in a non-TADA state.

In other states, the statutory language used may support an emergency physician's ability to determine ineffectiveness. For instance, California law states that "A health care provider or health care institution may decline to comply with an individual health care instruction or health care decision that requires medically ineffective health care or health care contrary to generally accepted health care standards applicable to the health care provider or institution."[18]

The most significant legal danger may not be an allegation of a violation of EMTALA, or of the standard of care, but instead, an allegation of infliction of emotional distress, or outrage, by acting in an insensitive or secretive manner.[19] Any decision not to provide requested treatment on the basis of ineffectiveness should be accompanied by a sensitive but candid disclosure of the medical rationale, with the positive message that everything effective, including comfort measures where appropriate, is being been done.

Some emergency physicians may conclude that, if they wish to avoid any possibility of legal liability, they should do anything and everything the patient or family requests under any circumstances, no matter how ineffective. Better a family satisfied that everything was done rather than having to explain, after the fact, why something was not done. However, the price paid for providing ineffective treatment for the benefit of family is abdication of professional judgment, infliction of unnecessary and often harmful treatment on the patient, and, as a side effect, increasing healthcare costs.

Responsibilities of emergency physicians with regard to determining futility

Emergency physicians have the professional responsibility to determine futility (lack of medical effectiveness) objectively. They should accurately assess the patient's current medical status. They should know disease and injury trajectories, including prognosis and outcomes with interventions. They should know and follow guidelines where appropriate, such as the *Guidelines for Not Starting CPR/Terminating Resuscitative Efforts.*[10] They should communicate with patients and families openly and effectively. They should also participate in (and collaborate with other national experts and medical specialties) in setting guidelines.

Emergency physicians can learn useful concepts and methods from the newest subspecialty of emergency medicine: hospice and palliative medicine. These techniques include giving and reinforcing information on prognosis, communicating bad news, assisting in advance care planning (e.g. discussing and writing DNR orders) and withholding or withdrawing treatment (where appropriate), or beginning the process through discussion.[20]

The emergency physician should explain that, despite withholding or withdrawing ineffective treatment, the patient will still be provided care and comfort until the end of life. This includes allowing families to be with the patient, treating the patient's pain, dyspnea, and other symptoms, and utilizing support personnel such as chaplains or social workers to help during this very difficult time.

In summary, whether to offer and perform an emergency medical treatment or procedure in a given situation is the responsibility of the emergency physician.

Physicians are under no ethical obligation to render treatments that they may judge have no realistic likelihood of medical benefit to the patient.[9]

"Ineffectiveness" as a standard for medical futility has the greatest ethical consensus and most utility in emergency medicine. Emergency physicians have the expertise and obligation to determine the patient's prognosis, communicate bad news, assist in advance care planning, and when appropriate, withhold or withdraw ineffective treatment, despite the patient or families wishes. When a cure is impossible, emergency physicians retain an obligation to care.[21]

Section IV: Recommendations

• Recognize the rare circumstances in which the issue of futility in emergency medicine arises—when a proposed intervention would be ineffective (or would not achieve the goals expressed by the patient, when the patient had decision-making capacity).
• Be cognizant of the professional codes, institutional policies, and case and statutory laws that support emergency medical determinations of futility in certain circumstances.
• Exercise well-grounded clinical judgment, based on scientific evidence, in making futility determinations based on ineffectiveness.
• Communicate openly and compassionately with patient, family, and caregivers about decisions to stop—or not to start—medical treatment based on clinical judgment.
• Continue to care for the patient with palliative measures when appropriate.

Acknowledgement

The author thanks Dr. John Moskop for his review and helpful comments.

References

1. Troug RD. (2010) Is it always wrong to perform futile CPR? *N Engl J Med.* 362, 477–9.
2. Junkerman C, Derse A, Schiedermayer D. Futility/unreasonable patient requests. In: *Practical Ethics for Students, Interns and Residents: Short Reference Manual*, 3rd ed. Hagerstown, MD: University Publishing Group, pp. 33–8.
3. Schneiderman LJ, Jecker NS, Jonsen AR. (1990) Medical futility: Its meaning and ethical implications. *Ann Intern Med.* 112, 949–54.

4. Beauchamp TL, Childress JF. (2009) Respect for autonomy. In: *Principles of Biomedical Ethics*. New York, NY: Oxford University Press, pp. 99–148.

5. Beauchamp TL, Childress JF. (2009) Beneficence. In: *Principles of Biomedical Ethics*. New York, NY: Oxford University Press, pp. 197–239.

6. Beauchamp TL, Childress JF. (2009) Nonmaleficence. In: *Principles of Biomedical Ethics*. New York, NY: Oxford University Press, pp. 149–96.

7. American College of Emergency Physicians. (2010) *Code of Ethics*. Section D(3)(c). The emergency physician's relationship with society: Central Tenets: Prudent Stewardship without Quality Compromise. Dallas, TX: American College of Emergency Physicians Press.

8. Council on Ethical and Judicial Affairs. (2010) Opinion 2.037 issued June 1997 based on the report, "*Medical Futility in End-of-Life Care*" adopted December 1996 (*JAMA*. 1999; 281, 937–41). Chicago, IL: American Medical Association Press.

9. American College of Emergency Physicians. (2008) *Non Beneficial (Futile) Emergency Medical Interventions Policy*. (Approved 1998; Reaffirmed 2002; Reaffirmed 2008). Dallas, TX: American College of Emergency Physicians Press.

10. Morrison LJ, Kierzek G, Diekema DS, et al. (2010) American Heart Association Guidelines for Cardiopulmonary Resuscitation and Emergency Cardiovascular Care Science Part 3: Ethics. *Circulation*. 122: S665–S675.

11. Raffin TA. (1992) Perspectives on clinical medical ethics. In: Hall JB, Schmidt GA, Wood LDH (eds) *Principles of Critical Care*. New York, NY: McGraw-Hill, pp. 2185–204.

12. Emergency Medical Treatment and Active Labor Act (EMTALA), 42 USC 1395dd (1986) Publication 99–272.

13. In re Wanglie, No. PX-91-283 (Minn. 4th Dist. Ct. Hennepin County, July 1, 1991).

14. Betancourt *v*. Trinitas Hospital, No A-3849-08T2 (N.J Super Ct., App Div Aug 13, 2010).

15. Gilgunn *v*. Massachusetts General Hospital. No. SUCV92-4820 (Supr. Ct., Suffolk County, Mass. April 21, 1995).

16. In re Baby "K," 832 F. Supp. 1022 (ED Va. 1993), aff'd 16 F3d 590 (4th Cir.), cert. denied, 115 S.Ct. 91 (1994).

17. TEX HS. CODE ANN. § 166.046. Procedure if Not Effectuating a Directive or Treatment Decision. Added by Acts 1999, 76th Leg., ch. 450, Sec. 1.03, eff. Sept. 1, 1999. Amended by Acts 2003, 78th Leg., ch. 1228, Sec. 3, 4, eff. June 20, 2003.

18. Cal. Prob. Code Sec. 4735 (2011).

19. Pope TM. (2010) The law's impact on the resolution of end-of-life conflicts in the intensive care unit. *Crit Care Med*. 39, 223.

20. Quest TE, Marco CA, Derse AR. (2009) Hospice and palliative medicine: new subspecialty, new opportunities. *Ann Emerg Med*. 54(1), 94–102.

21. Marco CA, Larkin GL, Moskop JC, et al. (2000) Determination of "futility" in emergency medicine. *Ann Emerg Med*. 35, 604–12.

Representing vulnerable populations

12 The care of minors in the emergency department

Chloë-Maryse Baxter

Pediatric Emergency Medicine Advanced Trainee, Sydney Children's Hospital, Randwick, NSW, Australia

Section I: Case presentation

A 5-week-old baby girl was brought to the emergency department (ED) by her mother. The baby had a fever and decreased feeding for several hours. The mother believed that the baby probably had the same respiratory virus as the other two young children in the family but had been advised to bring the baby in to the ED by her naturopath. Past medical history indicated that none of the children in the family had been vaccinated; the baby had a home birth, and had received most of her primary care from the naturopath. The emergency physician tried to convince the mother to allow a full septic workup since there were no focal signs of infection and a non-specific rash had developed in addition to a documented febrile spike in the ED. The mother agreed to urine and blood tests; results were negative for a urinary tract infection, and the white blood cell count was normal. Although she allowed intravenous (IV) fluids, the mother refused a lumbar puncture (LP) and antibiotics, stating she had been advised against these by the naturopath.

The emergency physician called child protective services, which removed the baby from the custody of the mother. The emergency physician followed the hospital protocol for febrile infants: LP, steroids and IV antibiotics. Once completed, the baby was admitted and the mother was permitted to be with the baby throughout the admission. The following day the baby was returned to the custody of the parents. Following the negative workup and improved course of the child, the pediatrician felt the baby was no longer at risk, and most likely had a viral infection.

Section II: Discussion

Dr. Peter Rosen: In our case, the mother filed a lawsuit against the state, against the emergency physician, and against the hospital. The emergency physician was worried about the child because on the night of admission, after a bolus of IV fluids, the child spiked a temperature to approximately 39 °C. He did not know whether this fever was bacteriologic or viral in origin, and was worried about the appearance of the child. Because of this, he decided a complete bacteriologic workup was necessary. There are real legal constraints on physician behavior in cases of child neglect and abuse. What are the physician's legal responsibilities?

Dr. Arthur Derse: In general, you do need the permission of the parent to be able to do diagnostic workups and procedures on a child. The law would protect any physician who took measures that a reasonable parent with an understanding of the situation would agree to. The situation is more complicated in the event a

Ethical Problems in Emergency Medicine: A Discussion-Based Review, First Edition. John Jesus, Shamai A. Grossman, Arthur R. Derse, James G. Adams, Richard Wolfe, and Peter Rosen.
© 2012 John Wiley & Sons, Ltd. Published 2012 by John Wiley & Sons, Ltd.

129

physician believes certain interventions are appropriate, but is simultaneously opposed by the parent. As a physician, your responsibility is to act in the best interest of the child. In the discussed case, there is a reasonable concern the child might have a bad outcome without an appropriate assessment for serious bacterial infections.

PR: I should add some additional information: the clinical team wished to speak with the naturopath, and the mother resisted, saying, "There is no point in doing that. I know what's best for my child. I keep a clean house, there is no way she could have a bacterial infection, and my husband will agree. My naturopath told me to come to the hospital for tests, but suggested that I refuse antibiotics and not allow you to perform an LP." She also added that she had done research on the internet, and referenced an article from the *New England Journal of Medicine* dated about 30 years prior about LPs causing meningitis.[1] The naturopath testified that if she had been contacted in this situation, she would have told the mother to go along with the doctor's recommendations. The parents filed the lawsuit because they felt the state did not have the right to remove the child from the custody of the parents, and prevent them from making medical decisions for their child. She also stated that this temporary transfer of custody had undermined her maternal feelings and her ability to bond with the child, and had destroyed her marriage. If you were seeing a child you thought probably had a viral infection, but the child was young and unvaccinated, how would you feel about not pursuing a workup?

Dr. Chloë Baxter: At 5 weeks this baby would not have had any immunizations (except for hepatitis B) based on the standard schedule with which I am familiar. At 5 weeks, babies like this are incredibly difficult to diagnose. Without really good reasons to the contrary, any 5-week-old baby who presents with a fever should undergo a full septic workup. One possible response to this scenario may involve some form of compromise. For instance, there have been studies that show a period of inpatient observation can allow for further parental counseling and education while awaiting laboratory and culture results that might confirm a viral etiology to the child's ailment.[2] Parents treated as such might be more inclined to agree to other interventions at a later date.

The physician could also contact the naturopath despite the mother's wishes to the contrary. Because the mother trusts the naturopath, it may be useful to tap into resources that may provide further information about the patient and family, and may better persuade the mother that a workup is necessary. The American Academy of Pediatricians refers to this parental comfort zone as the "medical home."

Dr. James Adams: Thinking about a compromise is important. As Aristotle would say, what is important is a golden mean; that is to say, in ethics what is most important is not simply a display of virtue, but also the struggle to find a middle ground. Going to child services should not be the first course of action. The initial strategy should not be direct opposition to the parents, but to try to find a cooperative stance. If the situation ends up necessitating the involvement of child services, the mother should understand that this was a last resort, and not something the physician wanted to do to demonstrate his superior knowledge or express power over the mother. I think it is important to emphasize that we are in a dilemma. The mother should understand that we have responsibilities to the child, and that if we believe there exists a significant risk to the child, then these responsibilities necessitate action.

PR: The physician in this case spent almost 2 hours trying to convince the mother to allow him to care for the child, and called the protective services when the child spiked the new fever. Have you ever had to call upon an outside agency to remove a child from the custody of the parents in order to protect the child from medical neglect?

Dr. Shamai Grossman: In the situation in which I facilitated removal of a child from the custody of the parents, it was clear the parents were not acting in the best interests of the child. It is worth acknowledging that the mother in our case sincerely believed that she was making decisions in the best interests of her child. The fact that the mother did not have adequate knowledge of disease processes and the necessary diagnostic tests is somewhat irrelevant; she had very different ideas of how children should be treated.

PR: I agree that this is not clear neglect. Parents often have beliefs about what is best for their child that conflict with medical opinion. We've all had to deal with this issue in treating children of Jehovah's Witnesses and Christian Scientists. Trying to convince parents that their own beliefs are trumped by our own is very difficult. How should a physician proceed in imposing the modern medical paradigm on parents who have a different belief system?

AD: There are some circumstances, in which we absolutely should not allow parents to adjudicate, and the law protects us in making that judgment. In a famous case in the 1940s, the US Supreme Court stated that parents are free to make martyrs of themselves, but not their children. In situations where a parent refuses a life-saving intervention for the child, I can't imagine a court preventing the physician from proceeding with the intervention. When the child's condition is not life- or limb-threatening, it's less obvious that physicians have a right to intervene. Essentially, as evidence of a true emergency increases, so too does the legitimacy of medical intervention a physician feels compelled to administer, even over the wishes of the parent.

PR: Some institutions have an ethics consultation service, which may be helpful in mediating physician–family disputes, because it gives the family members the opportunity to further articulate their concerns. If the mother trusts the opinion of a physician other than the emergency physician, it may be helpful to contact the trusted physician. Sometimes parents will relate better to one physician than another. If those options aren't available, you don't have a choice but to be aggressive in your treatment when confronted with an ill-appearing child.

AD: If you're going to be sued, you want to be sued for doing what you thought was right. You're in a much worse position if nothing is done for the child who subsequently has a bad outcome.

PR: That is a very important point to acknowledge. As far as I am aware, every [US] state has a statute protecting physicians from being sued for invoking child protective services where the physician has a concern regarding the child's safety. It is a difficult ethical position that most parents do not understand, but one which is omnipresent in our legal system.

Parents cannot withhold care for their children. This legal understanding stems from an increasing awareness of child abuse, and from the courts believing that children need legal protection until they are of the age to make autonomous decisions. The parents in this case did not understand that the conflict did not exist between the physician's ego and the mother's medical vision, but rather the state's choice. Without the child protective services' permission, the physician would not have been able to proceed with the workup.

AD: It is extremely rare for a physician to lose a legal suit when acting on concerns regarding a child's health interests. This is one of the few concepts over which there is widespread consensus among legislatures. Any judicial decision in favor of parental autonomy over a child's health interests as viewed by a physician would represent a move away from protecting children, as it may prevent physicians from acting on future clinical concerns.

PR: The emergency physician behaved in exemplary fashion. He tried to persuade the mother, and when that failed, he did not hesitate to act on what he knew to be in the child's best interests. I believe it is impossible to save a life negligently. That's what he was trying to do—save this child's life. I appreciate that it's an uncomfortable decision to strip parents of the right to have the final say about their children. It comes down to a question of which paradigm ultimately has greater positive impact on the child's best interests, and when a child is clearly sick the moral paradigm of saving human life takes precedence.

Dr. John Jesus: With that in mind, I'd like to raise a separate issue related to the discomfort we feel in going against parents' wishes. I believe some of this discomfort comes from a concern that if we act against what a parent wants for the child, we threaten the trust and respect the parent has for the medical establishment. Parental attitudes about the medical establishment may impact the child's safety, because parents may be more reluctant to bring the child to a hospital for future ailments. There is a body of literature attempting to link trust and respect of the medical establishment with effectiveness and compliance with medical care. The manner by which medical interventions are carried out may be as important as the interventions themselves.

131

CB: That said, there are recent trends in how the courts view the relationship between patients, parents, and doctors that are worth noting. It seems to me that courts have become less willing to simply go along with physician opinion. For example, I am aware of a case in Canada in which an anemic child of Jehovah's Witness parents needed a surgical procedure, and the child was going to need a transfusion. The parents took the case to court, because they had found another hospital willing to attempt the procedure without transfusions. The court allowed the parents to pursue this route even though the child's original doctors had insisted a transfusion was medically necessary.[3]

SG: It is my understanding that contradictory or competing medical opinions cannot be weighed equally by the court. The court itself cannot make medical decisions.

AD: The situation you raise is different in two important ways. First, the fact that the court weighed these opinions equally does not speak to how the ED physician comported himself in the scenario. Rather, it simply raised an alternative option for the family to pursue rather than to avoid surgery altogether. Secondly, the situation was not an emergency necessitating immediate action. Rather, there was sufficient time to obtain a different opinion and offer the parents a choice. In general, the courts will allow an intervention that is opposed to parental stated wishes if there is broad medical agreement on the indications of the intervention. The possible exception would be with a mature minor, or the patient under the age of 18 but whom the physician believes has decision-making capacity.

JJ: A child's ability to engage in medical decision-making is a gradual process. A 5-year-old cannot comprehend risks and benefits of medical therapy. To the extent possible, however, it is important to include the patient in the medical decision-making process and attempt to educate the child about the interventions that will be performed and why the physician feels the intervention is important. With the assistance of child life specialists, this role is becoming increasingly popular in certain pediatric EDs, because it lessens the anxiety young patients feel, increases their cooperation during the procedure, and changes an often traumatic and difficult intervention into a more pleasant experience with which everyone agrees and understands.

AD: The situation you just described is more applicable to the very young. What if the patient is older?

JJ: The situation is more complicated when the patient is older than 14, which is generally when some patients will begin to develop capacity to make reasoned decisions. Because there is no switch or arbitrary date that can identify when patients have developed the decision-making capacity, these situations need to be addressed on a case-by-case basis. We have already identified several categories of patients who can be treated without parental consent—those who are emancipated, those with sexually transmitted infections, and those who are pregnant, married, or serving in the military. In my opinion, the ethical justification of recognizing the ability of patients within those categories to make healthcare decisions autonomously is more arbitrary than recognizing the decisions made by a mature minor.

A very difficult situation would arise if a physician was faced with a mature minor who refuses a life-saving or life-lengthening intervention. The classic example involves the 17-year-old patient with metastatic lymphoma who has undergone radiation and chemotherapy for the last 10 years, recognizes the poor prognosis, and wishes to live out the rest of life without suffering through further radiation and chemotherapy. In this scenario, one could argue persuasively that the patient has a tremendous amount of experiential knowledge, and therefore may have a greater understanding of the benefits and burdens of the treatment and how they may fit with in the child's personal life goals and values, than any physician in the room. If a physician assesses and confirms a minor's decision-making capacity, then the physician should respect the patient's decision.

PR: The case was settled against the state, but dismissed against child protective services, but the appeals court returned the case to the lower court to let a jury decide the question as to whether the physician had exaggerated his concern for the child when communicating with the police and child protective agencies. The sad fact is that the physician was truly worried about the child, and tried to express that concern not only to the mother, but to child protective services and the police.

In June 2010, a jury found that the physician (in a compromise vote), had exaggerated his concerns to the child protective services and the police, but awarded the mother no damages. They unanimously rejected the mother's claims that the police, hospital staff, or the ED physician infringed on the mother's constitutional rights as a parent. It also freed the defendants from any liability for interfering with the mother's custodial relationship with her daughter.

Section III: Review of the literature

Treating children in the ED is often more complicated than treating adults because they may be too young to understand the implications of treatment, and cannot consent to certain procedures that need to be performed. Parents may be unavailable or unwilling to give consent, and physicians may have to use alternative means to ensure the child's best interests are upheld. This case is an example of what can happen when parents and doctors disagree on the best treatment for the child, and the difficulties that can arise when both parties believe they are acting in the child's best interests. Some ethical questions which arise from the case presented include:
• If the mother decided to leave after the urine and blood test results were returned, is the doctor under any obligation to treat the baby? Is the physician's duty of care to the family or the child, and when does this end?
• If parents and physician disagree on the best treatment for the child, how should this best be resolved?
• Why are parents allowed to refuse vaccination for their children but not medical treatment?

Duty of care

Duty of care is a legal concept that is based on an ethical consideration: that of "love thy neighbor," or in law, "do not injure thy neighbor." It imposes an obligation to prevent foreseeable harm to others through acts or omissions, and is grounded in the ethical concept of beneficence, to help those in need.[4,5]

A duty of care exists whenever there is an interaction between an expert and a novice, whether that is a realty agent and a house-buyer, or a doctor and a patient. No formal contract is required between the two parties for a duty of care to exist, and the larger the gap in expertise, the greater the obligation. Children are owed a greater duty of care than adults because they are less able to look after themselves or make reasonable decisions. The doctor's main obligation is to the patient, and all other parties come secondary. However, in considering the child, one has to also consider the parent who will be responsible for ongoing and future care outside the hospital. If a patient at risk leaves (or is taken from) the hospital, the doctor is still under obligation to take reasonable steps to minimize any potential harm to the patient. Establishing that a duty of care has been breached is the first step in finding that a physician has been negligent, and if the doctor in this case had failed to act and the baby had come to harm, then the physician could have been open to litigation for negligence.

Consent and refusal of consent to treatment

Requiring consent to treatment respects individuals' right to autonomy, but this is qualified by their capacity for self-determination. Legally, anyone under the age of 18 years is a minor with regard to medical treatment, and therefore parental consent is required before treatment can commence.[6] There are several exceptions to this rule that allow physicians to treat minors in the absence of parental consent[7-9]:
• Emergency treatment is required
• The minor is emancipated, e.g., married, in military service
• The minor is mature enough to understand the benefits and risks of the treatment proposed and able to make a voluntary and rational decision (usually from around 14 years of age)
• Certain medical conditions are involved, e.g., mental health, pregnancy, sexually transmitted infections.

Although the mature minor doctrine is not recognized by the US Supreme Court, some states such as Illinois, Pennsylvania, and Massachusetts have recognized this doctrine, and use it in determining the maturity of a minor in medical decision-making. In some states, there are some procedures that involve issues that are regarded as too complex, or consequences that are too enduring for even an emancipated or mature minor to give consent, e.g. abortion or sterilization. In such cases, the parents or the courts should be involved in order to make such decisions.[10]

Consent and assent

Underlying the concept of consent to treatment is the idea that the doctor–patient relationship is a partnership. Fostering an honest and trusting relationship will allow the most appropriate care to be given and enhance the quality and outcomes of treatment now and in the future. In this vein, the American Academy of Pediatrics (AAP) has recommended that assent from minors be obtained, even if this is not legally required.[7] This involves bringing the child into the partnership at the appropriate developmental level. Examples of how to do this include providing information and education of the child's condition, investigations and treatment; assessing the child's understanding and capacity to make treatment decisions; and assuring the patient that he or she has a choice with respect to alternatives in treatment (although if this is not the case then that should be communicated as well). All discussions with the child should be done using appropriate language and communication strategies, such as play.

When a minor refuses assent

In some circumstances a minor's refusal to consent should be respected, for example, in instances where the treatment can be delayed for a time, or if the child is being asked to join a research study. However, if the child refuses an investigation or procedure that the doctor feels is necessary, then a parent can consent on behalf of the child. On the one hand, this seems contradictory: if a child has the capacity to consent to treatment surely that must mean that there is also the capacity to refuse. However, while adults are allowed to refuse treatment on irrational grounds, or on no grounds at all, if both the physician and the parent are in agreement that a treatment is in the best interests of the child, it can be assumed that a child's refusal is not based on rational grounds, and is invalid.[11-13] The minor may have very good reasons for the refusal, e.g., fear of pain and side effects of

chemotherapy, but the cognitive stage of their development may prevent their making a truly informed or mature decision.

Research has shown that the cognitive development of children at 14 years of age is sufficiently approximate to that of adults as to enable them to make their own decisions.[14] At this stage, they are able to deal with abstractions, use deductive and inductive reasoning, apply reason to hypothetical situations, think about the future, and consider different options and their consequences.[15] However, making a mature decision depends on more than just cognitive development. A young person's social development is also important, and studies indicate that at 14 years, a young person may not have developed an internal capability for free, deliberate choice.[16] This results from emotional development and a sense of distinct personhood. In early adolescence, young people have a greater tendency than at any other time towards conformity, whether this is a desire to conform to authority or to their peers depends on prior experiences, individual qualities, confidence, prior relationships with authority, and emotional state. When determining young people's competence, it is not sufficient simply to consider their cognitive differences and similarities with adults, but also their maturity of judgment. It is argued that adolescents are more likely to differ from adults in their sense of responsibility (autonomy, identity, and self-reliance), their perspective (sense of morality and context) and their temperance (regulation of emotion, avoidance of extremes, and non-impulsivity).[17] However, the way in which these differences affect the young person's maturity of judgment has not been sufficiently subjected to empirical research to make a definitive assessment of the decision-making capacity with respect to medical treatment.

Most states have yet to address the issues accompanying the mature minor doctrine, while others either do not recognize it at all (Georgia), or have inadequately established its application. In those jurisdictions that recognize the mature minor, the minor has the same right as a competent adult to refuse life-sustaining treatment. In one case, a 17-year-old leukemic Jehovah's Witness was permitted to refuse a life-saving transfusion.[18] However, in another case a hospital petitioned a court for an order authorizing necessary medical treatment including blood transfusions for a 17-year-old patient, after the patient and parents refused blood transfusions based on religious beliefs.[19] While the court in that case gave credit to the "mature minor" doctrine, it found that the patient was not a mature minor, and therefore, his refusal to consent to blood transfusions was not based upon a mature understanding of his own religious beliefs or of the fatal consequences to himself. Only one state (Virginia) permits a 14-year-old to refuse life-saving treatment, if the parents also agree.[20]

When parents refuse consent

Even if a child assents to medical treatment, it is important to obtain parental consent. This is not only a legal requirement, but makes good sense, and is essential in fostering a strong doctor–family relationship that will benefit the child in the future. The AAP and the American College of Emergency Physicians recommend that EDs strive to provide patient- and family-centered care (PFCC), as this will optimize the child's care. PFCC considers the strengths, cultures, traditions, and expertise that all members of this partnership bring to the relationship.[21] It embraces the following concepts: (1) providing care for a person, not a condition; (2) the patient is best understood in the context of his or her family, culture, values, and goals; and (3) respecting that context will result in better health care, safety, and patient satisfaction.

As important as PFCC may be, any decisions must be in line with what the wider society would approve. There have been cases where the parents refused to consent to medical treatment on religious grounds. However, the courts have held that denying medical care to a child is not within the parents' First Amendment right of freedom of religion: "The right to practice religion freely does not include the liberty to expose . . . a child . . . to ill health or death. Parents may be free to become martyrs themselves. But it does not follow that they are free . . . to make martyrs of their children . . . "[22] Therefore, refusing consent to treatment on religious grounds is not necessarily a sufficient reason, although a court would aim to find a compromise if possible.

If the parents are able and willing to look after their child, then it is in the child's best interests to ultimately remain with that family. Removing a child from such a situation should only be a last resort. The right way forward may involve using the courts who will aim to establish what is in the child's best interests. Recently, however, there has been discussion that the optimal approach is that which causes the least harm non-maleficence may trump beneficence.

Prevention versus cure: parents refusing childhood vaccinations

Vaccination has been one the great public health successes of recent times, contributing to the eradication of infectious diseases such as polio, and reducing the incidence of others such as measles.[23] The United States, France, Italy, Croatia, Poland, and Taiwan are among the few countries in the world where some or all childhood vaccinations are mandatory. Other governments believe just as strongly in the immunization of children, but find that a satisfactory compliance rate results if vaccination is voluntary.

The anti-vaccination movement is nothing new, having accompanied the first compulsory immunizations in the nineteenth century. There has been a resurgence, however, due to publicity from celebrities and through the media.[24,25] Forty-eight of the 50 US states allow exemptions from vaccination for religious reasons, but only 20 states allow parents to decline immunization for "philosophic" reasons.[26] Although the number of children who receive no vaccines is low (<1%), around 85% of pediatricians annually will encounter a parent who refuses at least one vaccination.[27,28] As doctors, it is important to understand and work with such parents, if we are to stand any chance of helping our patients, their children.

Parents who refuse vaccination for their children tend to be white and of higher education and salary levels.[29] Vaccination is almost always refused because they fear that it may cause their children harm.[30–33] They believe, based on their knowledge and experience (however limited), that the risk of harm of vaccination outweighs the potential benefits. Vaccination has, in fact, become a victim of its own success: the diseases that it protects against are no longer prevalent in society. Parents do not see how ill children can become, let alone the complications that can sometimes arise from these diseases. On the other hand, possible links between vaccination and autism, multiple sclerosis, and sudden infant death are discussed in the media regularly, and there are stories of children who have been damaged by vaccination, and whose families have been compensated by the

National Vaccine Injury Compensation Program. It is not hard to see why parents exposed to such information, may decide that, despite the statistics, they would be placing their child at greater risk of harm by vaccinating than not. Something else to consider is that an injection is an action, and may be harder for some people to reconcile with if something goes wrong. Although ethically there may be no difference between an action and an omission when the intention and the outcome are the same, a parent may perceive an emotional difference between the responsibility that comes with agreeing to an action that could potentially cause harm versus an omission to act. This may be true even though the risk of harm may actually be greater in the latter instance.

One issue that is of particular concern when parents refuse to vaccinate their children, is the risk imposed on the greater community. Choosing to vaccinate not only protects the vaccinated child, but also helps to protect the whole society (even those who are unvaccinated) through the effect of herd immunity and the generally low incidence of the disease.[34] The required proportion of the population that needs to be immunized to establish herd immunity varies depending on the disease. For example, 85% of infants need to be vaccinated against *Haemophilus influenzae* type B disease, and 95% of children for measles.[35,36] Pertussis continues to circulate even with high levels of immunization, mainly due to diminishing immunity in adults. This is problematic since almost all deaths from whooping cough occur in babies under 3 months who are too young to be immunized.[37] There are some individuals who cannot be vaccinated (e.g., the immunocompromised or those allergic to a vaccine component) as well as others who, despite being vaccinated, have not mounted an appropriate immune response. These individuals rely on herd immunity to protect them from contracting illnesses the vaccines they are unable to receive are designed to prevent. Without sufficient herd immunity, these populations, in particular, are at risk for debilitating infections.

If vaccination is so important to society and to individual children, then should it not be compulsory, with no room for objections? There appears to be a conflict between the utilitarian goal of achieving the greatest good for the greatest number through vaccination, and the desire to respect the autonomy of parents to make decisions on how to best raise their children.

Refusing vaccination is not the same as refusing treatment for a disease. Vaccination involves taking perfectly healthy children, and exposing them to a risk of harm, albeit a small one, on the basis that it **may** provide some benefit in the future. Most physicians are not aware of all the potential complications of vaccines, and are unlikely to inform their patients of these, but there is no doubt that harm can result from vaccination. For example, rotavirus vaccination has been found to result in an increased risk of intussusception, and a flu vaccine in Australia was withdrawn for use in children under 5 years after it was linked to a significant increase in febrile convulsions and other complications in this age group.[38–40] Treating a child with a disease, in contrast, involves a child who is already at imminent risk of harm, and reducing that risk through administering therapy. It would, therefore, not be possible to ethically enforce vaccination unless situations arose such that there was clear benefit that outweighed potential harms as in a pandemic disease outbreak or bioterrorist attack. There are alternatives to compulsory vaccination such as education, inducements, and outbreak legislation.[41] These measures are employed in countries where vaccinations are voluntary, and achieve satisfactory success rates to avoid making them mandatory.[42]

There are some who would consider vaccine refusers as child abusers, and many doctors continue to decline seeing unvaccinated children in their practice.[28,43] The AAP advises against this since it is clearly not in the best interests of the child to close the door permanently on the family, and cut off any potential care for the child in the future.[44] Instead, it is recommended to respectfully listen to parental concerns, explain the risk of non-immunization, and discuss the specific vaccines that are of most concern to parents.[44] Refusing vaccinations is a risky decision to make, but we do not penalize parents for smoking near their children, or feeding them unhealthy food; instead we aim to help and educate them in making wiser choices.

Conclusion

Parents generally act in the best interests of their children and usually both physicians and parents agree on a proposed medical treatment. There are several circumstances where parental consent is not required, such as in cases of emergency treatment, an emancipated minor, or certain medical conditions.

Where parental consent is required, but parents and physicians disagree on the treatment plan, the doctor should take all reasonable steps to achieve an acceptable outcome or compromise. Ultimately, emergency physicians must recognize that their duty of care is to the patient without reservation; and failing to act in the best interests of the child could lead to charges of negligence. Legal recourse is only indicated if no suitable solution is achievable through negotiation and compromise.

A child's ability to consent varies with cognitive development and physicians must adapt their approach in respect of this. A child's assent to treatment should be sought wherever feasible, and in the case of the mature minor, their refusal of consent is considered equivalent to a refusal from an adult and should be respected. It is rare, however, that a mature minor is granted the ability to refuse consent to life-saving treatment, and such cases should be adjudicated by the courts.

Vaccination is one medical procedure that parents may refuse unless there is imminent danger from a vaccine-preventable disease. Parents who refuse childhood vaccinations are generally doing so because they fear vaccinations to be potentially harmful. Understanding the basis for their concerns is the first step in educating and supporting these parents in making wise health choices for their children.

Section IV: Recommendations

• In situations where parents and physicians disagree on medical care, whether it is preventive (i.e., vaccination) or curative (i.e., IV antibiotics), emphasize the common ground: both parties have the child's best interests in mind.
• Pursue all avenues to reach a compromise, if possible by involving both parents and the family's medical home; seek additional help from other physicians and specialists; involve the courts if no compromise is achievable.
• The "mature minor" is capable of providing appropriate informed consent for treatment. It is, however, unlikely that courts will uphold the rights of a minor to refuse life-saving treatment.
• In emergency situations, defined as conditions requiring prompt treatment, and not limited to potentially fatal or disabling conditions, any child may be treated without parental consent.
• Failure to provide treatment in emergency situations may constitute negligence.

References

1. Teale DW, Dashevsky B, Rakusan T, et al. (1981) Meningitis after Lumbar Puncture in Children with Bacteremia *N Engl J Med.* 305(18), 1079–81
2. Baker MD, Anver JR. (2008) The febrile infant: what's new? *Clin Pediatr Emerg Med.* 9(4), 213–20
3. Mian M. (2005) Ethics and law in paediatrics: Case 2. In: Baxter CM, Brennan MG, Coldicott Y, et al. (eds) *The Practical Guide to Medical Ethics and Law*, 2nd ed. Knutsford: Pastest, p. 266.
4. Jupin v. Kask, 849 N.E.2d 829, 835 (Mass. 2006).
5. McCall v. Wilder, 913 S.W.2d 150, 153 (Tenn. 1995).
6. Pipel HF. (1972) Minors rights to medical care. *Alb L Rev.* 36, 462–3.
7. Committee on Bioethics. (1995) American Academy of Pediatrics Policy Statement: Informed consent, parental permission, and assent in pediatric practice, (RE9510). *Pediatrics.* 95, 314–17.
8. Appelbaum P, Lidz C, Miesel A. (1987) *Informed Consent: Legal Theory and Practice.* New York, NY: Oxford University Press.
9. Consent for Emergency Medical Services for Children and Adolescents. (2003) Committee on pediatric emergency medicine. *Pediatrics.* 111(3), 703–6.
10. Guttmacher Institute. State Policies in Brief. *Parental Involvement in Minors' Abortions.* Available at: www.guttmacher.org/sections/abortion.php?scope=U.S.%20specific. Accessed June 1, 2011.
11. Cruzan v. Director, Missouri Department of Health, 497 U.S. 261 (1990)
12. McKenzie v. Doctors Hospital of Hollywood, Inc., (No. 90-6961-Civ U.S. Dist. CT S.D. Fl., June 24, 1991)
13. Sidaway v. Board of Governors of the Bethlem Royal Hospital and the Maudsley Hospital [1985] AC 871.
14. Piaget J, Inhelder B. (1969) *The Psychology of the Child.* New York, NY: Basic Books.
15. Weithorn LA, Campbell SB. (1983) The competency of children and adolescents to make informed treatment decisions. *Child Dev.* 9, 285.
16. Grisso T, Vierling L. (1978) Minors' consent to treatment: a developmental perspective. *Prof Psychol.* 9, 412.
17. Cauffman E, Steinberg L. (1995) The cognitive and affective influences on adolescent decision-making. *Temple L Rev.* 68, 1763–88.
18. Re E.G., 549 N.E. 2d 322 (IL 1989).

19. Re Long Island Jewish Medical Center, 557 N.Y.S. 2d 239 (1990).

20. Mercurio, MR. (2007) An adolescent's refusal of medical treatment: implications of the Abraham Cheerix case. *Pediatrics*. 120, 1357–8.

21. Committee on Pediatric Emergency Medicine. (2008) Patient- and family-centered care of children in the emergency department. *Pediatrics*. 122, e511–e21.

22. State *v*. Perricone, N. J. Rep., Vol. 37, p. 463, Atlantic Reporter, 2d Series, Vol 181, p. 751, 1962.

23. Plotkin SA. (2005) Vaccines: past, present and future. *Nat Med*. 11 Suppl, S5–S11.

24. Wolfe RM, Sharp LK. (2002) Anti-vaccinationists past and present. *BMJ*. 325, 430–2.

25. Kaufman M. (1967) The American anti-vaccinationists and their arguments. *Bull Hist Med*. 41, 463–78.

26. Johns Hopkins Bloomberg School of Public Health—Institute for Vaccine Safety. (2008) *Vaccine Exemptions*. Available at: www.vaccinesafety.edu/ccexem.htm. Accessed July 4, 2011.

27. Wooten KG, Kolasa M, Singleton JA, et al., Immunization Svcs Div, National Center for Immunization and Respiratory Diseases, Centers for Disease Control and Prevention.(2009) National, state, and local area vaccination coverage among children aged 19–35 months—United States. *MMWR Morb Mortal Wkly Rep*. 59(36), 1171–7. Available at: www.cdc.gov/mmwr/preview/mmwrhtml/mm5936a2.htm?s_cid=mm5936a2_w. Accessed December 14, 2011.

28. Flanagan-Klygis EA, Sharp L, Frader JE. (2005) Dismissing the family who refuses vaccines: a study of pediatrician attitudes. *Arch Pediatr Adolesc Med*. 159(10), 929–34.

29. Smith PJ, Chu SY, Barker LE. (2004) Children who have received no vaccines: who are they and where do they live? *Pediatrics*. 114(1), 187–95.

30. Gust DA, Darling N, Kennedy A, et al. (2008) Parents with doubts about vaccines: which vaccines and reasons why. *Pediatrics*. 122(4), 718–25.

31. Salmon DA, Moulton LH, Omer SB, et al. (2005) Factors associated with refusal of childhood vaccines among parents of school-aged children: a case-control study. *Arch Pediatr Adolesc Med*. 159(5), 470–6.

32. Fredrickson DD, Davis TC, Arnould CL, et al. (2004). Childhood immunization refusal: provider and parent perceptions. *Fam Med*. 36(6), 431–9.

33. Gust DA, Strine TW, Maurice E, et al. (2004) Underimmunization among children: effects of vaccine safety concerns on immunization status. *Pediatrics*. 114(1), e16–e22. Available at: www.pediatrics.org/cgi/content/full/114/1/e16. Accessed December 14, 2011.

34. Anderson RM, May RM. (1985) Vaccination and herd immunity to infectious diseases. *Nature*. 318, 323–8.

35. Plotkin SA, Orenstein WA. (1999) *Vaccines*, 3rd ed. Philadelphia, PA: WB Saunders.

36. Ada G, Isaacs D. (2000) *Vaccination: the Facts, the Fears, the Future*. Sydney: Allen & Unwin.

37. McIntyre P, Gidding H, Gilmour R, et al. (2002) Vaccine preventable diseases and coverage in Australia, 1999–2000. *Commun Dis Intell*. 26, S1–111.

38. Murphy TV, Gargiullo PM, Massoudi MS, et al. (2001) Intussusception among infants given an oral rotavirus vaccine. *N Engl J Med*. 344, 564–72.

39. Patel MM, Richardson Lopez-Collada V, Mattos Bulhoes M, et al. (2011) Intussusception risk and health benefits of rotavirus vaccination in Mexico and Brazil. *N Engl J Med*. 364, 2283–92.

40. Australian Government. Department of Health and Ageing. Departmental Media Releases. (2010) *Seasonal Flu Vaccine Remains Suspended for Young Children Without Risk Factors—Advice from the Chief Medical Officer*. Available at: www.health.gov.au/internet/main/publishing.nsf/Content/mr-yr10-dept-dept010610.htm. Accessed December 14, 2011.

41. Isaacs D, Kilham H, Marshall H. (2004) Should routine childhood immunizations be compulsory? *J Paediatr Child Health*. 40, 392–6.

42. Hull B, Lawrence G, MacIntyre CR, et al. (2002) *Immunisation Coverage: Australia 2001*. Canberra: Commonwealth Department of Health and Ageing. Available at: www.immunise.health.gov.au/report.pdf/. Accessed December 14, 2011.

43. Miller H, Ross G. (2011) *Immunity: When it's Smart to go With the Herd*. Available at: www.guardian.co.uk/commentisfree/cifamerica/2011/jun/13/vaccines-health. Accessed June 13, 2011.

44. Diekema DS. (2005) Responding to parental refusals of immunization of children. *Pediatrics*. 115, 1428–31.

13 Chemical restraints, physical restraints, and other demonstrations of force

Michael P. Wilson,[1] Christian M. Sloane[2]

[1]*Clinical Research Fellow, Department of Emergency Medicine, University of California San Diego, CA, USA*
[2]*Associate Clinical Professor of Emergency Medicine, Department of Emergency Medicine, University of California San Diego, CA, USA*

Section I: Case presentation

A 37-year-old man was brought to the emergency department (ED) for altered mental status. He had reportedly passed out in front of a local bar. The bar's owner called an ambulance due to the patient's inability to ambulate. The patient had been drinking alcohol and had an empty bottle of Jack Daniels in his pocket. On arrival at the ED, he had normal vital signs, his glucose level was normal, a strong odor of alcohol was on his breath, and he was able to speak with slurred speech. He was in a cervical collar (c-collar) and on a backboard. He had a large occipital hematoma with a laceration. The examination was otherwise unremarkable for trauma. He was belligerent, and repeatedly attempted to sit up and remove his cervical collar, stating, "Leave me the f— alone. I don't want to be here. Let me go." Verbal attempts to calm him were unsuccessful. An intravenous line was established, and the treating team medicated the patient with haloperidol. The patient continued to fight against the staff. He was subsequently intubated using rapid sequence intubation. A computed tomography (CT scan) of the head and cervical spine imaging studies were unremarkable. The patient later awoke, was extubated, and finally discharged from the ED clinically sober and with a steady gait.

Section II: Discussion

Dr. Peter Rosen: While there are many medical and ethical issues to consider, I would like to focus the conversation on how much force can and should be applied to patients when they are unable to make decisions for themselves.

Dr. Christian Sloane: When you approach these patients, you should begin with the least invasive means; begin with verbal interactions and gradually increase the severity of the interaction as necessary in order to pursue your workup.

PR: That is reasonable, but most intoxicated patients are somnolent and cooperative when they are left alone. They often become agitated when restrained with c-collars and back boards. If we don't supply the medical restraint, however, then we are not treating them correctly. Do you see that as an indication to escalate your force?

CS: Our obligation is to first do no harm. Since you cannot adequately assess the patient's injuries, removing some of the restraints may actually lead to a worse outcome than applying the force required to better examine the patient to rule out severe injury. The physician must always balance the risks and benefits of any restraint used on a patient.

Ethical Problems in Emergency Medicine: A Discussion-Based Review, First Edition. John Jesus, Shamai A. Grossman, Arthur R. Derse, James G. Adams, Richard Wolfe, and Peter Rosen.
© 2012 John Wiley & Sons, Ltd. Published 2012 by John Wiley & Sons, Ltd.

PR: What are the ethical and legal concerns when paramedics are called to a scene where they must restrain a patient in order to bring the patient to the ED? I've been involved in several lawsuits, in which I felt that the involved paramedics acted appropriately, but there was a bad outcome for which they were blamed. How do we provide medical coverage when we need to exercise force?

Dr. Arthur Derse: The opposite situation is also true. When there is a bad outcome, and the paramedics have left the scene, there is usually someone willing to testify that the patient should have been restrained, and taken to a hospital. Once they have arrived in the ED, there is an expectation that an emergency physician will do a screening examination, and try to determine if there is an emergent condition even in the midst of the patient's refusal of care. Ethically, people have the right to refuse treatment. Emergency physicians, however, have the right to determine whether the person making that refusal has decision-making capacity.

In the field, paramedics see many people who decline treatment. As an emergency physician who is serving as medical control, we need to know who called the paramedics, why they were called, and if the patient is capable of making decisions before allowing the paramedic to release the patient without treatment or transport to the hospital.

Once the person arrives, is evaluated, and then released, the worst that has happened is that they received a medical evaluation. The paramedics and the emergency physician have, at least, the responsibility to decide if this person is capable of refusing transport to the hospital. The standard used is what another reasonable paramedic would have done in a similar situation. To err on the side of caution by transporting a few people against their will is far better than allowing a few serious or fatal outcomes in people who were not transported.

PR: There are always issues of restraint: reported positional asphyxia, inappropriate use of haloperidol in combination with alcohol consumption, etc. If you decide that you do have to escalate restraint to include physical restraints how can you do it safely? Do tasers work for these patients, or would you just proceed to rapid sequence intubation and keep the patient paralyzed and sedated while you continue your assess-

ment? Once a patient has arrested in the midst of attempts to apply physical or chemical restraint, there frequently is a discussion as to whether it was positional restraint, positional asphyxia, or an inappropriate dose of haloperidol that caused the event. In the ED, we sometimes have to choose between two potentially bad outcomes. I'd prefer to defend my decisions made in an attempt to protect a patient, or evaluate the potential life- or limb-threatening injuries, than defend a decision in which I avoided the assessment because the patient was particularly difficult or aggressive.

CS: I would not use a taser in the ED since there are other tools available that are more effective. Again, I would like to emphasize that one should use only the minimum amount of force that is necessary to achieve one's goal. I have a systematic approach to addressing these patients. I first attempt to verbally reason with them. If that fails then I try medication. Only once I've tried all other options, do I then escalate to physical restraints. There are other patients where that approach wouldn't be appropriate, for example, with a wildly psychotic and violent patient. I still attempt to give patients like these a choice, and offer medication they can take themselves or medication the medical team can provide via an injection.

PR: I brought up the issue of tasers, because they've become popular on the [US] east coast with security forces. The reality is they are ineffective on patients who are drugged or significantly intoxicated. While I am unaware of any existing studies, I'm aware of a number of cases in which combative, incapacitated patients were "tasered" more than once without cessation of combative activity, some of whom went on to have a bad outcome. Do physicians have the legal grounds to force antipsychotic drugs onto patients when they are displaying behavior that is causing a danger to themselves or the people around them?

Dr. Mike Wilson: Patients who are a danger to themselves or others are exactly the patients we should chemically or physically restrain. Because it is legally required to demonstrate why we must restrain a patient, adequate documentation of the reasons and methods of restraint is important. Much of the reluctance to physically restrain patients comes from organizations like the Joint Commission that impose a number of reporting requirements once a patient is placed into restraints. According to the Joint Commission, physical restraints have the ability to cause both physical and psychological harm.

One of the few ED studies to look at the impact of physical restraints on patients in the ED was done by Zun in 2003.[1] In his study, the physical complications are fairly low (6.7%). Most of the complications were from patients who managed to free themselves of their restraints. In fact, only one patient in this study was injured by being in restraints due to his own violence, which were outnumbered by the cases of injuries to staff by combative patients. The physical complications of restraints, if properly monitored, are fairly low.

AD: In an emergent situation in which you feel there is a danger to the patient or others, most [US] states have an emergency treatment exception to informed consent that allows an emergency physician to act when the patient is not decisionally capacitated, a life- or limb-threatening injury occurs, no one is legally authorized to speak for the patient, or a reasonable person would consent to the treatment when time is of the essence. They also have statutes that dissuade the long term treatment of individuals with psychotropic medications as a result of legislative responses to the abusive use and complications of long term use of psychotropic medications. Many states allow patients to refuse psychotropic medication unless they are an imminent threat to self or others. When the imminent threat is over, they regain the ability to refuse psychotropic medications. Chemical restraints are sometimes less harmful to the patient than physical restraints, but there is no question that there is a stigma attached to the use of psychotropic medications for any long-term pacification or treatment of a patient.

Dr. John Jesus: I support the idea of giving patients a choice, and trying to respect what decision-making capacity they do have. Some patients have the capacity to make some, but not other decisions. For example, perhaps a patient does not have the capacity to decide about staying or leaving the ED, but is able to decide what type of restraint should be used. This approach attempts to give the patient some element of dignity, which is both important for the patient and the medical professionals attempting to care for the patient; this approach is likely to be a safer approach for both the patient and his caregivers.

Even in arguing for this approach, I also acknowledge that there are exceptions. One evening I was working in our lower acuity zone, and caring for a 38-year-old man who was actively psychotic. He was initially cooperative when I spoke to him, and seemed to calm down. As soon as I left his bedside, however, he quickly escalated, ran out of his room with security guards in pursuit. Before he could be tackled, he threw a computer screen at one of the attending physicians, and severely frightened several patients. He was also injured in the take down. I felt that I had an opportunity to chemically restrain him, but didn't successfully utilize the moment to ensure the safety of my staff from a potentially volatile patient—a mistake about which I've learned a great deal.

If you are going to physically restrain a patient, he or she should also be chemically restrained to prevent complications like rhabdomyolysis and other conditions associated with patients who struggle while they are physically restrained. Moreover, both chemical and physical restraints can be administered at a moment of maximum agitation, and the physical restraints gradually withdrawn as chemical sedation is established. Finally, if there is significant concern for spinal cord injury, it is appropriate to paralyze, sedate, and intubate these patients to prevent any further damage to their spine from their acutely intoxicated and uncooperative state.

PR: The concept of minimal restraints does not mean minimal use of appropriate medications, because many sedative drugs have an excitatory effect if given in small doses.

What about the patient who appears on the brink of becoming combative, but who hasn't yet declared himself with a violent act? Do we have the right to assume that these patients can quickly escalate, and based upon that assumption, should we proceed with sedating and restraining them before they demonstrate any violent behaviors? We're not allowing patients much margin for cooperation or for individual expression. That said, we have a duty to protect our colleagues, and we certainly have no reason to allow patients to hurt us if we can prevent it.

CS: You may justify chemical and physical restraints, if you deem that violent or dangerous behavior is imminent. Certain patients can act out unexpectedly and without warning, and you have to be careful with them. Caution may require that you continue their chemical sedation to prevent further agitation or escalation.

MW: The largest community study of this kind focused on severe mental illness, and was completed [in 2009] by Elbogen and Johnson.[2] They give empirical support to the idea that individuals who have a history of violence are at much higher risk for committing a violent act in the duration of that study. If we extrapolate that to the ED, it appears that we should have a lower threshold to restrain patients with a history of violence, either physically or chemically, especially if they are intoxicated or under the influence of illicit substances.

There is also some evidence that patients are less likely to commit violence when screened appropriately, and given some intervention in the ED. As such, ED physicians or specially trained staff may intervene and provide community resources, and explain to the patient how to avoid this kind of behavior in the future.

PR: In Denver, we could obtain a 30-day hold on patients who have had repetitive chemical-and alcohol-intoxicated behavior requiring recurrent presentation to an ED. Is there a way we can break the cycle in which many patients find themselves?

AD: Much depends upon the community in which one practices, because there are emergency physician statutes that allow patients to be restrained who are an imminent danger to themselves or others. A few states have statutes that allow for similar restraint when treating a person who can no longer take care of self. Often these patients have medical problems like dementia, alcohol dependence, or some other condition and the local community recognizes a need for inpatient treatment.

PR: Emergency physicians are at risk of becoming rather cynical, assuming that no alcoholic wants to address the addiction. We all have patients like this, and many physicians attempt to help patients through their acute intoxication, and try to discharge the patient before they slide into withdrawal. It does help to remember that sometimes, the emergency physician is able to break the cycle, and render the patient drug or alcohol free for a number of months. While ultimately there may be a relapse, at least we've given that patient some freedom from the repetitive, self destructive behaviors.

JJ: In addition to identifying who should be restrained and the manner by which it occurs, is the matter of how we treat those we've already chemically and physically restrained. I have witnessed nursing and ancillary staff members participate in behavior that I found ethically troublesome: taunting patients, calling them names, and being neglectful. I've also heard of patient take-downs that involve the administration of succinylcholine without simultaneous use of sedatives, which I would describe as a punitive measure at best. These acts of cruelty and disrespect shouldn't be tolerated on any level. It threatens our mission to provide medical care, and endangers the "good," broadly defined, that exists within each of us. It not only affects our own behavior, but has an impact on the behaviors of nurses, medical students and ancillary staff who look to their attending physician as a role model of what is appropriate.

PR: Education has an important role in these instances. Much of the sadism that is expressed towards patients who have been violent stems from our fear of being harmed by them. We are at risk of giving in to that fear, and treating those patients poorly.

AD: There is a natural inclination towards self-defense, especially if the patient has already been combative or assaultive. We have to be concerned about our response, and one of the most difficult challenges of teaching ED residents appropriate professionalism is emulating the very professionalism we hope to impart on the residents. Legally, if you are seen as someone who is always holding the best interest of the patient at heart, many legal reviewers and juries will be willing to overlook restraining a patient, using whatever method you deem appropriate. That said, at the point when they start viewing you as a physician who abuses patients, you will lose your moral standing and your legal argument for why the restraints were required in the first place.

Section III: Review of the literature

The use of restraints is frequent in medical institutions that care for behaviorally disturbed individuals, although rates vary widely depending on the particular hospital.[3] Ethicists and regulators have generally distinguished between two types of restraints: behavioral restraint, which represents an attempt to control behavioral dysregulation most often associated with psychiatric illness; and medical restraint, designed to permit medical care to continue. The review below mainly discusses the use of behavioral restraints. Use of restraints for medical reasons is less legally regulated, but presumably subject to the same sorts of ethical guidelines governing other emergent medical procedures.[4]

Although violent patients are commonly encountered in clinical practice in the ED, the use of restraints for behavioral control is now discouraged, with most professional societies and regulatory agencies now call for their use only as a "last resort." Nonetheless, emergency physicians are often required to make decisions about restraining patients in order to protect staff, other patients, or complete a medical workup. This review will discuss the current controversy over behavioral restraints, long-standing efforts to reduce use, restraint types, and the safe application of restraints if they are required.

The controversy over restraints

The use of restraints for behavioral reasons is controversial at best. There is a consensus among most regulatory agencies and professional societies that such measures are highly coercive, and so should be used as infrequently as possible. Coercive restraint has been compared in the literature and in court cases to the power of arrest, but a peculiar type of arrest in which the individual is deprived of liberty without benefit of a judge or jury.[5]

There are no randomized controlled trials that support the use of restraints, although there are now a large number of qualitative and retrospective studies documenting harm from restraint use.[6] Despite this, restraint use for behavioral reasons is generally viewed more positively by staff.[7] This may be because nursing staff in the ED are particularly susceptible to verbal and physical abuse, with slightly more than half of all nurses in a recent survey reporting verbal or physical abuse within the last 14 days.[8] Thus, restraint use has remained prevalent.

The benefit of restraining a violent patient seems obvious. There is a reduction in violence in psychiatric units that permit restraints, and at least one report has documented increasing levels of violence against staff in institutions that have minimized restraints.[9,10] However, much literature has also documented negative aspects of restraints. Although the risk of com-

plications of the restraint procedure are low in prospective studies in the ED,[1] restraint-related injuries, including asphyxiation, strangulation, and cardiac arrest, ranked seventh among the types of events reported to the Joint Commission from 1995 to 2005.[11] In addition, qualitative studies document psychological trauma after restraint episodes.[12–14] In addition, this procedure is almost always performed without the informed consent of patients, who generally find these forced measures unpleasant.[12]

Among professional societies and regulatory agencies, there is therefore fairly broad agreement that behavioral restraints are to be avoided if at all possible. At least one risk management guide on the subject of restraints has stated that[5]:

"(1) Each use of restraint or seclusion poses an inherent danger, both physical and psychological, to the individual who is subject to the interventions
(2) The decision to use restraint or seclusion nearly always is arbitrary, idiosyncratic, and generally avoidable."

A remarkable number of professional societies and regulatory agencies have subsequently agreed with this sentiment. Restraint use is viewed as "intrinsically unsafe" with a high propensity to cause injuries to staff and patients during forceful takedowns,[3,9] with calls for reducing or minimizing use from such diverse organizations as the Joint Commission, the American Psychiatric Association, the American Psychiatric Nurses Association, the American Academy of National Alliance for the Mentally Ill, Mental Health America, and the Child and Adolescent Psychiatry, the American Association of Community Psychiatrists, and the National Association of State Mental Health Program Directors.[5,15–18]

In Great Britain and other European countries, the use of physical restraint of any type is also strongly discouraged.[19] In the United States, restraints are permitted but heavily regulated by the Joint Commission. This organization imposes a number of requirements on institutions using restraints[20]:

"(1) A physician or licensed practitioner must see and evaluate the patient within 1 hour of initiating intervention.
(2) Seclusion or restraint can only be used when clinically justified, and after consideration of alternative treatment options.

(3) Seclusion and restraints must have time-limited orders: 4 hours for adults (older than 17 years), 2 hours for adolescents (9–17 years), 1 hour for patients younger than 9 years.

(4) Patients must have continuous monitoring with periodic evaluation with the intent to discontinue intervention at the earliest possible time.

(5) A face-to-face reevaluation must be performed before each renewal of initial time-limited orders.

(6) Clinical leadership (i.e., the medical director) must be notified after 12 hours of continuous seclusion or restraint and every 24 hours thereafter.

(7) With the patient's informed consent, family should be notified promptly when seclusion or restraint is initiated."

Failure to document safe restraint use is one of the most common reasons for Joint Commission citations.[20]

Reasons to restrain

The use of restraints is generally accepted only in an emergency situation when there is an imminent danger of harm to self or others.[9] Restraints in this instance are defined as either a mechanical method to restrict movement or a drug used to control behavior if not part of the patient's standard treatment for underlying psychiatric illness. The use of restraints to control behavior is thought not to have therapeutic value, and so clinicians must document that less restrictive interventions have been ineffective.[18] Restraints cannot be used for loud or disruptive nonviolent behavior, as a means of discipline, retaliation, or convenience on part of staff.[5] Patients may not be restrained for refusing medication.[9]

According to Joint Commission guidelines, physicians must make a face-to-face evaluation of restrained patients within 1 hour. This evaluation should document the need for restraints. In general, restraints should be removed as soon as the patient can commit to the safety of themselves or others.

Capacity

Competence is a legal term describing the determination by a court of law that the individual has sufficient ability to understand the legal proceedings on their behalf.[21] Decision-making capacity is a medical term that refers to the patient's ability to make informed

medical decisions on his or her own behalf, and it is possible that a patient is legally competent but lacks capacity to make a particular medical decision. Some authors have argued that the capacity to make medical decisions should be on a sliding scale. In other words, extensive capacity may not be needed for the refusal of minor treatments, but a correspondingly higher standard should be used for patients who refuse low-risk life-saving interventions.[22] In every instance, however, capacity is based on informed consent.[20] The basic elements of informed consent include: (1) the nature and purpose of the procedure; (2) significant risks of the procedure; (3) benefits of the intervention; (4) probable outcome if the procedure is refused; and (5) any possible alternatives to the test or procedure.

In general, restraints are necessary in situations in which there is an overwhelming risk of harm to the patient or others. Thus, these patients are generally thought to lack decision-making capacity. The need for restraints should be reevaluated in patients who are refusing treatments but nonetheless deemed to have decision-making capacity.

Types of restraint

When the physician makes a decision that some form of restraint is necessary, there are a multitude of options from which to choose. Broadly, there are two categories of restraints, either physical or chemical. Administration of medication is not considered a restraint unless it is a medication solely intended to control a patient's behavior, and is not part of treatment for an underlying illness. The choice of restraint should be individualized for each patient and situation.[23] Each type of restraint is discussed below.

Physical

Physical restraints usually consist of either containment strategies, known most often as seclusion, or manual devices to restrict movement, called restraints. Restraints are usually of two types, either soft or hard, depending on the type of material used to make the restraint. Soft restraints, also known by some manufacturers as quilted limb restraints (Posey®), consist of a soft blanket-like material that encompasses the limbs. This blanket-like material is surrounded by a strap which is tied to the gurney or bed, thus effectively preventing limb movement beyond the scope of the attachment strap. For violent patients, hard restraints are preferred.[23] These are typically made of nylon, plastic, or leather, and are similar to soft restraints. However, these restraints consist of more durable material, and so are nearly impossible to break or stretch. If violence towards staff is not a concern, more minimal soft restraints may be used. A Posey vest is a body type of restraint that leaves the limbs unrestrained. This is most commonly used in non-violent patients, such as in an elderly confused or demented patient at risk for falling out of bed.

Containment strategies to prevent flight risk may also be used, especially if the patient is not a danger to self. In this strategy, the patient is simply placed in a locked room and not allowed to leave. These rooms typically have a minimum of furniture and appliances, and have been cleared of anything that could be used as a weapon. This also offers the opportunity to provide a decrease in environmental stimulation.

Given widespread use in the prehospital setting of other methods such as tasers, some hospitals have begun to use this in the ED as well.[24] While the device is clearly effective at subduing violent patients, it has no role in the restraint of patients. Ethically, this violates the principle of using the least restrictive method possible. Legally, it also violates regulatory guidelines. According to the Center for Medicare & Medicaid Services (CMS), the use of weapons in the application of restraint or seclusion including the use of pepper spray, mace, nightsticks, and tasers, is never appropriate.[25] These weapons are reserved for law enforcement officials who are taking a patient or visitor into custody.

The process of applying physical restraints In general, physicians should not be part of the restraining team. This serves to preserve the therapeutic relationship between the physician and patient, which can be difficult if the physician is struggling to grab and restrain the patient.[26] On shifts with low numbers of staff or at smaller institutions, however, it may not always be possible to have a physician separate from the restraint process. Nonetheless, the emergency physician should be in charge of ordering the restraints and monitoring their safe application. Like other procedures, this requires a protocol that is agreed on in advance. Given the potential for injury to the patient or staff, all members of the restraining team should be well-trained in the procedures used. Security or police should always be informed if force is necessary, and

the restraint team should be large and well-organized to prevent injury to patients or staff. In practice, this usually means at least five people, one for each limb and one for the head. Another common technique is to use two mattresses in an attempt to encase the patient.

Throughout the restraining attempt, caregivers should remain calm, and attempt to explain to the patient the need for restraint even if the patient appears not to understand. If the patient attempts to leave before an adequate team is assembled, allow the patient to leave. This is especially true if the patient wields a weapon. The health of the caregiver should not be jeopardized in favor of the patient.

The use of restraint, when properly applied, can lead to avoidance of hospitalization if it allows psychiatric and pharmacologic interaction to occur. The removal of restraint is made on the basis of the patient's behavior and medical condition, and not as a result of bargains or threats. Removal of restraints is in reverse stepwise fashion: four limbs down to two limbs down to none.[26]

Although complications of restraints are generally low, deaths while in restraint have been reported with manslaughter convictions upheld for staff members who engaged in improper restraint practices.[5] Much research has concerned whether "positional asphyxia" could be a cause of death. Restraint of healthy human subjects does not seem to cause cardiorespiratory compromise either in a restraint chair or hobble-tie position,[27,28] but restrained patients are not often healthy subjects since they may have ingested toxic substances, have underlying cardiac disease, or both. A patient who is thrashing in restraints for hours may suffer from musculoskeletal injuries or rhabdomyolysis as a result of restraints. Close monitoring of these patients is therefore essential. In addition, many experts also recommend chemical calming whenever a patient is placed into physical restraints.[29]

Chemical restraint

The idea of chemical restraint is somewhat of a misnomer, as the correct goal of medication administration is calming instead of sedation.[29,30] There are three general classes of medication that are used for agitation, including the classical antipsychotics, the atypical or second-generation antipsychotics, and benzodiazepines. A fourth class of medication,

145

ketamine, has been recently recommended for excited delirium syndrome, a syndrome characterized by aggressive erratic behavior in a patient usually suffering from severe mental illness or under the influence of a stimulant drug such as methamphetamine or cocaine.[31]

Classical antipsychotics Conventional or first-generation antipsychotics such as haloperidol and droperidol are an older class of medications that tightly bind to dopamine receptors. Although they mainly affect this receptor subtype, these medications also cause sedation through an unknown mechanism. One possible explanation is that these medications are structurally similar to the inhibitory neurotransmitter γ-aminobutyric acid (GABA).[32] Alternately, these drugs may influence which environmental stimuli are found rewarding or salient by the patient, and thus help reduce psychotic symptoms.[33,34] Among the classical antipsychotics, haloperidol is perhaps the most widely used in the ED.[29,35] Since it has a number of important motor-related side effects, it should generally be used with a benzodiazepine to ameliorate some of the untoward effects unless there is a contraindication to benzodiazepine use.[36]

Atypical antipsychotics Atypical or second-generation antipsychotics are a later class of medication used in the treatment of psychiatric illness. The antipsychotics most often used in the ED include ziprasidone and olanzapine, which are available in both intramuscular or oral formulations, and risperidone, which is available in an oral formulation only. In general, these medications bind to a wider variety of receptor types than the first-generation antipsychotics. For agitation of psychiatric origin, second-generation antipsychotics are often preferred by many experts since they (1) can be given orally and (2) reduce agitation as well as intramuscular haloperidol, but with fewer side effects.[29,30,37] Nevertheless, their use still requires caution in intoxicated patients.[38,39]

Benzodiazepines Common benzodiazepines used in the ED include midazolam, lorazepam, and diazepam. Midazolam has a shorter duration of action than lorazepam and diazepam. As a class, benzodiazepines tend to cause respiratory depression as well as hypotension. In addition, they do not treat the underlying disease, and so are not recommended as a first-line agent alone for agitation.[30]

Ketamine Although typically used for procedural sedation, ketamine has recently received recommendations for use in excited delirium syndrome.[40,41] In part, this is because ketamine has a rapid onset of action, has minimal effects on respirations, and a long record of safety. Given that ketamine also tends to increase heart rate and blood pressure, however, more studies are needed before recommending its use in an agitated population that is presumably already tachycardic and hypertensive.

The continuum of force: how much restraint to use

In general, the emergency physician should use an approach similar to that of law enforcement, in that if coercive measures are needed, the minimum amount of force possible should be used. Unlike law enforcement, clinicians have an additional responsibility to maintain patient dignity. In practice, this means two things: (1) verbal de-escalation techniques should be used first if these can be done safely, and (2) oral medications should be used whenever possible. Once applied, every effort should be made to safely remove physical restraints as soon as possible. In general, restraints should be removed when at least one of the following conditions is met:

- When the medical workup is completed.
- When the patient is no longer a threat to self or others.
- When the patient is compliant with the treatment plan.

Conclusions

It is likely that as new medications arise, with even faster times of onset and improved safety profiles, there will be an even more intense push towards earlier chemical restraint and away from mechanical restraint and its numerous safety issues. Restraint is a forced procedure, and as with many procedures in medicine, as little force, or as minimally invasive an approach as possible, should be used to achieve treatment goals. Clinicians should maintain the higher ground, and avoid allowing personnel or themselves to be drawn into an emotional battle with an agitated patient. Clear documentation is of key importance whenever restraints are used, and frequent reassessment is necessary. Restraints should be removed as soon as they are no longer needed.

Above all, treat the patient with dignity. When the situation is unclear, it is better to err on the side of commonsense and do what is the best for the patient, thus maintaining a safe environment for all involved in patient care. There is no higher ethical obligation than treating a patient correctly in a humane dignified manner.

Section IV: Recommendations

• Clinicians should maintain the higher ground, and avoid letting the situation become personal or allow themselves to be drawn into an emotional battle with an agitated patient.
• Clear documentation is of key importance whenever restraints are used. Frequent reassessment is necessary.
• Restraints should be removed as soon as they are no longer needed.
• Do what is the best for the patient while maintaining a safe environment for all involved in patient care.
• Above all, treat the patient with dignity.

References

1. Zun LS. (2003) A prospective study of the complication rate of use of patient restraint in the emergency department. *J Emerg Med.* 24(2), 119–24.
2. Elbogen EB, Johnson SC. (2009) The intricate link between violence and mental disorder: Results from the National Epidemiologic Survey on Alcohol and Related Conditions. *Arch Gen Psychiatry.* 66(2), 152–61.
3. Sailas E, Wahlbeck K. (2005) Restraint and seclusion in psychiatric inpatient wards. *Curr Opin Psychiatry.* 18, 555–9.
4. Glezer A, Brendel RW. (2010) Beyond emergencies: The use of physical restraints in medical and psychiatric settings. *Harvard Rev Psychiatry.* 18, 353–8.
5. Haimowitz S, Urff J, Huckshorn KA. (2011) *Restraint and Seclusion: A Risk Management Guide.* Available at: www.nasmhpd.org. Accessed June 24, 2011.
6. Sailas EES, Fenton M. (2000) Seclusion and restraint for people with serious mental illnesses. *Cochrane Database Syst Rev.* 1, CD001163.
7. Stewart D, Bowers L, Simpson A, et al. (2009) Manual restraint of adult psychiatric inpatients: A literature review. *J Psychiatr Ment Health Nurs.* 16(8), 749–57.
8. Emergency Nurses Association Institute for Emergency Nursing Research. (2010) *Emergency Department Violence Surveillance Study.* Available at: www.ena.org. Accessed February 24, 2011.
9. Fisher WA. (1994) Restraint and seclusion: A review of the literature. *Am J Psychiatry.* 151, 1584–91.
10. Khadivi AN, Patel RC, Atkinson AR, et al. (2004) Association between seclusion and restraint and patient-related violence. *Psychiatr Serv.* 11, 503–8.
11. Ednie KJ. (2009) Aggression: Reducing risk in the management of aggressive patients. In: Jayaram G, Herzog A (eds) *SAFE MD: Practical Applications and Approaches to Safe Psychiatric Practice.* American Psychiatric Association. Available at: www.psych.org. Accessed June 24, 2011.
12. Frueh BC, Knapp RG, Cusack KJ, et al. (2005) Patients' reports of traumatic or harmful experiences within the psychiatric setting. *Psychiatr Serv.* 56, 1123–33.
13. Cusack KJ, Frueh BC, Hiers T, et al. (2003) Trauma within the psychiatric setting: A preliminary empirical report. *Adm Policy Ment Health.* 30(5), 453–60.
14. Robins CS, Sauvageot JA, Suffoletta-Maierle S, et al. (2005) Consumer's perceptions of negative experiences and "Sanctuary Harm" in psychiatric settings. *Psychiatr Serv.* 56, 1134–8.
15. American Psychiatric Nurse's Association. (2007) *Position Statement on the Use of Seclusion and Restraint.* Available at: www.apna.org. Accessed June 24, 2011.
16. Masters KJ, Bellonci C, Bernet W, et al. (2002) Practice parameter for the prevention and management of aggressive behavior in child and adolescent psychiatric institutions, with special reference to seclusion and restraint. *J Am Acad Child Adolesc Psychiatry.* 41 Suppl 2, 4S–25S.
17. National Alliance for the Mentally Ill. (2003) *Seclusion and Restraints.* Available at: www.nami.org. Accessed June 24, 2011.
18. Mental Health America. *Position Statement 24: Seclusion and Restraints.* Available at: www.nmha.org. Accessed June 24, 2011.
19. Gordon H, Hindley N, Marsden A, et al. (1999) The use of mechanical restraint in the management of psychiatric patients: Is it ever appropriate? *J Forens Psychiatry.* 10(1), 173–86.
20. Coburn VA, Mycyk MB. (2009) Physical and chemical restraints. *Emerg Med Clin North Am.* 27, 655–67.
21. Miller SS, Marin DB. (2000) Assessing capacity. *Emerg Med Clin North Am.* 18(2), 233–42.
22. Levinson JL. (2006) Legal issues in the interface of medicine and psychiatry. Available at: www.primarypsychiatry.com. Accessed June 24, 2011.
23. Rossi J, Swan MC. (2010) The violent or agitated patient. *Emerg Med Clin North Am.* 28, 235–56.

24. The Washington Post. (2010) *Hospital Experts Debate Wisdom of Using Stun Guns to Control Violent Patients, July 20.* Available at: www.washingtonpost.com. Accessed June 29, 2011.

25. Center for Medicare and Medicaid Services. CMS 482.13(e) Standard: Restraint or seclusion. In: *State Operations Manual Appendix A—Survey Protocol, Regulations, and Interpretive Guidelines for Hospitals.* Available at: http://cms.gov/manuals/Downloads/som107ap_a_hospitals.pdf. Accessed June 29, 2011.

26. Jacobs D. (1983) Evaluation and management of the violent patient in emergency settings. *Psychiatr Clin North Am.* 6, 259–69.

27. Vilke GM, Sloane C, Castillo EM, et al. (2011) Evaluation of the ventilator effects of a restraint chair on human subjects. *J Emerg Med.* 40(6), 714–18.

28. Chan TC, Vilke GM, Neuman T, et al. (1997) Restraint position and positional asphyxia. *Ann Emerg Med.* 30, 578–86.

29. Vilke GM, Wilson MP. (2009) Agitation: What every emergency physician should know. *Emerg Med Rep.* 30(19), 233–44.

30. Allen MH, Currier GW, Carpenter D, et al. (2005) The expert consensus guideline series: Treatment of behavioral emergencies. *J Psychiatr Pract.* 11 Suppl 1, 5–25.

31. Vilke GM, Debard ML, Chan TC, et al. (2011) Excited delirium syndrome (EXDS): Defining based on a review of the literature. *J Emerg Med.* March 24 [Epub ahead of print].

32. Richards JR, Schneir AB. (2003) Droperidol in the emergency department: Is it safe? *J Emerg Med.* 24(4), 441–7.

33. Howes OD, Kapur S. (2009) The dopamine hypothesis of schizophrenia: Version III—the final common pathway. *Schizophr Bull.* 35(3), 549–62.

34. Heinz A, Schlagenhauf F. (2010) Dopaminergic dysfunction in schizophrenia: Salience attribution revisited. *Schizophr Bull.* 36(3), 472–85.

35. MacDonald KS, Wilson MP, Minassian A, et al. (2010) A retrospective analysis of intramuscular haloperidol and olanzapine in the treatment of agitation in drug and alcohol-using patients. *Gen Hosp Psychiatry.* 32(4), 443–5.

36. Battaglia J, Moss S, Rush J, et al. (1997) Haloperidol, lorazepam, or both for psychotic agitation? A multicenter, prospective, double-blind, emergency department study. *Am J Emerg Med.* 15, 335–40.

37. Currier GW, Chou JCY, Feifel D, et al. (2004) Acute treatment of psychotic agitation: A randomized comparison of oral treatment with risperidone and lorazepam versus intramuscular treatment with haloperidol and lorazepam. *J Clin Psychiatry.* 65, 386–94.

38. Wilson MP, MacDonald KS, Vilke GM, et al. (2011) A comparison of the safety of olanzapine and haloperidol in combination with benzodiazepines in emergency department patients with acute agitation. *J Emerg Med.* May 19 [Epub ahead of print].

39. Wilson MP, MacDonald KS, Vilke GM, et al. (2010) Potential complications of combining intramuscular olanzapine with benzodiazepines in agitated emergency department patients. *J Emerg Med.* June 12 [Epub ahead of print].

40. American College of Emergency Physicians. (2009) *Excited Delirium Task Force. White Paper Report on Excited Delirium Syndrome.* Available at: www.ccpicd.com. Accessed June 29, 2011.

41. Roberts JR, Geeting GK. (2001) Intramuscular ketamine for the rapid tranquilization of the uncontrollable, violent, and dangerous adult patient. *J Trauma.* 51(5), 1008–10.

14 Capacity determination in the patient with altered mental status

Michael C. Tricoci,[1] Catherine A. Marco[2]

[1]*Resident, Department of Emergency Medicine, University of Toledo Medical Center, Toledo, OH, USA*

[2]*Professor, Department of Emergency Medicine, University of Toledo Medical Center, Toledo, OH, USA*

Section I: Case presentation

A 41-year-old man who was recently released from prison was brought to the emergency department (ED) by the emergency medical services (EMS), after his wife called 911. The patient was clearly agitated and intoxicated, and stated that he did not wish to be there, but his wife threatened to call the police if he did not go to the hospital. The wife was concerned about her husband after he showed up at their front door, drunk and bleeding. The patient stated that he got into a fight with a stranger. He said that he was stabbed in the left parasternal chest with a box-cutter. The patient repeatedly changed the subject, and made inappropriate jokes. He kept repeating that "I have had worse wounds," and he would rather go home and "close it with a hot iron."

Physical examination revealed: a normal blood pressure, heart rate 114 beats per minute, normal pulse oximetry, and a small amount of subcutaneous air near the wound. The patient's speech and balance were severely impaired. The patient was told of the possibility (in layperson terms) of pneumothorax, lung injury, or potential fatality. Despite listening to his doctor's concerns, the patient still wished to go home and treat his wound in his own way. He was eventually convinced to undergo a chest X-ray, which showed a very small pneumothorax.

Section II: Discussion

Dr. Shamai Grossman: How do we define capacity? What does it mean for a patient to be able to make a decision, and what criteria should we consider?

Dr. Richard Wolfe: To have decision-making capacity is to be in a mental state such that one is able to make the decisions the average person would make regarding one's care. In this case, the patient is in a temporary state of confusion given his alcohol use, which may lead to imprudent decisions he would not normally make. There is, therefore, good reason to say that the patient is incapable of making informed medical decisions. Such patients who lack decision-making capacity are very common in the ED population.

Dr. Arthur Derse: One must differentiate the legal terms competence or incompetence from our evaluation of decision-making capacity. Patients are assumed competent until a court finds them otherwise, a decision often based on the assessment of the evaluating physician. In such situations, the judge may appoint a guardian for the person. Decision-making capacity, on the other hand, is a medical determination about the patient's ability to make a proposed medical decision. The analogy I like to use is the patient as a working computer. Patients must be able to take in information, assess that information based on an internal set of values to reach a decision, and then present that decision coherently so as to communicate their preferences. If any of these abilities are compromised, the patient is incapacitated. The patient's decisions must also be fairly consistent over time. The law puts great trust in physicians in judging patients' capacity to make decisions.

SG: Should a patient's inconsistency matter when evaluating the capacity to make clinical decisions?

Dr. John Jesus: Patient inconsistency suggests the patient does not have reliable decision-making capacity, and should not be allowed to refuse treatment and leave the ED. The first step in addressing this situation is to explain to the patient what we are concerned about, as well as to provide explanations for why we insist on the patient remaining in the ED. It's important to respect the patient to the greatest extent possible, while attempting to maintain a productive relationship, even if the patient disagrees with physician's decision.

RW: I agree. Once there is reasonable doubt in the patient's decision-making capacity, I would make the judgment that the patient should be held for a period of observation, so that there may be reassessment once detoxification or sobriety is reached. If attempts to verbally convince the patient to stay fail, given my concerns, I am obliged to apply physical or chemical restraints.

SG: How was the situation handled in our case? What were the major concerns and why was capacity determination necessary?

Dr. Michael Tricoci: We were concerned the patient had an injury that would develop into a life-threatening condition, namely, a tension pneumothorax, if he did not receive appropriate treatment.

RW: The patient's intoxication alone should compel you to keep the patient in the department until he returned to his baseline mental status before he could be released, regardless of the presence or severity of wounds. Given the potential weight of the decision to leave without treatment, you might obtain an alcohol level in order to ensure that alcohol was the agent causing his intoxication, and to be certain that you've waited long enough to achieve clinical sobriety and restore decision-making capacity.

AD: That is a very important point. If a physician determines that a patient's decision-making capacity will change over time, and over time the patient does regain decision-making capacity by physician reassessment, then the physician may accept the patient's persistent refusal of medical care. Just saying "no" is not sufficient to properly refuse care; the patient has to be able to communicate the reasons for the refusal, the potential consequences, and how the decision is consistent with the patient's beliefs, in order to be deemed to have decision-making capacity.

JJ: Simply waiting for the patient to establish clinical sobriety does not necessarily resolve the question of whether he has the capacity to make clinical decisions. Decision-making capacity may be impaired by an underlying psychosis or delusional state. In addition, the patient's reliability is also an issue to consider when deciding on the ultimate disposition. As a recent prisoner who arrived intoxicated and injured from a bar fight, he probably did not engender an impression of reliability to the medical professionals caring for him. The physicians might have decided to admit him for continued cardiopulmonary evaluation if they didn't believe he would come back to the ED if his clinical status worsened.

SG: How much leeway do physicians have to hold a patient in the ED if the patient isn't intoxicated, but is clearly making an imprudent decision? Patients frequently leave against medical advice, and often seem to be ignoring significant risks.

AD: In the absence of a clear cause of incapacity, patients have the right to make an autonomous decision, even if it appears imprudent. In such situations it is important to be sure the patient and the family understand the risks involved, and that they may return for any reason. Documentation of the conversation is important, and one should try to get a signature on the "against medical advice" form.

RW: There are examples of situations in which a patient's judgment is impaired secondary to hypoxia, shock, or other forms of critical illness. In these situations, the physician must act in the patient's best interests.

AD: I agree. If you allow a hypoxic patient to refuse care and leave, only to have the patient die of hypoxic respiratory failure, you would face a lawsuit from family members who would argue that the patient shouldn't have been allowed to make an independent decision, and should not have been allowed to leave. This situation can be very stressful to the involved physician.

SG: There is a law in Judaism that precludes burying someone who committed suicide in a cemetery, as suicide is forbidden in Judaism. In actual practice, however, every person who commits suicide is buried in a cemetery in the usual fashion. The reason for this is because there's an assumption that any person who commits suicide is not of sound mind, and suffers from a degree of insanity that allowed him to commit suicide. When we encounter a patient who appears to have decision-making capacity, but who simultaneously makes decisions that might lead to death, should the physician deem the patient insane, at least temporarily?

Dr. Catherine Marco: The situations that are most vexing to emergency physicians are those where it is difficult to assess whether the patient has decision-making capacity. Cases of patients who obviously lack decision-making capacity versus those who obviously don't have this capacity are relatively simple to handle. We are, unfortunately, frequently faced with patients whose decision-making capacity is considerably less clear. We are forced to make a decision about whether to detain the patient or to accept the refusal of recommended care without any room for compromise. It is critically important to determine capacity in cases like this, even if it involves detaining the patient in order to make that determination. Most patients will voluntarily agree to some formal or informal testing of decision-making capacity when faced with the choice between doing so voluntarily, or doing so under the restraint of security personnel.

MT: It might also be useful to consider a sliding scale approach. In some cases, like this one, the situation is potentially life-threatening, and we do not hesitate to deem the patient's refusal as a sign of decision-making incapacity. Had that laceration been on the dorsal aspect of his forearm, however, and he wanted to go home without treatment, I doubt we would have been so quick to question his capacity to make decisions, and insist that the he stay in the ED.

AD: That is an important point. The level of capacity required to refuse treatment in a life-threatening situation is different from the level of capacity required to refuse non-life-saving care. In both cases you have to decide if the patient has decision-making capacity, but capacity is a very task specific choice.

JJ: It is perhaps a semantic point, but I don't believe capacity belongs on a sliding scale. A patient either does or does not have the ability to make choices based upon the patient's understanding of the benefits and burdens of the choice at hand. The **importance** of determining capacity, on the other hand, can and should change with the severity of potential consequences if the physician were to accept the patient's refusal. For example, physicians are more likely to demand greater proof of decision-making capacity of patients who attempt to refuse life-saving therapy, than if they attempt to refuse sutured closure of a superficial wound.

RW: Assessing the rationality of a patient's behavior is also influenced by our own biases as to what we believe is rational. One could certainly consider a Jehovah's Witness refusing a blood transfusion to be irrational, yet it is a personal religious belief that needs to be respected even though the physician disagrees with it, especially in the determination of whether the patient has decision-making capacity. Regarding our case, the patient's abnormal behavior would lead me to question the possibility of an underlying suicidal intent, and whether his wound may have been self-inflicted. The possibility of suicidality only gives further credence to the attempts made to prevent this patient from leaving the ED until his decision-making capacity could be better assessed.

JJ: The patient in our case seemed to have acted reasonably when he presented to the ED, albeit with the encouragement of his wife. I wonder if the patient's wife were included in the conversation about the need to keep him in the hospital, whether he might have made a more rational or intelligent choice.

SG: What happened to this patient?

MT: The patient was observed for several hours to ensure clinical stability and to assess decision-making capacity. The physician ultimately assessed adequate decision-making capacity based on orientation, deliberation, and communication that demonstrated his understanding of the potential consequences of his decision.

RW: What if the patient had announced that he was leaving before you had the chance to assess his decision-making capacity, and you simultaneously had an unstable patient who demanded your attention?

MT: I would have called security to prevent him from leaving. I wouldn't have been happy with the decision, but when forced into a corner, I would act in the best interests of the patient. That includes restraining him in order to assess his injuries and his decision-making capacity.

Section III: Review of the literature

Informed consent is a valued concept of utmost importance in the ED. A valid informed consent process includes the following elements: delivery of the relevant information, appropriate decision-making capacity to use this information to make and communicate a decision, and voluntary informed consent to a proposed medical intervention.[1,2]

Respect for patient autonomy is a fundamental principle of ethical medical practice. In most cases, when a patient possesses appropriate decision-making capacity, this is achieved by the patient's voluntary consent to medical interventions. Respect for autonomy is more difficult to honor in cases that involve patients who lack decision-making capacity.

Voluntary informed consent serves two functions, protecting a patient's wellbeing, and respecting patient autonomy, an individual's right to self-determination.[2,3] In some cases, these two functions may seemingly be in conflict. On the one hand, it respects patient autonomy but, on the other hand, voluntary informed consent may not correspond to what we believe is in the patient's best interests. This chapter will primarily assess decision-making capacity, a crucial element of the informed consent process.

What is decision-making capacity?

Decision-making capacity can be defined as a patient's ability to make informed decisions about medical care, at a particular point in time.[4] Another definition refers to a patient's cognitive and emotional capability to accept or refuse a proposed treatment, or choose between treatment alternatives.[5] There should also be

a distinction drawn between medical decision-making capacity, which is a judgment made by a physician, and legal competence, which is determined by a judge in the courts.[6] In some cases, a patient may have adequate capacity for medical decision-making, yet may lack legal competence, a far broader term of decision-making capabilities. The opposite may also be true in some cases.

During most routine patient encounters, there is no identifiable threat to the patient's ability to make a decision.[6] In other cases, however, a patient is not able to make reasonable decisions on his or her own, because the patient lacks decision-making capacity. Alternatively, the patient may disagree with recommended interventions, but has appropriate decision-making capacity, and the patient's autonomy should be respected. In such cases, the importance of the physician assessment of decision-making capacity is critical to appropriate medical decision-making.

In the ED, a physician is required to make many complex decisions during the course of each shift; many of them can be explained to the patient, but many cannot. When the patient has capacity to make decisions, it is important to include the patient in the decision-making process.[6] When a patient is fully alert and rational, the ability to participate in and consent to medical care is rarely questioned. A patient's lack of ability to consent to treatment is similarly assumed when the patient is clearly unconscious or frankly delirious. The need to specifically assess medical decision-making capacity is most significant in cases where a patient of any level of consciousness or mental acuity refuses a recommended medical intervention.

In recent years, the distinction between mental illness and impaired decision-making capacity has been better clarified.[7,8] In addition, the importance of respecting a patient's autonomy is rarely called into question when the doctor and the patient agree. When decision-making capacity is impaired or deficient, however, the beneficence of treatment is viewed as being more important than respecting an impaired patient's right to make decisions about his or her own body.

Threats to decision-making capacity in ED patients

When is a patient incapable of consenting to or refusing a medical intervention? Numerous potential barriers to decision-making capacity exist among ED patients, including (but not limited to), language and literacy barriers, cultural practices, mental illness, dementia, chemical intoxication, elderly patients, patients in extremis, severe pain, anxiety, minors, medication effects, metabolic disorders, and numerous other organic disorders causing cognitive dysfunction.[3,8–11] While these barriers must be identified and considered, they are not necessarily an indication of impaired decision-making capacity. Individuals with some impairment of decision-making capacity may demonstrate adequate understanding of a particular situation to make a reasoned choice.[7,12,13]

Assessment of decision-making capacity

Each assessment of capacity should be individualized to the patient and the particular situation in question. There have been many attempts to describe ways to assess decision-making capacity. In general, assessment of decision-making capacity is determined by clinical judgment. In difficult cases, an objective measurement may serve to support clinical judgment.[14] No tool can completely replace individual clinical judgment, which takes into account an array of medical, legal and social aspects of a patient's care.[5] A physician's clinical judgment, however, is not perfect. Therefore, the empirical basis for these determinations has progressed secondary to a number of clinical assessment tools designed to help evaluate decision-making capacity.[1,7,9,12,13,15,16] The following instruments have been suggested:

• A global assessment of a patient's ability to reason. This assessment is commonly performed through the patient interview. If there is not enough time for a full evaluation, simply asking the patient to express an understanding of short-term options and consequences may be used as evidence of intact or impaired cognition. More explicitly, there is widespread agreement that the ability to reason, as it pertains to medical decision-making capacity, consists of four parts: (1) The ability to receive information from the physician regarding the facts of the case; (2) the ability to process the facts and understand the implications of the illness; (3) the ability to deliberate between possible choices of treatment; and (4) the ability to make a choice between alternatives, and to communicate that choice effectively.[7,9]

Table 14.1 Mini-Mental State Examination

	Score	Maximum score
Orientation		
What is the (year) (season) (date) (day) (month)?		5
Where are we? (state) (county) (town) (hospital) (floor)		5
Registration		
Name three objects and ask patient to repeat		3
Attention and calculation		
Serial 7s (one point for each correct up to 5)		
Option: Spell "world" backwards		5
Recall		
Ask for the three objects repeated above		3
Language		
Name a pencil and watch (2 points)		9
Repeat "no ifs, ands, or buts" (1 point)		
Follow a three-stage command. (3 points)		
Read and follow the command "Close your eyes" (1 point)		
Write a sentence (1 point)		
Copy a design (1 point)		

• The Mini-Mental State Examination (MMSE; Table 14.1) consists of a brief standardized assessment of the patient's memory, speech centers, visuospatial ability, ability to calculate, and other executive cortical functions such as planning and judgment by presenting to the patient a brief series of questions and tasks. The assessment entails a series of questions for the patient to answer, the responses for which are then scored, with a maximum of 30 points. Some questions are simple, such as the patient's knowledge of the date, place, and self-identity. Others entail following directions to complete a complex or memory-driven task, testing visual fields, or attention-driven tasks. Few people scoring more than 27 have deficits in decision-making capacity, and few with a score less than 20 have decision-making capacity; the test, however, is inconclusive, especially for those with scores between 20 and 27.[17,18]

• "DECISION" is another clinical tool available to assist the physician. The acronym "DECISION" refers to the need to determine the need for capacity assessment; ensure the patient is not being coerced, and correct reversible medical conditions that might be responsible for impaired capacity; investigate cognition with standardized tests; survey the patient's goals, values, and fears; integrate gathered information searching for patient understanding; openly communicate assessment to involved parties; and note essential elements of capacity or its impairment in the medical record.[9]

• CURVES is another acronym that may be utilized to determine decision-making capacity. It reminds the physician to assess the patient's ability to choose between options and communicate the choice, assess the patient's ability to understand the details and consequences of alternative choices, assess the patient's ability to reason, assess if the decision is consistent with personal values, and if capacity is impaired sufficiently, identify if an emergency exists and seek a surrogate decision-maker.[13]

• ACE (aid to capacity evaluation) is a non-standardized semi-structured assessment tool focusing on seven aspects of capacity that evaluates a patient's ability to understand the medical problem, the treatment, the alternatives to treatment and the option of refusing treatment, ability to perceive consequences of accepting and refusing treatment, and ability to make decision not based on patently false beliefs.[3,14]

• McArthur Competence Assessment Tool (MacCAT) is a flexible yet structured interview with the patient to assess four cognitive abilities that relate to medical decision-making: understanding, appreciation, reasoning, and clear expression of a choice.[3,19]

The more experience a clinician has in assessing patient decision-making capacity, the greater is the proficiency gained in the use of clinical judgment as the primary assessment tool. Although standardized assessment tools may aid in the assessment of decision-making capacity, they should be used as supportive adjuncts and not as a substitute for overall clinical judgment, or the need to consult appropriate experts.

The sliding scale approach to assessment of decision-making capacity

Traditionally, the ability of a patient to make a proper informed decision has been considered and applied within a context of a risk/benefit analysis in which the choice made by the patient is weighed against its alternative. For example, a clinician should require a more definitive demonstration of a patient's ability to reason if the patient attempted to make a decision to accept an intervention with little benefit, but which carried with it a large degree of risk. In the opposite scenario, a clinician might not require a stringent test of a patient's ability to reason, if he chose a treatment that is highly beneficial and carried with it a low degree of risk. This would also apply to refusal of treatment.[7]

The "sliding scale" approach to decision-making capacity attempts to allow patients with capacity to participate in their care as much as possible while minimizing the harm from a decision made by a patient without decision-making capacity.[20] This approach suggests different levels of stringency for different risk/benefit situations. For example, "assent" is sufficient for a low-risk intervention, such as a phlebotomy for various blood tests. "Understanding" is indicated to recognize someone as decisional for those treatments or tests that carry more risk or that have alternative measures. The most stringent level, "appreciation" is required for when consenting or refusing a medical therapy that carries a high level of risk.[7] Both of the above frameworks still use a common and partially subjective understanding of rationality as the standard by which a patient demonstrates his or her thought process. A clinician should use any individual or combination of the above approaches while assessing the decision-making capacity of a patient.

Management of patients with impaired decision-making capacity

If a patient lacks appropriate decision-making capacity, whether due to chemical intoxication or other cognitive impairment, it becomes necessary to identify a surrogate decision-maker, or someone to make appropriate decisions on the patient's behalf. Documentation of patient values and desires, such as a living will, advanced directive, or a power of attorney, may be valuable in the determination of the best course of action. In most cases, the appropriate legal surrogate is the patient's next of kin, typically a spouse or first-degree relative, as defined by state law. There are situations, however, during which the patient's emergent condition is such that there is not enough time to identify and find the appropriate surrogate decision-maker. The appropriate decisions are then based upon presumed consent, defined as what a reasonable person in a similar position would consent to receive. Throughout this process, as the patient's condition changes, reassessment of the patient's decision-making capacity is indicated.

For patients lacking decision-making capacity, it is the physician's duty to prevent the patient from leaving the ED. Additional tact is often required when dealing with a patient who may become aggressive or combative. If the patient is refusing treatment, or lacks the capacity to consent for a simple small superficial laceration repair, some clinicians would determine that a lower standard of decision-making capacity be met to refuse such a procedure, representing a non-lethal injury with almost no morbidity. The case of a patient with a potentially lethal illness is quite different. If the patient does not have decision-making capacity, it may be necessary to have security officers physically restrain the patient, followed by chemical restraint. Attempts should be made to avoid the necessity for physical or chemical restraints, and if restraint is necessary, the least restrictive type of restraint should be used for the minimum amount of time. Ongoing empathetic communication, attempts to reason and discuss the best course of action, and listening to patient's concerns are important, regardless of the decisional state.

In the case of an intoxicated patient, simply observing the patient until there is clinical sobriety may be sufficient to reestablish decision-making capacity. It is also paramount that any reversible organic causes of the patient's decreased decision-making capacity be identified, and addressed as soon as possible. If an emergency exists, and the clinical team does not have the time to consult with family, a judge, or documents such as an advanced directive before an intervention is required, the physician should act upon the concept of presumed consent.

Documentation

Regardless of the patient's capacity, willingness to consent, or the outcome of the ED visit, all aspects of the case should be clearly documented in the medical record. A patient and family should also be given every available resource to address any additional psychosocial needs or concerns that they may have.

Case discussion

In the case of the intoxicated patient, as with any patient, assessment of decision-making capacity is the primary initial step. Simply analyzing the patient's capacity to reason through taking a medical history may be all the clinician needs to make a determination of the patient's decision-making capacity. Can he or she understand, consider, relate, and apply the relevant information in a cogent fashion? If decision-making capacity is uncertain, the physician should employ the use of any of the above clinical tools to assist his or her assessment. The physician may also consider input from other consultants, including family members, psychiatry, social work, ethics, or pastoral care.

Conclusion

Assessment of decision-making capacity is an essential skill for emergency physicians and should be done for all ED patients. For many patients who possess decision-making capacity, clinical judgment of intact capacity is sufficient. For patients who may lack decision-making capacity, management should include treatment of reversible threats to capacity, standardized tests of capacity, evaluation of the patient's previously expressed wishes, and a team approach which may include the patient, family, clergy, and social services. Assessment of decision-making capacity is an important expression of respect for patient autonomy.

Section IV: Recommendations

• Assess decision-making capacity for all patients.
• Correct reversible threats to decision-making capacity.
• Inform the patient of the risks and benefits, alternatives, and expected outcomes of the proposed medical intervention.
• If the patient makes a decision, assure that the patient is making an informed voluntary, autonomous decision.

• Document the assessment of decision-making capacity in the medical record.

• Reassess decision-making capacity as the patient's clinical status changes.

• Provide appropriate medical care, comfort care, psychosocial and spiritual support, and ongoing communication with the patient and family.

References

1. Moskop JC. (2006) Informed consent and refusal of treatment: Challenges for emergency physicians. *Emerg Med Clin North Am.* 24, 605–18.

2. Moskop JC. (1999) Informed consent in the emergency department. *Emerg Med Clin North Am.* 17, 327–41.

3. Tunzi M. (2001) Can the patient decide? Evaluating patient capacity in practice. *Am Fam Physician.* 64, 299–306.

4. Derse AR. (1999) Making decisions about life-sustaining medical treatment in patients with dementia: The problem of patient decision making capacity. *Theor Med Bioeth.* 20, 55–67.

5. Okonkwo O, Griffith HR, Belue K, et al. (2007) Medical decisional capacity in patients with mild cognitive impairment. *Neurology,* 69, 1528–35.

6. Magauran BG. (2009) Risk management for the emergency physician: Competency and decisional capacity, informed consent, and refusal of care against medical advice. *Emerg Med Clin North Am.* 27, 605–14.

7. Zaubler ZS, Viederman M, Fins JJ. (1996) Ethical, legal and psychiatric issues in capacity, competence, and informed consent: An annotated bibliography. *Gen Hosp Psychiatry.* 18, 155–72.

8. Welie SPK. (2001) Criteria for patient decision making (in)competence: A review of and commentary on some empirical approaches. *Med Health Care Philos.* 4, 139–51.

9. Larkin GL, Marco CA, Abbot JT. (2001) Emergency determination of decision making capacity (DMC): Balancing autonomy and beneficence in the emergency department. *Acad Emerg Med.* 8, 282–4.

10. Karlawish J. (2008) Measuring decisional capacity in cognitively impaired individuals. *Neurosignals.* 16, 91–8.

11. Fassassi S, Bianchi Y, Stiefel F, et al. (2009) Assessment of the capacity to consent to treatment in patients admitted to acute medical wards. *BMC Med Ethics.* 10, 15.

12. Kutner JS, Ruark JE, Raffin TA. (1991) Defining patient competence for medical decision making. *Chest.* 100, 1404–9.

13. Chow GV, Czarny MJ, Hughes MT, et al. (2010) CURVES: A mnemonic for determining medical decisional-making capacity and providing emergency treatment in the acute setting. *Chest.* 137, 421–7.

14. Moye J, Gurrera RJ, Karel MJ, et al. (2006) Empirical advances in the assessment of the capacity to consent to medical treatment: Clinical implications and research needs. *Clin Psychol Rev.* 26, 1054–77.

15. Pachet A, Astner K, Brown L. (2010) Clinical utility in the mini-mental status examination when assessing decisional capacity. *J Geriatr Psych Neurol.* 23, 3–8.

16. Okonkwo OC, Griffith HR, Copeland JN, et al. (2008) Medical decisional in mild cognitive impairment: A 3-year longitudinal study. *Neurology.* 71, 1474–90.

17. Etchells E, Darzins P, Silberfeld M, et al. (1999) Assessment of patient capacity to consent to treatment. *J Gen Intern Med.* 14, 27–34.

18. Dziedzic L, Brady WJ, Lindsay R, et al. (1998) The use of the mini-mental status exam in the ED evaluation of the elderly. *Am J Emerg Med.* 16, 686–91.

19. Grisso T, Appelbaum PS, Hill-Fotouhi C. (1997) The MacCAT-T: A clinical tool to assess patients' capacities to make treatment decisions. *Psychiatr Serv.* 48, 1415–19.

20. Howe E. (2008) Ethical aspects of evaluating a patient's mental capacity. *Psychiatry.* 6, 15–23.

15 Obstetric emergency: perimortem cesarean section

Kenneth D. Marshall,[1] Carrie Tibbles[2]

[1]*Resident Physician, Department of Emergency Medicine, Beth Israel Deaconess Medical Center, Boston, MA, USA*

[2]*Instructor in Medicine at Harvard Medical School, Department of Emergency Medicine, Beth Israel Deaconess Medical Center, Boston, MA, USA*

Section I: Case presentation

A 30-year-old woman, gravida 4 parity 2, who had said she was at 33 weeks gestation was brought by ambulance to the emergency department (ED) after sustaining stab wounds to the left chest. In the field, the patient was initially alert and oriented, and paramedics reported two stab wounds in the posterior chest and axilla. The last paramedic-reported vital signs were a heart rate of 140 beats per minute, blood pressure 85/40 mmHg, ventilatory rate 35 breaths per minute, and an oxygen saturation 80% on a 100% non-rebreather mask.

Upon arrival in the ED, the patient rapidly lost consciousness. During the patient's primary survey, diminished breath sounds were noted over the left lung field, and the patient was pulseless. A needle decompression of the chest yielded substantial air return while pads were applied to the chest. The monitor demonstrated asystole, and cardiopulmonary resuscitation (CPR) was initiated. Simultaneously, the patient was intubated, and a tube thoracostomy was placed on the left side, returning a large amount of blood. During the initial 2 minutes of chest compressions, the emergency physician running the code decided that an emergent cesarean section (c-section) would be appropriate given the late

stage of pregnancy, and requested that the ED c-section kit be readied.

A large midline abdominal incision was made with little bleeding evident from the incision, and no free blood in the abdomen. At 5 minutes into the resuscitation, a neonate was delivered with an APGAR score of 2 and 6 at the 1- and 5-minute marks, and the baby was taken to the neonatal intensive care unit (ICU). Resuscitation efforts were continued for 10 more minutes, with no signs of improvement in the patient's condition, at which point CPR was discontinued.

Section II: Discussion

Dr. Peter Rosen: I was involved in a medical malpractice suit several years ago. A mother was brought to the ED in the third trimester, and shortly after arriving, she arrested. Attempts were made to resuscitate the mother unsuccessfully, and a c-section was performed. The neonate was successfully delivered, but had some brain damage. The lawsuit was filed against the emergency physician for not performing the c-section sooner. Are there known indications for when the c-section should be initiated that are currently accepted?

Ethical Problems in Emergency Medicine: A Discussion-Based Review, First Edition. John Jesus, Shamai A. Grossman, Arthur R. Derse, James G. Adams, Richard Wolfe, and Peter Rosen.
© 2012 John Wiley & Sons, Ltd. Published 2012 by John Wiley & Sons, Ltd.

Dr. Carrie Tibbles: In this particular arena, we don't have the luxury of controlled trials or a large base of patients upon which to base our decisions. We must draw our conclusions based on a collection of case reports spanning two decades, and by using what we know about physiology and cardiac arrest. What we can surmise from the information we have is that the number one medical indication for doing a perimortem c-section is having a potentially viable fetus at the time one starts the c-section. If the fetus is previable or has already lost fetal heart tones, the physician should not proceed with the procedure. Once the decision is made to perform the procedure, the existing literature would suggest that starting within 4 minutes of arrest gives the fetus a much higher probability of surviving neurologically intact. Often emergency physicians will be pressured to make a very quick decision as time will have already been lost in the prehospital setting.

PR: Are there any medical criteria upon which an emergency physician would decide to avoid resuscitation of the mother, and focus exclusively on performing the c-section with the intention of delivering a viable fetus?

Dr. John Jesus: If an emergency physician finds himself within the time period that would allow a fetus to survive, they are also within the period of time during which the mother would receive the most benefit from continued resuscitation. A perimortem c-section can and should be considered part of the resuscitation of the pregnant patient as the resultant relief of the cardiac output burden the fetus places on the mother may allow better perfusion and better resuscitation of the mother.

CT: The resuscitation of the pregnant patient is not mutually exclusive of performing a c-section, but there is often a resource issue. If you have a single doctor and nurse running the case then there may well be a logistical difficulty: How many aspects of the resuscitation can one or two people do at the same time? In general, however, the resuscitation of the mother should proceed while the emergency physician makes the decision and performs the c-section.

PR: An emergency physician will generally resuscitate all patients arriving in cardiac arrest short of the patient who shows signs of decomposition, decapitation, or rigor mortis on a warm night. At what point

should the care of the mother be superseded by the care of the potentially viable fetus? From what I understand, the best chance for the child is achieved by the best care of the mother. Dr. Tibbles mentioned that when one doesn't hear fetal heart tones it diminishes the chances of a successful child resuscitation. I believe it is very difficult to determine active fetal heart activity with any accuracy in such a situation without an ultrasound, and I'm not so sure that I would rely upon it.

Dr. Kenneth Marshall: My understanding from the literature is that so long as the emergency physician believes the fetus had reached viability, there is no need to attempt obtaining a pulse by Doppler simply because this may take too much time.

CT: That said, if a patient presents to the ED after an overdose, and is found after a prolonged period of time in the field in asystole, **and** no fetal heart tones can be identified, then there is very little benefit to performing an emergency c-section. There are many situations in between the two outlined here that may be considerably more complicated, therefore if there is any question about the viability of the fetus, the emergency physician should proceed with the procedure.

JJ: I think there is a misperception among many physicians across the country that if they perform a perimortem c-section, they are "giving up on mom." There is an emotional affront to picking up a scalpel and cutting the abdomen of a healthy 25-year-old in cardiac arrest within 4 minutes of beginning the resuscitation. The emergency physician must begin thinking about the c-section the moment a pregnant patient hits the door.

PR: Most EDs don't have multiple physicians, and even if you call upon the paramedics or use the ED nurses to continue the CPR, chances are that if the physician embarks upon the c-section, performing the procedure will diminish the resources that would otherwise be directed at continued parental resuscitation. I also think that very few emergency physicians have ever performed a c-section, and probably believe that their surgical ignorance is the same as avoiding the surgery altogether once the risks and benefits are properly assessed. A c-section, per se, should not end anyone's life. They're not that hard to perform. That said, they are not part of the emergency medicine curriculum, and I think the internal turmoil involved in picking up the scalpel is powerful, particularly for a procedure that one has never performed, perhaps hasn't ever seen in person, and certainly doesn't feel confident in performing.

JJ: We've asked our residents and the obstetric attending physicians on service to include the emergency medicine residents in at least one c-section. I don't think it is impossible to have some exposure to the procedure as part of a residency curriculum, but I suspect that it is not common.

PR: Having performed one controlled c-section in an OR doesn't make you capable of doing an emergency c-section in the ED. Generally, most c-sections today utilize a low transverse incision, and crash c-sections in the ED will all be midline abdominal incisions. Furthermore, I doubt having performed one previously will instill a great deal of confidence when you undertake your first one in practice 20 years later.

CT: There are several procedures in emergency medicine that an EP will perform only once or twice during a career, and on that day the EP is expected to be spectacularly competent. It's hard to train for those types of procedures, and it's a challenge to know how much curriculum to devote to them.

PR: There are many procedures that we could teach but don't because the incidence of situations that require their performance is so low that it doesn't warrant taking the time from those procedures that we perform on a daily basis and truly require expert skill. I cannot fault a physician for saying, "My chances of successfully performing this procedure are so low that I don't see the point of inflicting unnecessary trauma to a patient who will not benefit from the procedure," and therefore I have to accept the reality that if somebody trained in that procedure were standing at my side, the patient might be salvageable. I also wouldn't fault someone who attempted the procedure believing that a very slim chance of delivering a viable baby is better than no chance. The appropriateness of the procedure depends on a combination of circumstance, equipment, and the individual physician. For example, I don't see any point in placing burr holes in a patient with a head injury if the nearest neurosurgeon is 500 miles away, and there is no way to care for the head injury without transferring the patient. Similarly, there's no point in undertaking a thoracotomy in the ED if you don't have a rib spreader.

KM: If one has easy access to in-house obstetric coverage it would be ideal to have them come in and lead the crash c-section while the emergency physician manages the resuscitation of the pregnant patient. On the other hand, if such coverage is not available, both patients have an extremely high chance of a poor outcome without an intervention. An emergency c-section ought to be considered a massive improvement over doing nothing no matter how extreme your level of discomfort with the procedure.

PR: Performing a c-section and ending the mother's life may not be synonymous, but if you're alone, one physician cannot resuscitate two people. When I no longer believe there is any further benefit to offer the mother through my attempts to resuscitate her, then I would turn my attention to attempting to deliver the child.

CT: We shouldn't underestimate the hemodynamic burden of the uterus and fetus on the mother. Up to 20% of a pregnant person's blood volume at a given time is going to the fetus, uterus, and placenta. Therefore, the removal of that hemodynamic burden improves the ability of your ACLS [Advanced Cardiac Life Support] drugs to circulate. If the physician doesn't consider that fact during the decision making, a c-section, which would have benefitted both the mother and the baby, might not be performed.

PR: One of the issues that came up in the lawsuit I reviewed was the child's neurologic impairment. The lawyers attempted to argue that the emergency physician was negligent because he did not perform the c-section the minute the mother hit the door. I argued that it was medically inappropriate to start the c-section before one has attempted to resuscitate the pregnant patient.

KM: Delivering children with neurologic impairment is the exception rather than the rule, at least as far as the published literature is concerned. In a 2005 review, there were 34 surviving infants from the 40-odd cases that were reported of emergency cesarean section (ECS).[1] Of those, five had neurologic impairment. In Great Britain, they published a list of perimortem c-sections limited to cases in which the mother died, and there were no reports of neurologic impairment in any infant that survived beyond about 2 weeks.[2]

159

CT: That 2005 review was unfortunately affected by a reporting bias, as physicians are less likely to report an unsuccessful procedure or a procedure that results in a bad outcome, such as severe neurologic impairment.

JJ: Performing an ECS is a heroic measure. I don't believe it is a sign of negligence or injustice if the procedure is not successful. In order to hold an emergency physician accountable for this procedure, you first have to prove that the procedure is within the standard of care by which all emergency physicians should operate. Because so few people have performed this procedure, I don't believe anyone could successfully argue that it is within the standard of care.

CT: I've looked at two medicolegal cases in which the argument was made that the emergency physician had an obligation to perform the procedure. I argued that the procedure was in line with a heroic intervention, and is a procedure emergency physicians should certainly feel empowered to perform if they feel capable. I argued further that any attempt to hold emergency physicians accountable to a standard of competency in this case was not realistic or fair.

PR: It is a very difficult situation to find oneself in, and I believe that if you don't consider and come to terms with the issues involved in advance, you may find yourself paralyzed by fear or the need to think through the issues at the very time in which you need to act.

KM: One aspect of the situation we haven't yet discussed is how to approach the family of the pregnant coding patient. Especially in light of the cultural issues that we've discussed, the physician should make an effort to reassure the family that as far as we know performing the c-section is in the best interest of both the mother and the child. At the same time, the EP should attempt to diffuse, to the extent possible, any misconception the family might feel that either the mother or the child is being favored over the other.

PR: There is one other point about family I would like to emphasize. I can think of almost no worse situation than to receive a newborn baby and simultaneously learn that my wife had died during the procedure. We will have a tremendous psychological impact on surviving family members, and should anticipate their emotional needs.

JJ: In summary, the perimortem emergency c-section is a procedure that needs to happen within 4 minutes of the start of the resuscitation. Preparation through participating in a controlled c-section and thinking through the ethical and logistical issues involved are absolutely paramount to prevent or lessen the tragedy and stress on the part of the family, the patient, and also on the physician and the medical personnel involved.

Section III: Review of the literature

Cases of the kind presented here, while uncommon, are fraught with anxiety for an emergency physician. Two lives, those of a woman and the fetus, hang in the balance, and the outcome depends on the physician making a rapid decision to provide treatment, a c-section and postnatal care. Complicating this situation further, the emergency physician may have reservations about whether performing an emergent c-section is indeed the clinically, morally, and socially correct course of action. Though the data available on such cases are imperfect, it appears to show that perimortem c-section within certain clinical guidelines is clinically the best hope of survival for mother and fetus. The purpose of this chapter is to provide reassurance that performing a cesarean in such situations is morally appropriate, and even laudatory, to comment on factors that may have an impact upon the physician's decision making about whether to perform this type of procedure, and to describe the need for augmented training of emergency physicians given the clinical utility of such procedures.

History

The case under discussion is an example of a perimortem c-section, which is a c-section performed when a pregnant patient is undergoing CPR. This concept was introduced in the 1980s to distinguish perimortem from postmortem c-sections, which had been historically done shortly after a mother had died, usually after succumbing to chronic disease or severe infection. This distinction makes sense in the light of a changing epidemiology of maternal mortality: prenatal care, infection control, and public health measures have made maternal mortality from chronic causes rare, and thus when maternal cardiopulmonary arrest does occur, it is generally from acute causes (e.g., trauma, pulmonary embolism, cerebrovascular accidents), leaving both mother and fetus more capable of successful rescue.

The concept of perimortem c-section was given its original impetus by a comprehensive review of world literature from 1900 to 1985, which shows that greater than 90% of neonates survive peri- and postmortem c-sections when delivered within 15 minutes of maternal death, and that the vast majority of these survivals are neurologically normal.[3] The authors of this review recommend that if CPR is being performed on a mother whose fetus has reached viability (roughly 26 weeks, or at which time the fundal height has reached 26 cm above the pubic symphysis), and the resuscitation is not successful within 4 minutes of loss of maternal vital signs, perimortem c-section should be initiated, and the baby delivered within 5 minutes.[3,4] This recommendation has since been adopted both in the United States and internationally.[5]

Who takes precedence: mother or child?

One major source of potential qualms about the morality of perimortem c-section is the idea that in pursuing this treatment, the physician turns the clinical focus from the mother to the fetus, and in so doing abdicates a responsibility to the mother, reduces the mother's likelihood of survival, or violates the mother's rights. The most crucial fact in overcoming such a worry is that in survivable cases of cardiac arrest, prompt c-section appears to be the best hope of recovery for the mother. Proof of this begins with consideration of the low survival rates for patients who arrive in the ED in cardiac arrest (6%–8% percent of patients) and those who arrest in the ED (perhaps closer to 20%).[6–8] Further, while overall survival rates specifically for pregnant women who arrest are unknown, it is well documented that the altered physiology of the pregnant patient complicates attempts at CPR.[9,10] Physiologic theory suggests that removal of the fetus and placenta may thus confer hemodynamic benefit to the mother.[2,3,11,12]

These observations amount to a prima facie case that suggests perimortem c-section is in the best interests of the mother as well as the child. Such a case is reinforced by the limited clinical data that are available. To date, the best data available is a comprehensive review of case reports of c-section after cardiopulmonary arrest.[11] In this review of 38 cases of perimortem c-section, 20 women were thought to have recoverable insults, and of these 13 were resuscitated. In addition, in 22 of the 38 cases, hemodynamic information was recorded, and of these 22 cases, 12 women showed dramatic hemodynamic improvement following perimortem c-section (e.g., return of spontaneous pulses), and two showed nonspecific improvement (e.g., change from asystole to pulseless electrical activity [PEA]). More recent case reports published since that review also report good outcomes.[13]

Nevertheless, such reviews and case reports are subject to a substantial publication bias, and there are clearly a number of unreported instances of perimortem c-section that have not led to survival of the mother. For instance, as part of its triennial report on maternal mortality (*Confidential Enquiry into Maternal and Child Health* [CEMACH]), the United Kingdom Department of Health keeps a record of peri- and postmortem c-sections not survived by the mother, of which there were 49 from 2000 to 2002, the latest triennium for which data are available. Unfortunately, the Department of Health does not compile data on perimortem c-sections that are survived by the mother, information which would be very useful in analyzing these issues.[14] Although, the data fall short of definitely proving that perimortem c-section is the optimal intervention for the arresting woman, they remain highly suggestive. Given the bleak outlook of cardiopulmonary arrest generally, perimortem c-section seems to be the most prudent strategy for effective resuscitation of the late-pregnant woman. Thus, the interests of the fetus and those of the mother appear to be aligned, and by performing a perimortem c-section, the physician is pursuing a course of action likely to be beneficial to the mother. The perimortem c-section should not come at the expense of a well-run resuscitation, which should continue during the procedure in order to maximize chances of maternal recovery.

Maternal consent and autonomy

A second source of concern that might trouble a physician about perimortem c-section is that it is a procedure to which the patient has not consented. In cases involving a potentially survivable insult to the mother, the answer to this worry is straightforward given the foregoing discussion: because perimortem c-section appears to be a potentially life-saving intervention for the woman during cardiac arrest, it would fall under the traditionally understood emergency exception to the need for informed consent to treatment. Briefly, such exception to the necessity of informed consent requires three conditions be met: that the person be unconscious or lack capacity to consent, that a life-threatening injury or disease requiring immediate treatment be present, and that under such circumstances, a reasonable person would consent to the treatment.[15]

The answer is not as straightforward in cases where cardiac arrest results from a non-survivable insult to the mother, for in such cases the perimortem c-section no longer confers benefit on the mother. Moreover, though it is tempting to say that the mother in unrecoverable cardiac arrest lacks rights or interests, this is an incorrect analysis. The woman maintains rights of dominion over her body even in this dire situation, so there could be, at least in theory, a conflict between maternal and fetal interests in such a case. However, while such conflict exists theoretically, in such emergent situations the clinician will, in all likelihood, not know the woman's wishes. Given the lack of any countervailing interest, saving the fetus is the right thing to do.

The most difficult case in this regard would be one in which the woman had indicated in advance that she would not want a perimortem c-section performed were she in extremis. Such cases are more difficult theoretically, but cases such as these that involve theoretical dilemmas are very unlikely to become reality. In the theoretical case, the physician would be confronted with a conflict between the woman's right to dominion over her body (using a principle-based approach to medical ethics, this would correspond to the principle of autonomy), and the good of saving the life of the fetus (corresponding to the principle of beneficence).[16] Suggestions regarding such a stark dilemma would require sophisticated and sensitive philosophic argument. However, we do not think this kind of stark choice will ever occur, and as a result, maintain that the physician's default should be to perform the perimortem c-section. This is because in order for a scenario of this kind to represent a true dilemma for the physician, several conditions would need to be met. The physician would need to be utterly certain of the woman's capacity to refuse such

an action, including her understanding of the procedure (its benefits, etc.), and also discern whether her refusal is borne out of some stable evaluative framework or plan of life. This burden of certainty will almost never be met by the physician in the pressured circumstances of this kind of emergency. Thus, even in such remote circumstances, the physician should perform perimortem c-section to save the fetus.

Fetal consent

The foregoing remarks have shown that there are no salient conflicts between the interests of the mother and fetus, and that performing perimortem c-section is consistent with optimal treatment for the mother. However, a second cause of hesitancy for the physician may be whether performing perimortem c-section is in the best interest of the fetus, or more accurately, the child the fetus may become. A physician may wonder whether delivering a neonate under such physiologically and operatively suboptimal conditions will produce a child with profound and tragic deficits. Katz's review includes 38 perimortem c-section procedures, of which 28 procedures yielded a total of 34 surviving infants.[11] Of these cases, the time of arrest to procedure information was available for 24 infants, and of these 24, 17 were normal, five had neurologic impairment, one had chronic respiratory problems, and one had hearing loss and retinopathy of prematurity. Of the 10 infants for whom the interval of time between maternal arrest and perimortem c-section was not recorded, four were normal, one had neurological impairment, and in five more the condition of the infant was not reported.

Further data comes from a review of the CEMACH studies (which, as mentioned before, only include cases in which the mother perished) in which all cases of perimortem c-section in the United Kingdom over 25 years up to the year 2000 demonstrates no cases in which a child survived beyond the early neonatal period with any neurologic sequelae, indicating that if the fetus survives the first several days of life, its chances of healthy survival are good.[17] Older data from the state of Michigan on **post**-mortem c-sections showed that while only 11% of post-mortem c-sections yielded long-term survivors, 100% of these were neurologically normal.[18] These data indicate that when a perimortem c-section is performed even under suboptimal conditions, a substantial number of surviving neonates are delivered. Two other points also emerge from the data. First, that increased rapidity of the procedure after loss of maternal vital signs is associated with better outcomes, and second, that long-term survivors have a fairly high likelihood of good function. Consequently, if a perimortem c-section is performed, the neonate has a fair chance of surviving, and if it survives long-term, it has a good chance of normal functioning. Comparing this range of possibilities to the outcome of foregoing perimortem c-section, which is assured death of the fetus, it seems clear that performing the procedure gives the fetus the best chance of developing into a healthy child, and so is in its best interest. This conclusion may ultimately vary from the particular circumstances of each case. Peri-mortem c-sections may end in tragedy depending on the mother's outcome, and the familial and social milieu into which even the healthiest infant is born through a perimortem c-section. However, these are tragic circumstances in which the emergency physician may at least offer the chance of life instead of death.

Familial consent

Another issue to consider is the preferences of the mother's family. Some suggest consulting with the family to obtain consent before performing the procedure.[19] We believe this is misguided for two reasons. First, as we have seen before, the evidentiary burden to establish a genuine countervailing reason not to perform the perimortem c-section to save the fetus is substantial: The physician would need to be certain who, if any, among the family present is actually the appropriate surrogate decision-maker, that the individual has capacity to consent or refuse, etc. Moreover, even if the family member refuses perimortem c-section, the physician's duty to attempt to save the fetus probably would outweigh such refusal. Given these problems with familial consent and refusal, and the enormous time pressures involved, attempting to obtain consent from a family member is the wrong approach. Instead, if the family is available, the physician should explain that a perimortem c-section will be performed, and that this procedure is in the best interests of mother and fetus.

Although we have argued here that a physician ought to try to attempt perimortem c-section within the abovementioned clinical guidelines due to the possibility of good outcomes both for mother and fetus,

the possibility of tragedy looms large. Even after technically perfect CPR and perimortem c-section, a wide range of tragic outcomes may ensue, from the loss of both mother and baby, to a surviving but neurologically crippled mother or baby, to the motherless infant. A physician should not be enchanted by the encouraging data in the review articles into expecting happy outcomes from perimortem c-section, but neither should they be dissuaded from acting decisively by fear of such tragic outcomes. As with so many other grave scenarios in the ED, the tragedy in such situations occurs independently of the physician, even if the attempts to help ultimately do not change the character of the tragedy.

Clinical judgment

To this point, we have primarily dealt with the ethics of perimortem c-section within narrow clinical guidelines. However, to the extent that the situation an emergency physician faces deviates from this "ideal" scenario, the physician will need to use one's clinical judgment as to whether to perform a perimortem c-section. Cases could deviate from this ideal in a number of ways, such as mothers arriving at the ED who have been coding more than 4 minutes, grossly inadequate operative conditions, lack of capability to perform the procedure without interrupting the code, and lack of capability to properly care for the delivered neonate. In these circumstances, the physician will need to weigh a number of factors: the prior health of the mother and fetus, the type and degree of injury to the mother, the duration and quality of the code, the availability of equipment and personnel to care for the neonate, etc. As the data indicate, chances of maternal and fetal survival are small but real even outside of ideal conditions. Thus, performing perimortem c-section outside the ideal clinical situation certainly falls within the range of ethically permissible approaches for the emergency physician. However, insofar as a circumstance deviates from the ideal, the prognosis for mother and fetus diminishes. Ultimately it will be a clinical judgment based on the particular circumstance to decide whether perimortem c-section is in the best interest of mother and fetus. The emergency physician should feel reassured that in this vexing situation, the only clear ethical requirement is to try to do what one thinks is best for the patient.

Conclusion

We have argued in this chapter that it is ethically permissible for an emergency physician to perform perimortem c-section within certain clinical parameters, and that in such cases it is likely the ethically correct course of action. However, it must be acknowledged that perimortem c-section is a therapeutic measure at the extreme limit of the emergency physician's range of practice. While it is a procedure with definite indications, it remains a rare and heroic measure, reserved for situations which most emergency physicians will never face, and which those who do will experience likely once only. As such, an emergency physician may feel wholly unqualified for such an undertaking, and as a result, we believe that the factors favoring perimortem c-section even within idealized conditions fall short of making its performance an ethically obligatory action. Emergency physicians should be reassured that performing perimortem c-section is ethically permissible. On the other hand, physicians should also realize that if they believe themselves to be unable to perform perimortem c-section, their decision not to undertake the procedure will not represent an unethical act of omission.

Section IV: Recommendations

• A perimortem c-section is a procedure for which emergency physicians receive little if any training but because it is a procedure that clearly falls into their domain, this dearth of training is inappropriate. Even a small amount of training, such as assisting with a small number of non-emergent cesareans during required obstetrics rotations in residency, or simulator training of perimortem c-section, could be easily accomplished and be potentially helpful for an emergency physician who encounters this kind of emergency.

• As emergency medicine physicians receive little if any training on performing perimortem c-sections, emergency staff may not be familiar with the equipment required for the procedure, and the ED may not have the necessary equipment. Physician training should be expanded, and EDs should have protocols and kits in place to help staff in performing well in these emergencies.

• A perimortem c-section should be thought of as a potentially life-saving procedure for mother and fetus. Thus, the procedure should not interfere with or take precedence over a well-run resuscitation.

• More data are needed about outcomes for perimortem c-section. Health departments that keep data about maternal mortality should consider expanding data collection to include cases in which mothers are resuscitated, including perimortem c-section cases.

• Without a medical countervailing reason, perimortem c-section should be done in cases that fall within the 4-minute guideline. Cases falling outside of this window will require the clinical judgment of the physician guided by the details of the situation.

• A perimortem c-section represents a uniquely stressful and emotional event, even compared with the already stressful environment of the ED. The family of the mother and fetus will be under great strain, and the ED staff are likely also to be profoundly affected as well. A coordinated crisis response is critical to support the emotional needs of patients, family, and staff.

References

1. Katz VL, Balderston K, DeFreest M. (2005) Perimortem cesarean delivery: were our assumptions correct? *Am J Obstet Gynecol.* 192(6), 1916–20; discussion 1920–1.

2. Warraich Q, Esen U. (2009) Perimortem caesarean section. *J Obstet Gynaecol.* 29(8), 690–3.

3. Katz VL, Dotters DJ, Droegemueller W. (1986) Perimortem cesarean delivery. *Obstet Gynecol.* 68(4), 571–6.

4. Stallard TC, Burns B. (2003) Emergency delivery and perimortem C-section. *Emerg Med Clin North Am.* 21, 679–93.

5. American Heart Association in collaboration with the International Liaison Committee on Resuscitation. Guidelines 2000 for cardiopulmonary resuscitation and emergency cardiovascular care: International Consensus on Science, Part 8: Advanced Challenges in Resuscitation: Section 3: Special Challenges in ECC: Cardiac Arrest Associated With Pregnancy. (2000) *Circulation.* 102 Suppl (8), I247–9.

6. Sasson C, Rogers M, Dahl J, et al. (2010) Predictors of survival from out-of-hospital cardiac arrest: A systematic review and meta-analysis. *Circ Cardiovasc Qual Outcomes.* 3(1), 63–81.

7. Nichol G, Stiell IG, Laupacis A, et al. (1999) A cumulative meta-analysis of the effectiveness of defibrillator-capable emergency medical services for victims of

out-of-hospital cardiac arrest. *Ann Emerg Med*. 34(4), Part I, 517–25.

8. Kayser RG, Ornato JP, Peberdy MA. (2008) Cardiac arrest in the emergency department. A report from the American Heart Association National Registry of Cardiopulmonary Resuscitation. *Resuscitation*. 78, 151–60.

9. Lee RV, Rodgers BD, White LM. (1986) Cardiopulmonary resuscitation of pregnant women. *Am J Med*. 81(2), 311–18.

10. Mallampalli A, Guy E. (2005) Cardiac arrest in pregnancy and somatic support after brain death. *Crit Care Med*. 33 Suppl 10, S325–31.

11. Strong TH, Lowe RA. (1989) Perimortem cesarean section. *Am J Emerg Med*. 7(5), 489–94.

12. Dildy GA, Clark SL. (1995) Cardiac arrest during pregnancy. *Obstet Gynaecol Clin North Am*. 22(2), 303–14.

13. McDonnell NJ. (2009) Cardiopulmonary arrest in pregnancy: two case reports of successful outcomes in association with perimortem Caesarean delivery. *Br J Anaesth*. 103(3), 406–9.

14. Lewis G. (2007) *Saving Mother's Lives: Reviewing Maternal Deaths to Make Motherhood Safer: 2003–2005*. The seventh report on Confidential Enquiry into Maternal Deaths in the United Kingdom. London: The Confidential Enquiry into Maternal and Child Health (CEMACH).

15. Derse AR, Rosen P, Friedman JB. (1995) Consent: explicit and presumed. In: Iserson KV, Sanders AB, Mathieu D. (eds) *Ethics in Emergency Medicine*, 2nd ed. Tuscon, AZ: Galen Press, pp. 95–105.

16. Beauchamp TL, Childress JF. (2001) *Principles of Biomedical Ethics*. New York, NY: Oxford University Press.

17. Whitten M, Montgomery L. (2000) Post-mortem and perimortem caesarean section: what are the indications? *J R Soc Med*. 93, 6–9.

18. Behney CA. (1961) Cesarean section delivery after death of the mother. *J Am Med Assoc*. 176(7), 617–19.

19. Meyer HB. (1986) Postmortem cesarean section: Removing and resuscitating a fetus from a dead patient. In: Iserson KV, Sanders AB, Mathieu DR. (eds) *Ethics in Emergency Medicine*. Baltimore, MD: Lippincott Williams & Wilkins, pp. 126–9.

Outside influence and observation

16 Non-medical observers in the emergency department

Joel Martin Geiderman

Co-Chairman, Department of Emergency Medicine, Professor of Emergency Medicine, Cedars-Sinai Medical Center, Los Angeles, CA, USA

Section I: Case presentation

You are the emergency department (ED) chairperson of a large, not-for-profit teaching hospital. In this capacity, over a several-month period you receive requests from four different parties who would like to "observe" in the ED. What are the ethical issues, and how would you respond to the following situations: (1) a Sheriff's chaplain trainee would like to spend several evening nights observing; (2) a board of directors member's niece has a guest star role as an emergency physician in a television medical drama, and would like to spend a day shadowing an emergency physician; (3) a colleague's daughter, a college student, is not sure if she wants to pursue a medical career or not. He asks you if she can spend a few hours in the ED; and (4) the chief of staff of one of your US senators would like to spend a day in the ED to better understand public policy issues in healthcare. In addition, some staff members have raised concerns about Joint Commission members observing patient encounters as well as nurse epidemiologists who are surreptitiously observing whether staff wash their hands between patents. How should you respond to these situations?

Section II: Discussion

Dr. Peter Rosen: In part, we owe the thirst for visiting the ED to the television show *ER*, which has both helped develop the specialty and to sensationalize it. Perhaps we've created our own monster. Important to the analysis of those who would like to spend time in the ED is their motive. We're not afraid to use the ED as an educational site, but there is a clear difference in my mind between allowing a chaplaincy student or medical student in to the ED to obtain a feel for what the actual life of an emergency physician is like, versus the friend of a trustee or colleague, or a fledgling actress. I also suspect that the decision to allow film crews into the ED is made by someone in administration, rather than by the emergency physician working in the ED. When I was departmental chair, I had little say in those decisions. As much as I tried to protect patient confidentiality when I worked in Denver and San Diego, we constantly had television crews in the ED.

Dr. Joel Geiderman: There is a sense of theater that has developed around the ED, and it has been fueled by *ER* and other television dramas and reality TV hits

Ethical Problems in Emergency Medicine: A Discussion-Based Review, First Edition. John Jesus, Shamai A. Grossman, Arthur R. Derse, James G. Adams, Richard Wolfe, and Peter Rosen.
© 2012 John Wiley & Sons, Ltd. Published 2012 by John Wiley & Sons, Ltd.

that have aired throughout the years. The cases described are drawn from real-life examples, and I included them because they speak to the spectrum of ethical acceptability of non-physician observers in the ED, with the chaplaincy student being on one end and the actor being at the other end.

I have talked to emergency physicians who work in a variety of geographic areas and found that requests to film patient–physician encounters in the ED are not at all uncommon. When I have turned down such requests, a common response is that, "I guess I will have to go try another hospital." Because of the popularity of shows like *Trauma: Real Life in the ED* and the seemingly natural human desire for fame and recognition, I am sure that they easily found someone and somewhere else to consent to their requests. Nevertheless, I believe it is important for chairs to stand up and say that part of our professional duty is to say "No," and to refuse requests to violate patient privacy, than to potentially exploit patients, by allowing this type of filming in the ED. Having said this, when it comes to some observers, there are also significant gray areas. What about the college student who is earnestly interested in pursuing a career in medicine and successfully completed the course work to do so? What about the high school student who has made no commitment but merely expressed a potential interest? The question then is where do we draw the lines between who should be and should not be allowed to observe patient interactions within the ED?

There is almost never any direct benefit to the patients themselves. As such, any argument defending the presence of non-physician observers in the ED must be framed in terms of societal benefit. Because members of society may benefit from the experiences of some non-physician observers, one could argue that as a matter of distributive justice, patients and emergency physicians are burdened with the responsibility of training non-physician observers. Nevertheless, as physicians interested in medical ethics, we must choose between situations in which we believe this is permissible and justifiable and when it is not.

PR: The possibility that another emergency physician will grant permission to a request that you refuse is ubiquitous to any ethical decision we make. We can't control the world. I am most comfortable, however,

with the concept described by Voltaire when he said, "We have to cultivate our own gardens." Just because many of my colleagues agree with a decision of which I disapprove, it doesn't make it right for me to ignore my misgivings and accede to the will of my colleagues. College or high school students can be included in the ED educational observation programs depending on how much of an educational program your department is running. We had programs in San Diego, in which we chaperoned high school students through the ED. With careful guidance and consideration, we were able to both provide the students with an interesting experience while protecting patient privacy. There is no question that it is important to facilitate the observation of people considering a career in medicine. In fact, one of the questions all students applying to medical school will be asked is: "What do you know about the practice of medicine?" We demand that students applying to medical school have significant exposure to the clinical setting through observation, research, or volunteer work.

Dr. James Adams: I have also banned the television crews based on what I find to be ethically appropriate or inappropriate. Our job is to be the advocate for the individual patient. I have to ask "What are we trying to accomplish?" We can achieve many of the objectives of those who seek to know more about the ED with a tour and an in-depth discussion. It is important that we protect our professional role, protect the interests of the patient, and protect their privacy.

Dr. Arthur Derse: It is tempting to use televised recording of ED encounters to communicate and educate the public about issues that affect the ED. At the same time, we have to be careful that we don't achieve the goals of public education while sacrificing patient privacy and dignity. We have to resist the trend to have everyone drop in to see what's going on. The Health Insurance Portability and Accountability Act (HIPAA) has a great impact on clinicians today. HIPAA prevents clinicians from allowing a colleague's daughter or a college student from observing medical encounters, but does provide an exception for chaplains. There is not a lot of educational benefit in having a chief of staff of a US senator observe individual physician–patient encounters. It might be better to say, "We emergency physicians would be happy to meet with the senator to talk about the issues that affect our discipline. We will give you more than a day's experience; we'll give you our collective professional lifetime experience to inform your judgment." We do have, however, a responsibility to inform and mentor the next generation of healthcare professionals forward in their careers.

PR: I will never forget the television crew that I was trying to chaperone while simultaneously trying to run a very busy shift in the ED. We had a patient with a gastrointestinal bleed who was undergoing an emergent sigmoidoscopy. The television crews let themselves into the room, and were setting up to film the procedure before I had the chance to stop them. It was absolutely infuriating, and I had a long meltdown in the public relations office at the end of that day.

Dr. John Jesus: Perhaps it is because I have been a patient in the ED on two separate occasions that I am strongly opposed to having commercial television crews in the ED. I presented to the ED once for chest pain that was quickly diagnosed as a spontaneous pneumothorax. I remember the presence of many students and EMTs [emergency medical technicians] during the chest tube insertion, and remember feeling no discomfort with their observation of the procedure. That said, the idea of someone filming me in respiratory distress for public consumption I believe to be inappropriate. Though admittedly anecdotal, I also recently asked my friends, family, and neighbors how they would feel if they knew they would be filmed during a trauma resuscitation. I received uniformly negative responses from everyone with whom I spoke.

The literature on the topic of patient perceptions of having their interactions with the ED recorded demonstrates that many patients don't notice that they are being filmed, and most of those people who do notice don't seem to mind. Between 15% and 20% of people, however, are aware of the cameras, and are made uncomfortable by them. I believe that it is our responsibility to protect those people who would feel their privacy violated by the recording of their interactions with the ED, no matter how small the percentage of patients they represent. I acknowledge the need to balance the principle of public beneficence through education and demystifying the ED with the principle of respect for persons. There isn't any question,

however, that the balance of principles in this instance favors the protection of patient privacy over the provision of public education and entertainment. In the era of reality TV, the typical approach to televising patient encounters is to record them during their resuscitation without patient consent, but only airing them when retroactive consent can be obtained later in the course of the patient's recovery. This is a perfect example of how clinicians and television crews can "wrong" patients without actually "harming" them. The simple act of recording patients without their consent during trauma resuscitations violates their right to privacy. Even though no harm is inflicted on the patient, the public perception of unwanted violations of privacy represents a real threat of public trust in the specific institution and the broader discipline of emergency medicine.

PR: The photographer Gene Richards took photographs of patients in the ED and published them in a book entitled *The Knife and Gun Club*. He originally came to Denver General at the request of *Parade Magazine*, so that they could produce a weekend issue on the ED. The decision to allow Gene Richards to go ahead with this project was made by administration, and then foisted upon us. Gene is a wonderful man and a terrific photographer. The reporter who wrote the original *Parade Magazine* article was very professional and did a very nice job. Though I was opposed to the whole idea and had no say over it, I was happy to know that the people involved were decent human beings. An unintended consequence of publishing one of the photographs in *LIFE* magazine occurred. Somebody in Denver thought he identified himself in one of the photos and sued Denver General and *LIFE* magazine. The case went to settlement even though the picture didn't really look like him. There really are people who don't like the idea of their privacy being invaded.

Dr. Shamai Grossman: The appropriateness of having chaplain observers in the ED depends on what the role of clergy is in a particular ED. This will vary with the institution, and it may also vary with the individual. There are institutions where clergy are truly part of the care team, and so a training chaplain would be thought of in the same way as a medical student or nurse in training. Then there are other institutions, in which clergy are thought of as outsiders, somewhat foreign, whose presence would be seen as inappropriate as the presence of news crews or television cameras. In those institutions it would be much more difficult to allow clergymen or clergy students into the ED for observation. Each institution truly needs to set up guidelines that set limits on who can observe patient encounters in the ED. It behooves us to create these up front. As such, when we are confronted with administrators who want to send down their own people to observe, we have preestablished guidelines that dictate who is able to do so and how it will be done.

PR: We had a wonderful chaplaincy program when I worked at the University of Chicago, and they helped me initiate a design to help rape victims feel less exposed and more supported. They were a tremendous asset in the management of bereaving relatives, and I wouldn't hesitate to allow one of their students to observe in any ED. The other side of that coin was articulated in an article that I rejected not long ago. This study mandated asking people about their religious attachments, and whether they wanted to have religious support while they were in the ED. I think that this is a true slippery slope. There are many institutions to which patients are brought without any choice of their own, such as Catholic hospitals that are part of destination policies for city ambulances. To institutionalize a religious undertone to medical care and force it on patients has been one of the ethical problems of patient distribution. Not being permitted to advise abortion for rape victims and other controversial conflicts between religion and medical care are among the reasons I am so opposed to having a mandatory religious experience for patients. The reality is that there are significant numbers of our population who are atheist and for whom religious mandates are just as unacceptable as asking a Jewish patient to accept a Muslim or Catholic orientation. While the bottom line is the protection of our patients' privacy, I think that we also have to accept the reality of the pressures under which every ED runs. If we have a structure in place, we may be able to reject some of these requests more readily, and offer alternatives to direct patient observation that may achieve the same educational goals.

JG: The decision to allow certain observers into the ED may become a political question. In some of these cases you may feel forced. In those instances, you have to make sure that the observers stay out of patient activity areas, where they can observe patients directly or are able to read names and patient details. In cases where a non-medical observer does go into a room to observe a patient–clinician encounter, the patient should be introduced to whoever it is and ought to be asked for consent for the observer's presence. Of course, some of our patients are unable to give consent, and observers probably don't belong in their rooms.

Some people would argue that non-medical observers are trying to gather information for the public good. Those of us who are more cynical believe that this isn't actually true. For example, I had a US senator come through our ED about 6 months ago just before he spoke at Grand Rounds on the subject of healthcare reform. I was asked to give him a tour. Though I kept him out of the patient rooms, and I covered up patient names, I tried to counter the myth that most patients who come to the ED don't really need to be there based on chief complaint. To prove the point, I used our computer system to go through 40 patients and their chief complaints. These included chest pain, altered mental status, SOB [shortness of breath], "waiting for ICU," "hypotensive on pressors," etc. I showed him all of this and argued that the vast majority of these people really needed to be there because they had bona fide emergencies and were very sick, not because they had the sniffles. Thereafter, he addressed the packed auditorium to give his speech, and posited that healthcare reform would provide a benefit to "all these people" in EDs who "didn't need to be there" by affording them with an alternative place to go. All I could think of was that I had wasted my time and breath, giving him the tour and trying to educate him. He was going to want to say and believe what he wanted, no matter what kind of evidence I put in front of him. The relevant point for this discussion is, despite our best efforts, some observers will use their experience to further their own self-interests rather than those of patients. We have little control over it.

I also worry that some of these requests really devalue our specialty. Other disciplines don't receive the same requests. What is it about emergency medicine that makes people think that it is okay to ask ridiculous questions of us? There is a role for us to play in upholding the dignity of our specialty, even apart from protecting our patients' privacy.

JA: In one sense, the ED is approached because it is inherently compelling and interesting. As much as surgery would be interesting, as much as walking through an OB/GYN [obstetrics/gynecology] or medical clinic would be interesting, the care we provide and the context in which we provide it is compelling, which is why many of us pursued this specialty in the first place. Furthermore, we are often the interface between the community and the hospital in a way that other specialties are not. It is this interface that many people are interested in, and that may be why we're approached so frequently with requests to allow non-medical observers in to the ED.

JJ: Protecting patient privacy in the ED is already a very difficult task. The burden of proof should always lie with those who want to impinge upon patient rights and patient privacy rather than with those who seek to protect them. Without careful consideration about the situations in each case, we may take steps in the direction of patient privacy attrition. Rather, we should seek to move toward a culture of greater patient protection.

PR: It has always amazed me that the people who are most willing to invade our patients' privacy are the same people who insist on maximum privacy when they themselves are patients. Sometimes, you just have to say "No."

Section III: Review of the literature

There is surprisingly little published literature on the issue of non-medical observers in the ED. For many of us in administrative roles, such requests seem unending and ubiquitous. Perhaps some of this stems from the aforementioned sense of theater that has developed in EDs due to exposure on television, the sense of openness that exists in the ED, and the sheer drama of what occurs within our halls on a daily basis.[1] Requests for observers in other areas appear less common. There seems to be little demand to observe what happens on a typical medical-surgical floor. However, from time to time there are requests by legislators or community leaders to be present in

the inpatient care setting, allegedly to better understand various aspects of healthcare operations. When reporters take on emotionally charged subjects such as pediatric illness or breast cancer, or when pharmaceutical representatives want to "shadow" physicians, most often in procedural areas such as operating rooms, they appear to do so for their own purposes, usually to increase sales and revenues for their employers and ultimately to profit themselves. Obvious evidence for this is when observers offer to pay physicians for the privilege of observing.[2] It would seem more logical to offer payments to the patients rather than the caregivers or institutions. For the purposes of this chapter, non-medical (outside) observers will be defined as follows:

> Outside observers are individuals who are present during patient-physician encounters and are neither members of a health care team nor enrolled in an educational program for health professionals such as medical students.[2]

This chapter will examine the various types of individuals who request observation privileges in the ED, and the ethical, legal, and other considerations that should be considered in weighing such requests. Some of these requests may be honored if certain conditions are satisfied, whereas in other cases, requests should be rejected a priori based on conditions that are generally extant in EDs and the inherent vulnerability of ED patients. Box 16.1 lists some types of observer who might seek to be present during patient care activities in EDs.

Autonomy

The ordering principles of modern Western medical ethics are often viewed through the lenses of autonomy, non-maleficence, beneficence, and distributive justice, with autonomy being the prima facie consideration.[3] Under this model, individual patient choices as to whether or not to participate when observers request to be present (especially when refused) should be honored. However, physicians must be sensitive to the vulnerability of certain patient populations when even considering such a request. In many circumstances, patients undergoing treatment are not well positioned to be able to refuse participation out of fear of being treated less well if they refuse.

Box 16.1 Examples of individuals seeking observation privileges in the ED

- High school or college pre-med (or potential pre-med) students
- Emergency medical services (EMS) or potential EMS personnel
- Chaplaincy personnel (or students)
- Surveyors
- Quality assurance personnel
- "Secret shoppers"
- Consultants
- Trustees
- Financial donors
- Actors
- Writers
- Politicians/legislators or their staff
- Commercial film crews
- News crews
- In-house public relations staff
- Device manufacturers' representatives
- Pharmaceutical manufacturers' representatives
- Patients' families/visitors
- Physicians' friends
- Physicians' families

Patients in EDs, especially minorities or indigent populations, may feel even more vulnerable because of their inherent feelings of inferiority or indebtedness. Patients in elective situations are less subject to such pressures. Since we can never be sure of the effect of these pressures, we should apply a sliding scale when considering asking patients to participate, depending on the weight of other principles that may be present in the situation. When there is little societal benefit at stake, we should not even place the patient in the position of having to choose; when there is more societal benefit at stake, we may lessen the standard.

One instance in which it is rarely permissible to accept a lower standard is when the patient lacks decisional capacity.[2] Surrogate decision-makers may occasionally be employed in such circumstances (e.g., cases involving minors or when there is a compelling public interest) but in general, since the presence of observers has been deemed to represent a "substantial invasion of privacy" it should not be permitted, and if done, only with the consent of the legal guardian.[2]

Non-maleficence

In some circumstances, great harm can be done to patients by the presence of observers in the ED. In others, great harm can be done to the medical profession as a whole, or the specialty of emergency medicine in particular. It stands to reason that most patients treated in EDs are treated in the communities in which they reside. As such, the likelihood that they will be recognized or known by other members of the community during a visit to the ED cannot be minimized. In addition, the presence of non-medical observers may inhibit the willingness of patients to disclose necessary information to their caregivers. Overall, such an environment may feel less safe to patients seeking care and could even deter them from visiting the ED.

When non-essential observers are allowed to participate, even with the patient's permission, it can be argued that the patient is being exploited. When the observer is doing so for personal gain, such as a drug representative, or the actor in the opening example of this chapter, one can make an even stronger case for patient exploitation. Since the treating physician has a duty that is first and foremost to the patient, it is his or her duty to protect the patient from this form of harm. It is assumed that healthcare professionals are versed in and will observe the tenets of confidentiality. Such individuals can also be held to account by professional organizations, employers, and under the law. When non-medical observers are allowed to observe, it is the duty of the supervising physician to assure that the observers understand and are committed to the same medical standards of confidentiality as are health professionals.[1] In practice, however, this may be difficult to assure.

The concept of non-maleficence generally applies to patients (rather than the medical profession) since the notion of professionalism demands that medical care be patient centered. However, it can be argued that the ability to reliably deliver patient-centered care can only be assured if the profession is trusted by the public at large. Thus, anything that harms this relationship is bad for patients and the medical profession at the same time.

Beneficence

In general, it is nearly impossible to argue that the presence of non-medical observers provides any direct benefit to patients. For patients who are unable to express a preference, or whose desires were not clearly stated in advance, this can never be assured. In some cases in which consent can be obtained, it can be posited that the inclusion of observers (for instance, for commercial filming) may provide a psychological benefit. However, as already emphasized, patients may feel under psychological duress or be so cognitively impaired by their illness or the unexpectedness of their circumstances that they are not to be able to make an informed decision that they otherwise might make.[4–6] In such cases, although patients may subsequently regret their choices, often they cannot undo the invasion of their privacy or confidentiality.

Distributive justice

Society has an interest and a right to well-trained and well-meaning health professionals including physicians, nurses, social workers and chaplains. They also have a right to caregivers who will, for instance, wash their hands, follow established standards, and treat them with courtesy and respect. In this regard, since the benefits will accrue to all members of society, the burden of fielding observers falls on all of society, as long as autonomy is preserved and other principles (such as not re-disclosing confidential information) are not violated. Even trustees and donors may occasionally be accommodated, as long as it is for patient-centered purposes, and they are properly supervised. However, the burden of proof is high when allowing such access. In contrast, societal interests in commercial filming, acting careers, or the profits of drug- and device-makers (or their representatives) are limited, if any. Thus, the inclusion of observers for these endeavors should be viewed with skepticism, and generally be avoided, especially in the emergency setting.

Legal and regulatory considerations

Legally, patients are entitled to a reasonable expectation of privacy. In order for a civil suit (a tort) to succeed in this regard, the activity must be deemed "highly offensive to a reasonable person." The courts have recognized this right in the context of a medical setting as early as 1881. *DeMay* v. *Roberts* involved a family doctor, John DeMay who brought a nonprofessional friend, Alfred Scattergood, "an unmarried male," to witness a childbirth without disclosing to Alvira Roberts, the plaintiff, the fact that Mr. Scattergood was not employed in a professional capacity.[7] The Michigan Supreme Court upheld a jury verdict in the case that found both the doctor and his friend liable for damages. The court ruled that the plaintiff had "a legal right to the privacy of her apartment at such a time, and the law secures to her this right by requiring others to observe it, and to abstain from its violation."[7]

Cases have more recently been successfully brought against hospitals and producers over the presence of commercial film crews employed during the filming of reality television shows.[8,9] Some courts have even ruled against television news organizations and their parent companies, despite the fact that reporters enjoy special protections in the Constitution under the First Amendment.[10–13]

Miller v. *NBC* specifically dealt with the issue of a television crew entering a private home during a "ride along" with paramedics.[11] In this case, the family of a man who was filmed during a failed attempt at cardiopulmonary resuscitation sued NBC for invasion of privacy under an intrusion claim. The family further alleged trespass and infliction of emotional distress. The trial court initially denied all three claims. However, in an opinion that reversed the lower court, the Court of Appeals noted:

> There is little California case law . . . to assist us in making this determination, probably because even today most individuals not acting in some clearly identified official capacity do not go into private homes without the consent of those living there . . . not only do widely held notions of decency preclude it, but most individuals understand that to do so is either a tort, a crime, or both.[11]

Following this ruling, the family entered into a confidential settlement agreement with the television network.

Shulman v. *Group W Productions* involved an action for invasion of privacy brought by an accident victim against a television production company that videotaped, voice recorded, and aired a documentary showing her rescue from the scene, without consent.[12] In this case, the California State Supreme Court ruled that the case could proceed on an intrusion claim, resulting in an out-of-court settlement.

The presence of drug or device manufacturers' representatives during patient encounters can also trigger lawsuits. In *Sanchez-Scott* v. *Alza Pharmaceuticals,* the plaintiff sued over the presence of a drug salesman during a breast examination during an oncologic visit.[14] Interestingly, in ruling in favor of the plaintiff, the court cited *Shulman,* the case involving emergency treatment by EMS personnel.

Although the legal burden is high for intrusion lawsuits to succeed, the unwanted publicity and negative community perceptions that accompany such claims should also serve as deterrents to allowing indiscriminate access to observers. As well should be the legal and human costs of defending even unsuccessful claims. HIPAA, enacted by Congress and signed into law by President Clinton in 1996, established the "Privacy Rule" as Federal Law.[15] As such, the rule has far reaching consequences. It is beyond the scope of this chapter to explicate all the consequences of HIPAA, some of which are yet to be determined. Nevertheless, it should be pointed out that civil and criminal penalties may be levied on covered entities that knowingly violate the rule. For violations that occur after February 18, 2009, the cap on civil penalties has risen to US$ 1.5 million per calendar year.

The Joint Commission and other regulatory bodies also have standards that regulate the rights of patients to privacy, some of which are tied to HIPAA and other statutes. In order to maintain a safe harbor in surveys by such organizations, healthcare workers and administrators should be skeptical of requests by observers without a clearly established "need to know."

Existing policies, guidelines, and best practices

Interestingly, neither the American College of Emergency Physicians (ACEP) nor the Society for Academic Emergency Medicine (SAEM) or the American Academy of Emergency Medicine (AAEM) have policy recommendations regarding the presence of observers in the ED. The American Medical Association (AMA) has an excellent document that deals with this subject, which was promulgated through its Council on Ethical and Judicial Affairs in 2005. Much of this was prompted by the presence of pharmaceutical and device manufacturers' representatives who "shadowed" physicians during patient encounters, often involving remuneration for physicians.[2,16]

In 2007, in Canada, Fraser Health, British Columbia's largest health authority banned sales visits or "clinical preceptorships" with staff or physicians in clinical areas.[17] According to one account, "the days when a pharmaceutical or medical equipment representative could . . . wander through the emergency room [sic] . . . are now over."[17]

In the interest of full disclosure, according to publically available websites as of this writing, both Cedars-Sinai Medical Center and the Feinberg School of Medicine at Northwestern (the home institutions of the author and a senior editor of this chapter) offer shadowing experiences for premedical students.[18,19] Presumably, adequate safeguards are in place, and there has been a decision that on balance, the societal interests in this activity outweigh other ethical concerns. Clearly, in cases where this is deemed to be true, it is up to all physicians involved in the activity to assure that it is.

Much of the discussion at the beginning of this chapter centered upon the issue of commercial filming in the ED. Since this subject has received much attention in the past 10 years, the conclusions drawn from a preponderance of opinions in this example may inform other considerations.[1,20-22] Commercial filming is perhaps the ultimate challenge to our concepts of privacy, confidentiality, and respect for patient choices with regard to the notion of modesty. The archetype of this activity, the reality show *Trauma: Life in ER* routinely filmed patients during their very first moments of emergency resuscitation and treatment (for the purposes of this discussion, the terms "filmed" and "videotaped" are used interchangeably). The approach the producers took was to obtain consent from the patient or surrogate before the airing of any film obtained during the encounter. The problem with this approach is that by the time the patients were asked for their permission, their privacy had already been violated by the very presence of the film crew during the recording. Also, clearly, the patient's own feelings and values as to modesty had not even been considered. Even when patients or their surrogates (e.g., parents) could consent, they might have lacked adequate decisional capacity or felt under duress to agree; in some cases it was later claimed that they feared that their care would be negatively affected if they refused.[23] In other cases, patients later regretted their decisions to participate but lacked the ability to control the use of their images and depictions of their experiences afterward.

The ACEP and the SAEM, through their respective ethics committees have adopted restrictive policies with regard to commercial filming as has the AMA Council on Ethical and Judicial Affairs. In all cases, the consent of patients who are not under duress and who possess adequate decisional capacity is required. The principles underlying these various policies may be referred to in making decisions regarding other types of observers. As previously mentioned, commercial filming has also resulted in successful lawsuits on the basis of invasion of privacy. This knowledge should also guide decisions regarding the inclusion of non-medical observers in the ED.

Section IV: Recommendations

• Requests for observers should be reviewed and approved by individuals in positions of authority who understand the concept of professionalism and the ethical principles germane to the decision.
• Societal interests should be considered, but not at the expense of individual patient rights.
• If observers are present, they should only be allowed to observe intimate patient care encounters with the knowledge and consent of patients. Patients must have the capacity to consent, and not be in positions of status inferiority or under duress.
• By definition, patients who lack decisional capacity can generally not be observed during their care, except in rare circumstances and with the consent of a parent or legal guardian.
• Physicians or institutions should not accept payments from outside observers.

References

1. Geiderman JM. (2001) Fame, rights, and videotape (editorial). *Ann Emerg Med.* 37, 217–19.

2. Council on Ethical and Judicial Affairs, American Medical Association. *Patient Privacy and Outside Observers to the Clinical Encounter.* CEJA Report 4-A-05. Available at: www.ama-assn.org/resources/doc/code-medical-ethics/50591a.pdf. Accessed August 29, 2011.

3. Beauchamp TL, Childress JF. (1994) *Principles of Biomedical Ethics*, 4th ed. New York, NY: Oxford University Press, pp. 120–88.

4. Smithline HW, Mader TJ, Crenshaw BJ. (1999) Do patients with acute medical conditions have the capacity to give informed consent for emergency medicine research? *Acad Emerg Med.* 6(8), 776–80.

5. Schaffer MH, Krantz DS, Wichmann A, et al. (1996) The impact of disease severity on the informed consent process in clinical research. *Am J Med.* 100, 261–8.

6. Schmidt TA, Salo D, Hughes JA, et al. (2004) Confronting the ethical challenges to informed consent in emergency medicine research. *Acad Emerg Med.* 11(10), 1082–9.

7. DeMay v. Roberts, 46 Mich. 160, 9 N.W. 146 (Mich. 1881).

8. Kinsella v. Welch, A-2985-02T2 (N.J. Super. 7-15-2003) No. A-2985-02T2. Available at: http://caselaw.findlaw.com/nj-superior-court-appellate-division/1005892.html. Accessed August 28, 2011.

9. Fisher D. *The Real Reality TV.* Available at: www.forbes.com/2005/06/21/privacy-lawsuit-televison-cz_df_0621documentary.html. Accessed August 29, 2011.

10. Dietman v. Time, Inc., 449F, 2d 245,249 (9th Cir, 1971).

11. Miller v. NBC, 232 Cal Rptr. 668, 678–679 (1986).

12. Shulman v. Group W Productions, Inc., Supreme Court of California, SO58629 (1998).

13. Wilson v. Lane, US Supreme Court, 119 S Ct 1692 (1998).

14. Sanchez-Scott v. Alza Phamaceuticals, 86 Cal. App 4th 365 (2001).

15. HIPAA Privacy Rule. Available at: www.hhs.gov/ocr/privacy/hipaa/administrative/privacyrule/. Accessed April 15, 2011.

16. Leibman M. (2003) *AMA: Shadowing Violates Privacy.* Medical Marketing and Media August 2003. Available at: http://allbusiness.com/government-bodies-offices/10608074-1.htlm. Accessed April 24, 2011.

17. Jones D. (2007) Health authority bans physician shadowing. *CMAJ.* 177(11), 1339–40.

18. Independent Student Volunteers. Available at: www.cedars-sinai.edu/About-Us/Volunteer-Opportunities/Volunteer-Groups/Independent-Student-Volunteers.aspx. Accessed August 29, 2011.

19. White E. (2011) *A Day in the Doctor's Shoes.* Available at: www.northwestern.edu/newscenter/stories/2011/03/

doctor-shadowing-program-feinberg.html. Accessed August 29, 2011.

20. Geiderman JM, Larkin GL. (2002) Commercial filming of patient care activities in hospitals. *JAMA*. 288(3), 373–9.

21. Iserson KV. (2001) Film: Exposing the emergency department. *Ann Emerg Med*. 37, 220–1.

22. Geiderman JM. (2003) Saying no to cameras in the emergency department. *Cal J Emerg Med*. 4, 16–18.

23. Mathieu J. *Reality TV Bites*. Available at: www.houstonpress.com/2002-09-05/news/reality-tv-bites/. Accessed August 29, 2011.

17 Religious perspectives on do-not-resuscitate (DNR) documents and the dying patient

Avraham Steinberg

Professor and Director, Medical Ethics Unit, and Senior Pediatric Neurologist, Shaare Zedek Medical Center, Jerusalem, Israel

Section I: Case presentation

A relatively healthy 80-year-old man presents with acute respiratory distress secondary to pneumonia with preexisting orders of do-not-resuscitate (DNR) and do-not-intubate (DNI). The physician believes that if the patient is placed on a ventilator for several days, while receiving treatment for the pneumonia, he would likely survive to be extubated without long-term residual effects. The patient's family wishes for patient comfort measures only, and would like to withdraw intravenous fluids, vasopressors, and mechanical ventilation.

The physician's religious beliefs tell him he cannot allow a patient who could otherwise survive his illness die without an attempt at resuscitation. Must the physician abide by the DNR/DNI order and withdraw all interventions while the patient is in the emergency department (ED)?

Section II: Discussion

Dr. Peter Rosen: Before we begin our discussion of the ethical issues involved in the physician's decision-making, we must clarify if the patient is able to communicate his own preferences, or if we must base our discussion on his DNR/DNI document and family understanding of his wishes alone.

Dr. Avraham Steinberg: If the patient is able to communicate and refuses treatment in real time when a decision has been reached, then there is no ethical dilemma. We are obligated to respect the patient's decision. Hence, if he is able to say that he doesn't want to be treated, then he should be allowed to go home. Therefore, for the discussion to be meaningful, we should assume that the patient cannot express his current wishes.

PR: In the United States, a signed document DNR carries weight, and is nearly identical to the patient refusing care. Let's assume that there is no signed document, and that we must rely on the patient's relatives to express a preference for the patient's care. Legally, a relative cannot withhold life-saving care from any relative unless he or she has court-appointed guardian status and is deemed to be acting in the patient's best interests. If the physician concludes that the relative is not acting in the patient's best interest, the physician need not comply with the relative's wishes, when that relative is not the legal guardian.

AS: I suggest that we include the assumption that there is a signed DNR document. We should also explore, however, the ethical meaning of this document: does the DNR/DNI document apply to this particular situation? DNR/DNI documents and advanced directives are designed to guide clinicians'

Ethical Problems in Emergency Medicine: A Discussion-Based Review, First Edition. John Jesus, Shamai A. Grossman, Arthur R. Derse, James G. Adams, Richard Wolfe, and Peter Rosen.
© 2012 John Wiley & Sons, Ltd. Published 2012 by John Wiley & Sons, Ltd.

interventions at the **end** of patients' lives. I believe the important issue here is how to interpret an advanced directive when the patient presents with a condition that doesn't necessarily represent the patient's last hours.

PR: The interpretation of a DNR/DNI document and an advanced directive is somewhat dependent on what its contents specify. If the directive states that the patient does not wish to be intubated, then the physician doesn't have the right to intubate the patient, even if he believes it will be medically efficacious. Most advanced directives are not so task-specific, however.

AS: I believe we must interpret DNR/DNI and advanced directives within the clinical context in which patients find themselves when they present to the hospital. If someone has an advanced directive, and loses consciousness on arrival at the ED from a developing epidural hematoma, wouldn't you intubate and drain the hematoma despite the DNR/DNI status? The circumstances I've just described don't appear to represent the patient's intent when he first signed the DNR/DNI document. Given that he cannot articulate his preferences, we must rely on what the family knows of his end-of-life preferences, and on what we believe is in the patient's best interests.

PR: In this situation, the physician would attempt to address the family, and explain the difference between life-ending illness and illness that can be treated with a reasonable expectation for recovery. The physician can, and perhaps should, give a recommendation as to what the family should decide, given the physician's experience with and knowledge of the disease process. The ethical dilemma only occurs when the family disagrees with the physician despite the explanation and recommendations, persistently refusing life-saving medical care.

AS: I would first attempt to address what was the patient's intent when he signed the DNR/DNI or advanced directive. The situation behind a patient's intent, I would go on to explain, is not one that precludes intubation and resuscitation for highly reversible disease processes—it is highly likely that he will resume a normal life after this procedure. DNR/DNI documents and advanced directives ought to be open to interpretation, based on whether the treatment

represents routine medical treatment or end-of-life interventions with little hope of benefit.

PR: I don't disagree with that concept. The difficulty, however, lies with the prediction of the outcome, and in the analysis of when age-related comorbidities should influence your treatment decisions. The patient's chance of surviving pneumonia as an 80-year-old is, all things being equal, not going to be the same as it would be if he were 20 years old. If, however, you are willing to commit to the notion that his condition is survivable, then I agree that you don't have to follow the DNR/DNI document or an advanced directive that would otherwise preclude intubation. The problem we have created is trying to tie decision making to a medical action rather than a strategy. We must attempt to distinguish between the stages of disease and the utilities of the medical actions.

Dr. John Jesus: Agreed. I am, in fact, studying this very question. I found myself faced with a number of patients with active DNR/DNI documents who presented to the ED with highly reversible medical conditions. After a relatively short clarifying conversation about their code status, it quickly became clear to me that these patients never intended to preclude intubation and resuscitation for highly reversible conditions, angioedema being the prototypical example. Subsequently, I initiated a study to further clarify what patients' understood about their own DNR/DNI documents, and whether there were any conditions under which they would prefer a reversal of their code status.

Dr. Shamai Grossman: The situation can be taken even further: What should a physician do if there is no other physician available, and the family is still insistent that they don't want their relative treated—should the physician honor the DNR document even if it is illogical and perhaps counter to the ethical principles by which the physician conducts himself?

AS: In the United States, it seems that the solution is simpler, as the physician can attempt a trial of resuscitation or intubation and admit the patient to the ICU. If the patient does not improve, withdrawal of care already administered is more easily accomplished. However, in my view, the relatives' position is not necessarily always equivalent to the best interest of the patient, and it definitely does not represent an autonomous decision. In fact, this is a clear form of a paternalistic decision, giving the relatives the prerogative to decide what is best for someone else. Hence, given the situation described by Dr. Grossman, I see no ethical problem should the physician act in the best of the patient's interest as he sees it, and legally he has the option to turn to the court for support.

AS: The position that there is no moral difference between omission and commission is well accepted in secular medical ethics. This however is not accepted by Jewish law, and the Israeli Dying Patient Act 2005 adopted this distinction.

SG: I would argue that proactively initiating care should give one the moral upper hand, particularly where the condition is reversible; and withdrawal of care can only be considered morally appropriate when the treatment is not found to sustain life, but merely prolongs the patient's suffering.

AS: If the family also disagrees with the decision to attempt a trial of resuscitation or intubation, then the treatment decision must be based on whether the treating physician believes the family is acting in the patient's best interests, and whether the family members presenting this request have the legal authority to refuse treatment. If neither of these considerations is applicable, then the physician does not need to heed their input.

PR: While the physician does have the legal right to act in the patient's best interests, ignoring the input from the patient's family is sure to eventuate a lawsuit, regardless of the final outcome. The threat of lawsuit is separate from what the physician should do, however, and unless the family present consists of legally appointed guardians, the family is not legally permitted to refuse treatment the physician deems life-saving for a condition that is highly reversible. In this circumstance, I would recommend that the physician document his or her position well. It would be difficult to defend resuscitation and intubation of a patient with a DNR/DNI patient in septic shock; if the patient has an early case of pneumonia, however, and has a probable chance of survival, then the physician has the right to proceed.

AS: The case presented is a relatively healthy 80-year-old man with pneumonia. From this description, I would feel very comfortable with my attempts to convince the family to agree to intubation; if they disagreed with me, I would also feel comfortable with intubating the patient against the family's wishes. The reason for this position is that the value of life stands on its own, separate from the quality of one's life. When I am in doubt, I err in favor of life. Many American physicians appear to weigh the quality of their patients' lives, in addition to life in and of itself, when considering whether to provide certain medical interventions. In the four principles of US medical ethics, life is not mentioned. The four principles are: autonomy, beneficence, non-maleficence, and justice—but where is life? There seems to be something very important missing. Hence, it seems to me that there are some US physicians who would doubt whether the quality of life of this 80-year-old man would be sufficient to disobey the DNR/DNI documentation of the patient.

PR: That's an interesting problem that requires a definition of life, which is a topic full of controversy. Decisions on quality-of-life issues are difficult for a physician to make, because the perception of a satisfactory quality of life is not universal, being dependent upon culture, age, general health, and innumerable sociologic parameters. Without the input from the patient, it can be near impossible to decide what is considered a "good" quality of life. I believe life is a qualitative and not a quantitative event. I can't define life precisely enough to be able to know what I am preserving without introducing a statement of quality. Ethically, however, it's wrong for the physician to impose a personal definition of quality on the patient.

A second problem I have in this case in particular, is the medical definition of "simple pneumonia." Pneumonia, per se, is a disease that has a wide spectrum of activity. An early pneumonia is treatable, survivable, and curable, even in an 80-year-old. Pneumonia that has advanced to become septic shock, however, is probably not treatable even in a 20-year-old, and the statistical survival of a pneumococcal septic shock is the same with and without antibiotics once the blood pressure drops.[1-3] When physicians give ethical advice to patients, they have to be clear that it is based on what they understand to be reasonable medical evidence.

The issues we've just discussed came to a head in an argument I had recently regarding a patient who came to the ED with an active DNR/DNI order, but who had a bowel obstruction. The surgeons refused to operate on the patient without first reversing the patient's code status. Is it possible to maintain a DNR order while treating reversible disease? If resuscitative measures were needed, then the DNR order would be enforced.

AS: The Israeli Dying Patient Act 2005 allows a physician to treat an incompetent patient for whatever is reversible, and once complications occur such that there is an irreversible situation, further treatment can be withheld. Most people do not mean to dismiss treatment for a reversible condition when they sign DNR/DNI orders. Life is worth saving.

PR: The problems with DNR/DNI documents and advanced directives have arisen for two reasons. First, we have too many people who want to interpret rules rigorously, and who use no judgment when interpreting the code status and DNR/DNI documents. Secondly, while in the United States it is possible to withdraw treatment when it becomes futile, it is actually a very difficult task. In the ED, however, withdrawing treatment is not the same as never having started it. The reality is that it's much harder to withdraw treatment than to commence it.

JJ: Reversing a DNR order and not starting treatment is very different in the ED setting, because we often must act with incomplete information, and under the pressure of time constraints that preclude further understanding of patient preferences. It is more appropriate to initiate care in the ED, and then withdraw care in the ICU [intensive care unit] where there is more time to determine if care is truly futile or contrary to patient wishes.

PR: Perhaps we can shift our focus to a new situation: a Jehovah's Witness with a massive GI [gastrointestinal] bleed that would, by any medical standard, necessitate blood transfusions. Imagine that the patient is confused, thus is unable to communicate whether or not he wishes to uphold his restriction against receiving blood, but his family claims that his religious beliefs are devout, and that he would not want to receive blood.

AS: I feel that I should give him life, and then allow him to struggle with the life I gave him. According to my value system, the value of life overrides everything except for killing someone for giving life. I would, therefore, seek to give him life despite his preference to avoid life-saving treatment. To me, a decision to withhold life-saving measures in a totally reversible situation is conceptually a form of suicide. This is similar to someone threatening to commit suicide by jumping from a roof. I would try to stop him.

PR: When I first became involved in medical ethics most medical students and residents would agree that physicians should not allow someone to die if there was something that could be done to save them. More recently, however, ethicists have convinced us that we are interfering with patients' autonomy, and that we should permit patient death when the patients have documented their preferences in some form or another. As a physician, I find it difficult to accept that position. It doesn't bother me that I might get sued for keeping someone alive, rather, it troubles me a great deal to allow someone to die whom I could have saved.

JJ: DNR/DNI documents have been studied for 30 years, and recently, there are several papers that reveal a significant percentage of patients who change their mind soon after they have signed a DNR/DNI document. Put simply, people change their minds. That is especially true if presented with an acute illness. If the Jehovah's Witness cannot communicate his wishes, it is reasonable to administer blood products, and then readdress his beliefs and transfusion preferences when the patient has regained decision-making capacity. That said, if a physician is convinced that receiving blood products is not permitted because of the patient's devout religious beliefs, then I do not believe anyone would fault the physician for withholding blood products. It is important to document what the physician considered before making his decision.

PR: Many years ago I was a surgeon and had a patient with a gunshot wound to the abdomen who was a Jehovah's Witness. He said, "You can do anything you want to save my life but . . ." It was at that very moment that I intubated him, and I never let him get out the rest of his sentence, which I presume would have been, "but do not give me blood." I didn't deliberately interrupt him, but he was dying and I didn't think there was time to listen to him any longer. He survived his surgery and thanked us for saving his life, although he was not happy about receiving blood.

SG: This begs the question of whether patients are really able to autonomously make decisions with inadequate knowledge. Are patients ever able to understand all the possible medical outcomes of intubation, transfusion, or treatment for angioedema? I'm not sure they are able to understand the medical complexities enough to determine whether or not a particular decision might place them in an unacceptable position. Patient autonomy alone is inadequate to guide physicians in making treatment decisions with unconscious patients, and must be balanced with other ethical principles.

AS: I agree that many patients and families do not completely comprehend DNR/DNI status or medical management decisions. I fear that we go too far if we take DNR/DNI documents at face value. We should not interpret a DNR/DNI document as precluding intubation in any and all circumstances. This is not what is meant by patient's autonomy. Moreover, even autonomous wishes by competent patients cannot always be taken at face value. Often patients express certain wishes, but after second thoughts they may change their minds or modify their requests, especially if they are provided with additional information or better explanation of their situation.

PR: Even as a physician I often do not know the medical details of a procedure that I may personally need, and I don't care to. What I care about is the outcome. It is our obligation as physicians to understand that we know more than our patients, and it's not being paternalistic to think that they can't possibly understand the ramifications of particular decisions they make. You have to decide for yourself whether you can live with the ramifications of your own belief system. At some point you have to recognize that you are doing the best you can to provide the best possible outcome.

Section III: Review of the literature

Good ethics start with good facts. Hence, in order to discuss the ethical issues related to the case at hand we should ascertain the detailed facts of the case:

- Elderly person (80 years old)
- Relatively healthy
- At real-time for decision-making capacity (assumed that the patient is incompetent)
- Diagnosis at admission—pneumonia (assumed without septic shock)
- Without treatment will surely die; with treatment very likely to survive without long-term residual effects (highly probable but not certain)
- Preexisting orders of DNR/DNI; however, no indications as to the intentions for the described situation when he certainly is not a dying patient in the moral-legal sense, i.e., has no terminal illness with no chance to survive despite treatment
- Family wishes to withdraw care, allowing the patient to die.
- The attending of record, on personal religious grounds, disagrees with allowing the patient to die without appropriate treatment.

Values and principles

Value of life
Secular ethics has recently diminished the importance of the value of life per se, and attributes significantly higher weight to the quality of life and to autonomy.[4] Using the four principles approach, the value of life is not listed.[5] In the world outside of medicine, we currently find diametrically opposing attitudes to the value of life. On the one hand, people who commit acts of terrorism do not appear to regard life as precious, neither for themselves or for the innocent bystanders they may injure. On the other hand, those who participate in disaster relief seem to spread with abundance their compassion and efforts to safe lives, even while endangering themselves.

Religious ethics continues to place a very high value on life itself in all circumstances, including medical situations. As a result, this perspective may oppose actions to actively hasten death. This approach is mutually accepted by the three large monotheistic religions (i.e., Judaism, Christianity, and Islam). In Judaism, for example, it is clearly stated that life is of supreme value, taking precedence over almost all other values, and overrides almost all other legal-religious commandments.[6]

In our case, accepting the DNR/DNI document at face value might seriously jeopardize the value of life, since it is very likely that the patient will die without treatment, whereas if treated aggressively, including intubation, he may survive without long-term residual effect. From the perspective of those who value the preservation of life above almost all other responsibilities, the physician ought to treat the patient. Because the patient is unable to exercise his autonomy in real time, in addition to the highly questionable applicability of the preexisting DNR/DNI document to the actual medical situation at hand, even from a secular point of view, it seems wrong to let this patient die in the circumstances described in our case.

Autonomy

In current secular ethics, autonomy seems to have become the overriding principle in almost all instances.

This principle seems to be the centerpiece of principlism. It is cited more frequently than the others. The concept of autonomy has come to dominate discussions of medical ethics; nevertheless, there is a growing and focused opposition to its predominance.[7]

The principle of autonomy is a particularly important principle when two conditions are met: (1) The person expressing autonomous wishes is fully competent to make prudent decisions at the time of decision-making; and (2) it is clear that the patient fully comprehends the situation and the meaning of the autonomous wishes, and clearly and explicitly expresses the wishes. DNR/DNI orders and advance medical directives are forms of "extended" autonomy, which might, indeed, represent patients' wishes. The document, however, may also misrepresent patients' end-of-life care preferences. Patients may change their minds since the time of signing a DNR/DNI document. Moreover, they may not have been aware that the signed DNR/DNI document would pertain to the actual medical situation at hand. When the patient lacks decision making capacity, it is impossible to verify with certainty what the patient's true preferences are. Family members may also act as an "extension" of the patient's autonomy through making decisions on behalf of the incapacitated

patient. This extension may also be morally problematic, as even the closest of family members may only approximate a patient's true preferences and may not understand how these translate to the medical emergency at hand. Furthermore, families may have ulterior motives, and may not always represent the patient's best interests.

Although the concept of autonomy is respected by multiple religious perspectives, it is not given the same value as is attributed to it by current secular ethics. This is true for Judaism as well as for Christianity.[8,9] As a result, clinicians of similar religious perspectives may place the value of life over and above personal autonomous wishes in certain circumstances.

In our case, denying treatment to the patient will certainly lead to his death, whereas providing treatment may prolong his life without long-term residual effects. It is possible, if not probable, that the patient did not realize or intend to deny himself life-saving therapy for the given circumstances when he signed the DNR/DNI document. Providing the necessary treatment may not constitute a violation of autonomy. It seems clear that overriding the family's wishes may not constitute a violation of autonomy either, since the family's position also represents an approximation of what they believe the patient would decide, without any better understanding of the DNR/DNI document. Moreover, healthcare providers also have a duty to act according to their moral-religious beliefs, and hence they cannot be compelled to act against their consciences.

Other moral principles

Beneficence is one of the four moral obligations of the four principles approach. In general, the continuation of life is more beneficial than dying, unless the quality of life is very poor, and entails significant pain and suffering. In the case described above, there is a reasonable chance that the patient will recover and enjoy life after the treatment, and hence there is a moral obligation to treat him based on the principle of beneficence.

From a **distributive justice** point of view, it seems clear that saving the life of this patient will not add any outstanding economic burden on his family or on society, and despite the fact that he is 80 years old, he has the right to receive the needed treatment in order to prolong his life.

The ethical meaning of advanced medical directives

A competent person can express his or her end-of-life care preferences in the event that he or she becomes incapacitated. This can be done by documenting the personal wishes in a written and signed advanced medical directive. This form represents "extended" autonomy, and is legally and morally binding. It may give a person confidence about the future, and provides the treating medical team a morally defensible mode of action in what are often difficult situations. Such documents, however, have significant problems: Do they really represent the patient's autonomous wishes in real time, and do they account for the possibility that the patient changed his or her mind? Did the person who signed the original advanced directive realize or comprehend all the possible medical emergencies in which he or she might find themselves thereafter? The answers to these questions are not at all clear, and as a result, cast serious concerns over the moral status of advanced medical directives and DNR/DNI documents. Advanced directives ought to be viewed as an approximation of the patient's autonomy, rather than fully expressed autonomous wishes. This leads to the conclusion that although advanced medical directives are, in principle, binding, they should be evaluated on a case-by-case basis.

Section IV: Recommendations

• If an emergency physician believes that a patient would consent to life-saving treatment if he or she had the ability to communicate, then they should consider disregarding preexisting DNR/DNI orders as irrelevant to the situation at hand.
• The emergency physician may disregard family wishes if he or she does not feel that they represent the best interests of the patient.

• If family members are legal guardians for the patient and are not acting in the best interests of the patient, a physician can consider obtaining a court order to overrule their wishes.
• If legal advice or court order compels a physician to uphold a DNR/DNI document, a physician whose religious beliefs lead him or her to oppose the ruling has a moral right to remove himself from the case, and appoint another physician to take his place.

References

1. Kramer MR, Rudensky B, Hadas-Halperin I, et al. (1987) Pneumococcal bacteremia—no changes in mortality in 30 years: analysis of 104 cases and review of the literature. *Isr J Med Sci.* 23, 174.
2. Mufson MA, Oky G, Hughey D (1982) Pneumococcal disease in a medium sized community in the USA. *JAMA.* 248, 1486–9.
3. Mufson MA, Kruss DM, Wasil RE, et al. (1974) Capsular types and outcome of bacteremic pneumococcal disease in the antibiotic era. *Arch Intern Med.* 134, 505–10.
4. Thomasma DC. (1999) The sanctity-of-human-life doctrine. In: Pellegrino ED, Faden AI. (eds) *Jewish and Catholic Bioethics.* Washington, DC: Georgetown University Press, pp. 54–73.
5. Beauchamp T, Childress J. (eds) (2009) *Principles of Biomedical Ethics,* 6th ed. New York, NY: Oxford University Press.
6. Jakobovits I. (1959) *Jewish Medical Ethics.* New York, NY: Bloch, pp. 45ff.
7. Clouser KD, Gert B. (1994) Morality vs. principlism. In: Gillon R. (ed.) *Principles of Health Care Ethics.* Chichester: John Wiley & Sons, p. 254.
8. Steinberg A. (1994). A Jewish perspective on the four principles. In: Gillon R. (ed.) *Principles of Health Care Ethics.* Chichester: John Wiley & Sons, p. 65ff.
9. Finnis J, Fisher A. (1994) Theology and the four principles: A roman catholic view. In: Gillon R. (ed.) *Principles of Health Care Ethics.* Chichester: John Wiley & Sons, p. 31ff.

Non-physician influence on the scope and responsibilities of emergency physicians

Laura G. Burke,[1] Jennifer V. Pope[2]

[1]*Clinical Instructor of Medicine, Harvard Medical School, Harvard Affiliated Emergency Medicine Residency, Beth Israel Deaconess Medical Center, Boston, MA, USA*
[2]*Clinical Instructor of Medicine, Harvard Medical School, Assistant Residency Director, Harvard Affiliated Emergency Medicine Residency, Beth Israel Deaconess Medical Center, Boston, MA, USA*

Section I: Case presentation

A 42-year-old woman presented to the emergency department (ED) with right-sided chest pain after moving large boxes. The pain was not pleuritic, and the review of systems was negative. She had no significant past medical history, took no medications, and had not traveled recently. The family history was non-contributory. The vital signs were: blood pressure 110/70 mmHg, heart rate 80 beats per minute, respirations 14 breaths per minute, temperature 37 °C. Oxygen saturation was 100% on room air. The physical examination was normal except for palpation tenderness over the right anterior chest wall in the mid-clavicular line over the fourth, fifth and sixth ribs. The patient had clear breath sounds. There were no murmurs, and the rate and rhythm were normal. The emergency physician concluded that the pain was from musculoskeletal strain. A chest X-ray study was performed that was unremarkable. The plan was to discharge the patient with rest and mild analgesia. Prior to discharge the emergency physician received a phone call from the hospital chief executive officer (CEO), who told the physician that the patient was the wife of a board member and that her husband was concerned about a pulmonary embolus (PE). He wanted the emergency physician to order a chest computed tomography (CT) scan. The emergency physi-

cian explained the medical decision-making, and communicated that in his opinion, a CT scan was not indicated. The CEO then came down to the ED, and demanded the CT scan be performed to be sure there was no PE.

Section II: Discussion

Dr. Peter Rosen: This is not an ethical dilemma; rather it is a political problem. It seems to occur in the ED with greater regularity than on other medical services. Perhaps this has to do with the history of emergency medicine, when the ED was run by untrained and, perhaps, incompetent physicians. Additionally, many clinicians have rotated and spent some time in the ED, which leads them to feel as though they know something about emergency medicine. If the CEO is a physician, the situation easily resolves itself as you can simply transfer the responsibility for caring for the patient to the CEO. If the CEO is an administrator however, then it becomes a much more difficult issue to navigate.

Dr. Arthur Derse: In our case, someone who isn't a professional clinician requests a study that harbors some risk that the emergency physician doesn't feel is warranted. Moreover, if this same non-professional has the ability to threaten the physician's job security,

Ethical Problems in Emergency Medicine: A Discussion-Based Review, First Edition. John Jesus, Shamai A. Grossman, Arthur R. Derse, James G. Adams, Richard Wolfe, and Peter Rosen.
© 2012 John Wiley & Sons, Ltd. Published 2012 by John Wiley & Sons, Ltd.

the physician's decisions may be affected by these requests, threatening the clinician's professionalism. Emergency physicians ought to have professional autonomy. There are some hospitals that cater to "VIPs," offering special privileges, such as staying in special rooms, or record restriction from certain physicians. Alternatively, you may have patients who demand certain interventions they may not need. While it is certainly the goal of the physician to have a happy patient, it presents a challenge to the ability of the physician to be autonomous.

PR: Every hospital has VIP care, and it generally is not the best care available. When a VIP appears, senior physicians who have remained relatively removed from clinical medicine suddenly decide to make all medical decisions for the patient. This approach may be one way to resolve issues like these. I would rather avoid conflict with a patient or superior, and allow a more senior member of the medical staff to relieve me of the responsibility. If that option is not available, then I would attempt to convince the patients of my assessment and treatment plan. If they are not receptive to hearing the logic behind my judgment, then usually I will agree to the additional testing, so that I may go on with my business in the ED. Often times it isn't the patient demanding something; rather, it's the patient's referring physician who hasn't seen the patient, but has told the patient to come to the ED to get a specific test, for instance, a CT scan for a possible pulmonary embolism. The physicians should first call and discuss the case with me, but they rarely take the trouble to do that.

Dr. Shamai Grossman: I believe that there are, in fact, ethical issues concerning our case. There is growing data to suggest that radiation from frequent CT scanning or repetitive scanning, especially in relatively young women, has some long-term detriment. Since the goal as physicians is to first do no harm, then the patient's request poses an ethical challenge. Is it permissible to expose this patient to radiation that I actually believe the patient does not require, especially in light of the evidence that suggests that it may be detrimental to the future health of the patient? Sometimes, there are compromises physicians can make with the family that are not potentially harmful. Sending a D-dimer level, for example, would be an appropriate test in regards to our case. The situation,

however, may have involved a medical decision in which there existed no compromise. In this circumstance, the clinician would then be faced with the decision—either perform the unnecessary and potentially harmful test or lose employment.

Dr. Laura Burke: I had a 77-year-old woman with chest pain that had lasted all night long, was fairly reproducible with no other associated symptoms, normal vital signs and a normal EKG [electrocardiogram]. The pain resolved after ASA [acetylsalicylic acid] and ibuprofen. We thought there was low probability of an acute coronary syndrome, but given her age and the fact that she had never had a cardiac work up we opted for two sets of cardiac enzymes and a provocative cardiac stress test. A family friend who was also a cardiologist requested an echocardiogram secondary to changes he perceived on the EKG. I reviewed the EKG again, but did not appreciate any of the changes the cardiologist claimed. I repeated the EKG, after which the cardiologist felt more comfortable with the original plan. Although we ended up doing the standard of care, I felt the pressure of an outside influence on our medical decision-making that I didn't feel was indicated.

PR: The solution to handling outside political pressures is to decide when the political pressure is greater than the professional standards under which you want to practice. We've all had situations when political pressures have become intolerable. It is inappropriate to argue and refuse to tolerate a political decision and its associated pressures, however, in front of patients or their families. Medicine is a science, but it is hardly an exact science. We do our best to make sound clinical judgments. What we are asked to do in emergency medicine is a logical impossibility: to prove a negative—that the patient does not have a particular pathology. We all develop a style, becoming comfortable with what we consider adequate negative evidence. The reality is that there are times when I am comfortable in agreeing with differing medical opinions. My ego is strong enough to consider other medical opinions and to amend my original assessment and treatment plan in light of the opinions of others.

Yet another issue that has come up in our conversation is doing something for a patient that you find dangerous. The risk of radiation from a CT scan is a hypothetical risk based on computer predictions that I don't have the mathematical background to challenge. There are other situations when a treatment presents obvious danger to the patient. How do we ensure that the person applying the pressure for such treatment be held responsible for the outcome? For example, when I was a surgical resident I assisted an attending surgeon in a case of perforated sigmoid diverticulitis. The attending said, "This poor lady—I've known her for 30 years. I'm just going to close the incision and hope the antibiotics prevent potential complications." I was taught that the appropriate surgical treatment in the setting of a perforation is to bypass the fecal stream with a colostomy. I inquired as to whether he would perform a temporary colostomy, since it was obvious to me that she would die without one. The attending declined on the basis that she was used to a certain standard of living, and that she would not want a colostomy if she were able to make the decision for herself. Since I was a resident, I had no power to alter his position. I could do something afterwards, but I couldn't change the outcome for that patient. If you are of equal rank, I would argue that you are obliged to take charge as the physician responsible for the patient care. That is the only professional stance.

SG: Yet, I could make a cogent ethical argument that you had an obligation to protest on this patient's behalf even as a resident. It may not have been successful, but that doesn't mean you were exempt from trying.

AD: There are some legal concepts that may help you think about situations like these. If you provide an intervention you don't think is indicated, and the patient has an untoward consequence that can be reasonably connected by proximal cause to the intervention, you will be legally responsible. From a legal perspective, it is much easier to defend why you avoided a particular intervention, than trying to defend a treatment you didn't believe would hold any benefit. In a case where you foresee a terrible outcome due to poor clinical decisions with which you do not agree, you must make clear that the responsibility for the action was not your own. State your disagreement, and withdraw yourself from the patient's care or the case.

Dr. Jennifer Pope: Do you think it's easier to avoid some of the non-physician influences in emergency medicine because we don't do as many "elective" procedures, like plastic surgery, or even orthopedic procedures?

PR: It depends on the case. I often receive a lot of pressure from people who come in with advice they have received. The advice may have originated from an unreliable source, yet the patients may be adamant about following the advice, because they trust the person who gave it to them more than they trust you. We tend to get lots of unwanted help from referring physicians, who don't call us, but want to impress the patient that they're doing a job for them. In so doing, the patient is sent to the ED for a specific test, which leaves you with an expectation that you may not be able to meet. This situation is far more common than pressures from administration. Many physicians have had instances where they had to modify their personal desires based on rank. For instance, a house officer who is asked to order a test or perform a procedure by an attending physician, but is convinced that the attending is wrong. I believe residents have some protection under the law, because they are not the responsible attending physician.

AD: In general, the captain of the ship theory holds that the attending physician would be responsible for any decision, unless the task is so egregiously wrong as to be obvious to any rank. An example would be following orders from an intoxicated attending. Generally, the residents' understanding of the standard of care evolves as they progress through residency, but their decisions may be trumped by the physician ultimately responsible for the patient. There are some rare cases in which an attempt is made to prove that a resident's actions fell below the standard of care for their level of training. Those attempts are generally not successful, because juries are very sympathetic to the situation in which residents find themselves, and hold the licensed physician ultimately responsible.

PR: Most of these situations are capable of compromise. The biggest error that you can make as a young physician is to allow your ego into the middle of the situation. Recently, there was a case in an ED where a rape victim presented. The emergency physician wanted to administer the "morning after" pill. At this particular institution, however, there existed a policy to avoid administering this intervention from the ED, and instead refer the patient to the gynecology clinic the next morning where there were gynecologists on staff who would be happy to see the patient and provide the appropriate medications. The ED physician decided he wasn't going to allow a policy to dictate how he should practice medicine. The chief administrator of the hospital the next day reminded him that there was a policy against giving the pill in the ED, and that if he didn't abide by that decision he could resign from his position. The ED physician filed a lawsuit, and he was ultimately terminated from that institution. In reviewing the case, he made an issue over a decision on which it would have been easy to settle the dispute without compromising his professional standards.

SG: What you are describing is truly the art of medicine. I was an attending cardiologist while simultaneously an emergency medicine resident. I was constantly confronted by cases of patients whose pathology I clearly understood far better than the attending. A lot of tact went into my relationship with these attending physicians, but ultimately I found a way to work with my attending colleagues and provide the best care for the patient.

PR: When I was a resident, we provided care under the supervision of the surgical attending physicians who were assigned our services as teaching attendings. One evening I was asked to see a 10-year-old boy, which was unusual because the hospital didn't usually admit children. He had originally been admitted for gastroenteritis. On my evaluation, however, he clearly had appendicitis. I attempted to call the family medicine attending on call that evening, and told him as diplomatically as I could that his patient had changed since he had examined him that morning. I informed him that the boy had clearly developed appendicitis, and I asked if he wanted me to call a surgeon for the patient. He thanked me for the information and said he'd take care of it—nothing happened. Later that evening, I was called to start an IV [intravenous line] on the patient, but no surgeon had been asked to see the patient. In my judgment he was on the verge of rupturing his appendix. I called the attending back, and his son informed me that he had just gone to the movies. I was just in a terrible dilemma, because I couldn't stand the thought of just walking away from the case.

A cardiothoracic surgeon came by, to whom I was also assigned. I told him about the case, and that I was considering taking the patient to the operating room myself. He advised me not to, because the hospital wouldn't allow me to perform surgery without an attending, and because the mere attempt would end my career. He told me to walk away from the case, and assured me that he would take care of it. He called the chief of staff, and he left a message with the attending and with the chief of staff that the patient should have a surgical consult. I continued to follow the patient, and I discovered that the attending of record didn't have a surgeon see the child for two more days, at which point the boy had ruptured his appendix. I was devastated at the time, because I did not know what I could have done differently to stop this from happening. Subsequently they removed the hospital privileges from the family physician, who had refused to come and see the child.

House officers, in particular, get into situations where we know what's right and wrong, but we don't have the power to make a change. We have to accept that as a part of the reality of our training program. Subsequent to our graduation, we similarly will forever have political pressures that we have to accept. If, and when those pressures become unbearable, it is time to change jobs.

PR: It is critical to have a strong structure in your ED that can alleviate some problems associated with these cases. For example, a strong chairman has the power to explain to a CEO that the requests being forced upon the emergency physician to perform are inappropriate, unprofessional, and not good for administration. He can keep it on a professional level, and keep you out of trouble. If you don't have a chief who will fight for you, you should strongly consider finding new employment. If you do resign, do it in a thought out manner by finding a job and obtaining a good recommendation, rather than with turmoil, lawsuit, and expulsions behind you. The same thing is true as you develop more experience and expertise as a physician. Remember that there is no place for arrogance and ego when it comes to your practice, no matter the amount of experience. I believe in trying to achieve compromise as opposed to unwaveringly defending your position.

Dr. John Jesus: What makes me most uncomfortable about this case is that, the forces that influence administrative bodies, the CEO, or the non-physician, include factors other than what is medically appropriate (e.g., money, power, politics, etc.). It is true that we are often going to have to order a test that isn't indicated. If this patient were to have an anaphylactic reaction to the IV dye that we administered, however, and this were to go to court, I would rather be in the position of doing something I thought was medically appropriate, rather than what someone told me to do. It's a particularly difficult position for a young physician, who is generally more vulnerable to the influence of superiors.

PR: Most of the tests we order have a low incidence of negative consequences, unlike an angiogram, which has a true risk of contrast nephropathy. You have to fight for those instances where the risk is greater, and that makes it a judgment call. If you are subjecting the patient to a test or intervention you think is absolutely wrong, that is when you need to share the responsibility with your chief of staff, and challenge the decision.

Section III: Review of the literature

In addition to the ethical challenges emergency physicians face in their interactions with other clinicians and patients, there are a number of non-physician influences that affect the practice of emergency medicine. Whether they involve industry, regulatory agencies, or administrative officials, these situations may blur the lines between ethics and politics. This chapter explores the nature of these influences and the considerations that should guide how a physician responds to these pressures under a given set of circumstances.

Administration and family influences

The case narrative illustrates the ethical dilemmas posed by involvement of a non-clinician administrator in the physician–patient relationship. Little data exist on the frequency of such dilemmas or the effect of these influences on clinical outcomes. When such outside influences lead to testing that may be harmful to a patient, the principle of non-maleficence may be at risk. However, the risk of harm may be difficult to determine prospectively, and may be underestimated in the face of the political pressures of the workplace.

Beauchamp and Childress summarize philosophers' interpretation of justice as "fair, equitable and appropriate treatment in light of what is due or owed to persons."[1] There are a number of material principles of justice that specify how resources should be fairly or equitably distributed, including the principle of need. If the physician is driven to use scarce resources on a particular patient for whom they are not indicated, this may violate the principle of need, "which declares that distribution of social resources based on need is just."[1] Such temptations exist in daily clinical practice. For example, seeing a less critical patient first who happens to be a friend of the board of trustees may be seen as a violation of the justice principle. This practice may be especially egregious if it delays care for an indigent patient who may be sicker or have fewer resources that can support the particular case. In this scenario, the patient with greater need has been given lower priority in the allocation of a limited resource (time with a physician). Alternatively, the physician may take the utilitarian view that the board member's experience in the ED may have repercussions for the financial health of the institution, and undermine its ability to care for many indigent patients, and thus justify the differing standards of care. In addition, if the wishes of the administrator are not congruent with those of the patient, there may be pressure to take a course of action that undermines patient autonomy.

Similar ethical tension may exist when families insist upon a particular diagnostic or treatment plan for a patient that may be of debatable benefit. The decision of whether to yield to a family's demands similarly depends upon the risk associated with the diagnostic or therapeutic modality, the likelihood of benefit, and the cost to the individual and the healthcare system. While there are guidelines and algorithms for various medical conditions, few are known to be perfectly sensitive or specific. The Ottawa ankle rules may dictate that a patient with an injury does not need an X-ray study. If the certainty of the diagnosis eases the mind of an insistent patient or family member, however, the physician may consider its benefit well worth the cost of the test and the minimal risk of radiation. Yet, if that same family was to demand magnetic resonance imaging (MRI) or an arthrocentesis, the risk/benefit and cost/benefit profiles may shift in favor of denying the request, even if it leads to dissatisfaction and workplace political ramifications. Consequently, it may be acceptable for the physician to be driven to alter his or her practice for reasonable requests that do not jeopardize patient wellbeing, autonomy, or reasonable standards of professional practice.

Industry: influence of the pharmaceutical industry on emergency medicine

One controversial ethical issue facing emergency medicine is the influence of gifts from the pharmaceutical industry to physicians. An analysis conducted by Marco and colleagues in 2006 examined the ethical arguments for and against physician gifts from the pharmaceutical industry.[2] Drug samples are one of the more debated gifts from pharmaceutical representatives because they provide a potential benefit to patients. Drug samples allow some patients to obtain medications that they otherwise could not afford. Some might consider it unethical for an emergency physician to deprive an indigent or uninsured patient access to free medications. An alternative viewpoint as outlined by Marco et al. is that availability of drug samples may alter a physician's choice of which drug to prescribe, perhaps leading to the prescribing of a more costly or less efficacious drug.[2] This practice could lead to an adverse health outcome when an inferior drug is prescribed simply because it is free, and more readily available. It may be easier for a busy EP to prescribe this sample drug rather than investigating a means to obtain a more appropriate medication. Marco and colleagues also describe the controversy of whether a drug sample is a gift to the patient or the physician, as the physician may obtain benefits such as a patient's gratitude.[2]

In view of the conventional wisdom that nothing is truly free, one must consider who is actually bearing the cost of drug samples. Presumably pharmaceutical companies provide these samples to maximize their revenue in some way. Perhaps a drug sample will lead to long-term use of a more expensive medication

when another less expensive drug is sufficient, potentially increasing healthcare costs.[2] Also, the cost of manufacturing and providing drug samples is presumably passed on to the consumer in the form of higher drug prices. Whether this cost burden is justified is subject to debate.

An area of particular concern for academic emergency medicine is the influence of the pharmaceutical industry on medical research. There have been prominent examples of conflicts of interest in clinician–researcher and industry interactions that have come to media attention.[3] Modifying research for one's own professional gain violates the ethical principle of beneficence. Berger cites Howard Brody's *Ethics, the Medical Profession and the Pharmaceutical Industry*, which describes the process by which well-intentioned researchers become indebted to industry funding their research.[3,4] When researchers are dependent on industry for financial support, they may be influenced to conduct their research in a way that maximizes industry benefit rather than scientific integrity.[3,4] Other authors have taken a more pragmatic approach, and acknowledge the degree to which emergency medicine research relies on industry funding. Newgard and colleagues argue for greater involvement of emergency medicine leaders in industry-sponsored clinical trials to ensure that ethical guidelines are followed and conflicts of interest are minimized.[5]

In addition, the Society for Academic Emergency Medicine has a published set of guidelines aimed at helping physicians and researchers maintain conduct that respects the ethical principles of justice, patient autonomy, and beneficence.[6] Ongoing discussion, education, and vigilance of individual physicians, however, are crucial to maintaining an ethical relationship between industry and emergency medicine.

Regulatory agencies

A commonly encountered example of non-physician influence on the practice of emergency medicine is typified by regulatory agencies that oversee opioid prescribing. Pain is the most common chief complaint of patients presenting to the ED.[7] The Oath of Maimonides calls on physicians to "never see in the patient anything but a fellow creature in pain."[8] Rosen lists the following "responsibilities of trying to achieve the missions of medicine" as curing disease, alleviating the ravages of disease and providing comfort.[9] While emergency physicians may be frequently unable to cure the ailments of ED patients, Rosen reminds us that we are always able to provide comfort. Unfortunately, emergency physicians have been notoriously poor at providing pain relief in the ED, a phenomenon known as "oligoanalgesia."[10] In 1989, Wilson and Pendleton found that only 44% of patients in the ED with pain received analgesic medication.[10] Although this study ignited a discussion of oligoanalgesia in the ED, and elevated our focus on patients' pain to include it as the "fifth vital sign," five studies over the past 20 years demonstrate that only 30%–64% of patients in the ED with pain receive analgesia.[11–15]

So why is oligoanalesgia such an issue among physicians including emergency physicians? Hill proposes three main reasons: societal barriers to appropriate opioid use, lack of education on the pharmacology of opioids, and influence of disciplinary boards on prescribing practices.[16] This discussion will focus on the ethical considerations of regulatory agencies' impact on physicians' prescribing practices.

Background

Although many barriers contribute to the inadequate treatment of pain, fear of disciplinary action for prescribing opioids for cancer and non-cancer-related pain has been described in the literature. A survey of oncologists finds that 18% cited excessive regulation of analgesics as a barrier to optimal pain management.[17] A survey of Wisconsin physicians reveals poor knowledge of controlled substance regulations and sufficient fear of regulatory discipline to alter opioid prescribing practices.[18] Of the 90 questionnaires completed, 50% of the responses on controlled substance regulations were incorrect. Additionally, 54% of the physicians indicate that fear of disciplinary action would affect their prescribing practice by reducing the drug dose, decreasing the number of refills, or choosing a drug in a lower schedule.[18] This study triggered a movement in Wisconsin focused around physician education, and improving the clinical and regulatory environment around pain management. Yet another survey of Wisconsin physicians finds that 40% did not understand state and federal opioid prescribing laws. Although 59% report no concern of being investigated, 19%–46% use other methods like limiting the number of refills or prescribing a smaller quantity to avoid investigation by a regulatory agency.[19]

In response to these early surveys, the Pain and Policy Study Group surveyed members of the state medical boards regarding the legality and medical acceptability of prescribing long-term opioids for cancer and non-malignant pain.[20] Most respondents feel that long-term prescribing of opioids for cancer-related pain is legal and acceptable. Only 12% find this practice legal and acceptable for chronic, non-malignant pain while most respondents do not find it medically acceptable and would investigate it.[20] These results prompted an educational series for the medical board members on appropriate pain management. This survey of the state medical board members demonstrates that physicians' fear of prescribing opioids may be well founded. In 1997, a survey of New York state physicians finds that 58% are moderately concerned or very concerned about a possible investigation by regulatory agencies if they are to write prescriptions for opioids for patients with chronic, non-malignant pain. In addition, 41% are apprehensive about prescribing opioids for patients with acute pain.[21]

There are little data in the emergency medicine literature on the impact of the fear of disciplinary action for prescribing opioids. Most studies are based on providers' beliefs and not outcomes; McErlean and colleagues conducted a study examining the impact of an opiate prescription diversion sanction on the frequency of opiates prescribed in a single ED.[22] Opiate prescribing rates were compared around the time of a physician arrest for diversion of opiate prescriptions. The study finds that patients with moderate pain are less likely to receive opiates in the ED and at discharge, but this effect had diminished by 90 days. McErlean and colleagues conclude that factors outside the physician–patient relationship may influence pain management; specifically the fear of discipline from a regulatory agency.[22] This study suggests that influence from regulatory agencies potentially undermines physicians' autonomy to treat pain adequately.

Should physicians be fearful?

While most of the above data are based on physicians' attitudes and not outcomes, the fear of discipline from regulatory agencies does exist. The question then arises: Is this a legitimate fear? Studies have looked at the actual risk of disciplinary action for opioid prescribing at the state and federal level.

Richard and Reidenberg examined disciplinary action against New York State physicians by the state board.[23] Of the physicians' disciplined for overprescribing opioids, 56% had other charges of misconduct including self-prescribing, failure to maintain adequate medical records, or having had sexual relations with the patient.[23] This study finds that there is no actual risk of disciplinary action for prescribing opioids if the physician documented a doctor–patient relationship, and was treating a painful condition.[23]

In addition, Jung and Reidenberg examined the risk of disciplinary action by the Drug Enforcement Agency (DEA) against physicians prescribing controlled substances, including opioids, for pain. The reason for disciplinary action included fraud, sex in exchange for prescriptions, and prescribing without seeing the patient.[24] Similar to the state level, when adequate documentation of a doctor–patient relationship exists and treatment is initiated for a painful condition, the risk of disciplinary action by the DEA is negligible. These studies suggest that the actual risk of physician discipline for prescribing opioids when medical records document a doctor–patient relationship is non-existent. These studies do not take into account claims made against physicians that were subsequently dropped.

Pain management plays an important role in most ED interactions. Emergency physicians should be well versed in the pharmacology of pain management, and be able to treat their patients' pain according to their clinical judgment and experience. Influence from fear of disciplinary action from regulatory agencies may be a barrier to adequate pain management and undermine the principle of beneficence. However, the actual data suggest that if physicians maintain appropriate medical records when treating painful conditions, no such risk exists.

Conclusion

Non-physician influences on emergency medicine may come from a variety of sources. Whether it is industry or regulatory agencies that alter prescribing practices, these outside influences may undermine the physician–patient relationship. Emergency physicians must be aware of the potential for these factors to change their practice, alter clinical outcomes, and threaten academic integrity. There are also times when it is prudent for physicians to adjust their practice in order to accommodate outside influences. Nevertheless, it is crucial that these influences do not undermine patient care. In an ideal world, protocols involving each outside influence and their ability to influence the emergency physician would be readily available as a reference. Such resources, however, rarely exist. Instead, physicians must develop their own sense of when they should challenge an administrator, influential body or other interest, and when it is best to walk away from their position altogether.

Section IV: Recommendations

• It may be reasonable to adjust one's practice to accommodate non-physician influences in certain circumstances when there is potential for patient benefit, or at the very least, minimal risk of patient harm.
• The physician must strive to respect professional norms and above all, patient wellbeing in the face of pressure from non-physician influences.
• The potential for conflicts of interest is especially great at the intersection of medicine and industry. This common ethical conflict is being increasingly recognized in academic emergency medicine, and a greater number of physician organizations are developing guidelines to help emergency physicians navigate this challenge.
• It is important that physicians do not let fear of regulatory action compromise patient care. This is especially true for pain management, a condition for which inadequate treatment is considerably more common than inappropriate physician sanction.

References

1. Beauchamp TL, Childress JF. (2001) *Principles of Biomedical Ethics*, 5th ed. New York, NY: Oxford University Press.
2. Marco CA, Moskop JC, Solomon RC, et al. (2006) Gifts to physicians from the pharmaceutical industry: an ethical analysis. *Ann Emerg Med*. 48(5), 513–21.
3. Berger E. (2008) Leak: Avandia and the integrity of the peer review process. *Ann Emerg Med*. 51(5), 636–8.
4. Brody H. (2007) *Ethics, the Medical Profession and the Pharmaceutical Industry*. Lanham, MD: Rowman and Littlefield Publishers.
5. Newgard CD, Kim S, Camargo CA. (2003) Emergency medicine leadership in industry-sponsored clinical trials. *Acad Emerg Med*. 10(2), 169–74.

6. Schears RM, Watters A, Schmidt TA, et al. (2007) The Society for Academic Emergency Medicine position on ethical relationships with the biomedical industry. *Acad Emerg Med.* 14(2), 179–81.

7. Burt CW, McCaig LF. (2001) Trends in hospital emergency department utilization: United States, 1992–99. *Vital Health Stat* 150, 1–34.

8. Johns Hopkins University Sheridan Libraries. Bioethics: Guide to finding information about bioethics and related subjects. Oath of Maimonides. Available at: http://guides.library.jhu.edu/bioethics. Accessed January 1, 2012.

9. Rosen P. (2009) No opiates for headache. *J Emerg Med.* 36(3), 3.

10. Wilson JE, Pendleton JM. (1989) Oligoanalgesia in the emergency department. *Am J Emerg Med.* 7(6), 620–3.

11. Fosnocht DE, Swanson ER, Bossart P. (2001) Patient expectations for pain medication delivery. *Am J Emerg Med.* 19(5), 399–402.

12. Lewis LM, Lasater LC, Brooks CB. (1994) Are emergency physicians too stingy with analgesics? *South Med J.* 87(1), 7–9.

13. Petrack EM, Christopher NC, Kriwinsky J. (1997) Pain management in the emergency department: patterns of analgesic utilization. *Pediatrics.* 99(5), 711–14.

14. Selbst SM, Clark M. (1990) Analgesic use in the emergency department. *Ann Emerg Med.* 19(9), 1010–13.

15. Brown JC, Klein EJ, Lewis CW, et al. (2003) Emergency department analgesia for fracture pain. *Ann Emerg Med.* 42(2), 197–205.

16. Hill CS, Jr. (1990) Relationship among cultural, educational, and regulatory agency influences on optimum cancer pain treatment. *J Pain Symptom Manage.* 5 Suppl 1, S37–45.

17. Von Roenn JH, Cleeland CS, Gonin R, et al. (1993) Physician attitudes and practice in cancer pain management. A survey from the Eastern Cooperative Oncology Group. *Ann Intern Med.* 119(2), 121–6.

18. Weissman DE, Joranson DE, Hopwood MB. (1991) Wisconsin physicians' knowledge and attitudes about opioid analgesic regulations. *Wis Med J.* 90(12), 671–5.

19. Wolfert MZ, Gilson AM, Dahl JL, et al. (2009) Opioid analgesics for pain control: Wisconsin physicians' knowledge, beliefs, attitudes, and prescribing practices. *Pain Med.* 11(3), 425–34.

20. Joranson DE, Cleeland CS, Weissman DE, et al. (1992) Opioids for chronic cancer and non-cancer pain: A survey of state medical board members. *Fed Bull.* 79(4), 15–49.

21. Pantel ES. (1998) *Breaking Down the Barriers to Effective Pain Management.* Report to the Commissioner of Health, Barbara A De Buono, MD MPH, from the New York State Public Health Council. Albany, NY: New York State Public Health Council, Appendix E.

22. McErlean M, Triner W, Young A. (2006) Impact of outside regulatory investigation on opiate administration in the emergency department. *J Pain.* 7(12), 947–50.

23. Richard J, Reidenberg MM. (2005) The risk of disciplinary action by state medical boards against physicians prescribing opioids. *J Pain Symptom Manage.* 29(2), 206–12.

24. Jung B, Reidenberg MM. (2006) The risk of action by the Drug Enforcement Administration against physicians prescribing opioids for pain. *Pain Med.* 7(4), 353–7.

19 Privacy and confidentiality: particular challenges in the emergency department

Jessica H. Stevens,[1] Michael N. Cocchi[2]

[1]*Clinical Instructor, Harvard Affiliated Emergency Medicine Residency Program, Beth Israel Deaconess Medical Center, Boston, MA, USA*

[2]*Instructor of Medicine, Harvard Medical School, and Attending Physician, Department of Emergency Medicine and Department of Anesthesia Critical Care, Associate Director, Critical Care Quality, Beth Israel Deaconess Medical Center, Boston, MA, USA*

Section I: Case presentation

A 56-year-old woman presents to the emergency department (ED) for atypical chest pain. When a resident approaches the patient to obtain a history, the patient complains that not only has she given her story three times, she could also give the history of the patient next door because she's heard that three times too. Next, a 65-year-old man with pancreatic cancer has a cardiac arrest in the ED. The patient's wife is contacted by phone during the resuscitation, in order to verify the patient's prior do-not-resuscitate (DNR) status, but says she cannot think clearly. Ultimately, resuscitation is unsuccessful, and the patient expires before the family has an opportunity to arrive and verify the patient's DNR order. A little later, an 80-year-old man with hematemesis and concerns about an upper gastrointestinal bleeding is brought in. The patient is awake and alert and in no apparent distress. The patient's daughter, a former nurse, calls the ED demanding information, adamantly insisting that the emergency physician pretreat the patient with lorazepam before inserting a nasogastric tube, because of a prior bad experience with a nasogastric tube placement. The patient, on the other hand, appears calm, and apologizes for his daughter's behavior. He does not request sedation for nasogastric tube placement.

Section II: Discussion

Dr. Peter Rosen: The reality is that there are many parts of the hospital that are not designed for optimal patient care. I can remember being a patient in the CCU [coronary care unit]. There is nothing worse than having to go to the toilet in the middle of the CCU. Just because there are curtains drawn around you doesn't make it more private for someone who is used to being alone for such personal hygienic activities. The ED isn't any better. No matter how well designed the ED is, there are going to be opportunities to overhear conversations; I don't really see this as an ethical issue.

Dr. John Jesus: I believe that logistical concerns can be ethical concerns. The underlying principle behind the importance of privacy and confidentiality is that of treating people with dignity. Although there will always be a tension between optimal treatment and consideration for patients in the ED and the resources available, there also are varied spectrum of interventions and approaches that consider patient privacy and confidentiality. In our first scenario, I would try to lower my voice so that I'm not overheard so easily, and perhaps apologize for the fact that we can't provide better confidentiality and privacy.

Ethical Problems in Emergency Medicine: A Discussion-Based Review, First Edition. John Jesus, Shamai A. Grossman, Arthur R. Derse, James G. Adams, Richard Wolfe, and Peter Rosen.

Dr. Michael N. Cocchi: There are definite challenges to maintaining patient privacy and confidentiality in the ED. Specifically, the ED tends to be a busy place, often times with a great deal of congestion within a relatively small space. I'm not sure it is ever possible to protect the privacy of patients assigned to the hallways, where even curtains are missing. Nevertheless, I do agree that there are little things that we can do, like trying to keep our voices down and being mindful of closing the curtain. I wonder if it is even reasonable to expect complete privacy and confidentiality in a setting like the ED. The ED is clearly not a physician clinic where all patients can be interviewed and examined behind a closed door. There are instances in the ED during which we must sacrifice privacy for patient care. For example, we often like to keep the curtains open when treating an unstable patient, so that the ED team is more quickly aware of any changes in the patient's status. This sort of consideration spills over into the ICU setting as well.

PR: It seems to me that we want it both ways. Here we are talking about making it private for the patient so that nobody but the patient interacts with the medical team, and yet there are many who would argue in favor of bringing patient relatives into the trauma bay during resuscitations to watch people die.

Dr. Shamai Grossman: As physicians, our primary goal is to take the best possible care of patients. It is helpful to note that our discussion focuses on a secondary agenda. Privacy and confidentiality is a matter of comfort, and although we want to make patients as comfortable as possible, comfort often takes a back seat to taking the best possible care of a patient. We could increase patient privacy and confidentiality dramatically if we kept patients out in the waiting room, rather than filling the hallways and adjacent rooms separated by curtains. If we did this, however, we wouldn't provide great patient care, we might even ignore potential life threats in our efforts to protect patient privacy. Clearly, there is a balance. If, in your pursuit of providing the best possible care of patients in the chaotic environment that is the ED there is a breach of confidentiality, well then, so be it.

PR: I worked with a director of an ED at UCLA [University of California at Los Angeles] years ago, who was enamored with the touchy-feely issues in the ED. One day he decided that his nurses weren't

concerned enough with patient privacy and patient comfort. He decided to serially take every nurse in the department, have them go into a patient's room, strip off all their clothes, put on a patient gown and sit there for 2 hours. The nurses in the department thought that everybody was talking about them.

I wonder if a lot of patient comfort needs aren't in fact dependent on how ill they are. I've never heard a patient complain about privacy, comfort, pain issues when he or she was seriously ill.

Dr. Jessica H. Stevens: Yet, there are certain intimate details of a patient's history and experience that have important clinical implications and need to be uncovered in the ED, for example, HIV [human immunodeficiency virus] status, sexual history, or substance abuse history. I worry that patients will be less likely to honestly reveal details about issues such as these if they are not in an environment that fosters and engenders a sense of privacy and confidentiality. If a patient presents with severe hypertension and chest pain, it would be very important for the clinicians to know whether the patient has just been using cocaine. What do you feel are common patient expectations for privacy and confidentiality in the ED?

PR: In most EDs in the United States, there is no place in the department that you could take a patient where you can guarantee the patient complete privacy and confidentiality. No matter how much you lower your voice, sound will carry to some one who can overhear it. I believe people's expectations have a lot to do with what kind of ED they frequent. If they go to a city hospital ED they don't expect a lot in terms of privacy or comfort. Patients may complain, but they actually complain less than many patients who go to the expensive private community hospital and encounter conditions that don't meet their expectations for privacy. I've found over the years that the importance of privacy is manifold and includes visual privacy and auditory privacy, and last but not least, it should provide a degree of smell privacy. One of the real problems in taking care of patients is that we have become desensitized to actions that patients consider an invasion of their privacy. Take a rectal examination: it's impossible to have a rectal examination and not be embarrassed. Yet, it's impossible to perform a rectal examination more than once, and feel embarrassed about doing it. If patients knew how little concern we had about their private parts, they would probably experience a great deal less humiliation.

JJ: I agree that patients rely on us to keep their information confidential when they disclose sensitive and embarrassing information. The next rational conclusion one may draw from this fact is that consideration of patient privacy and confidentiality **is** good patient care, as this is part of what allows patients to trust us with their care. It is impossible to separate completely the primary and secondary goals of patient care. While I agree that acutely ill patients care little for their own privacy and confidentiality concerns, those patients encompass the vast minority of patients who present to the ED.

PR: While we would all agree that privacy and confidentiality are good for patient care, you will find EDs where you can't achieve those goals to the degree you would like. The question is then, "What do you do about it?"

JJ: There are significant challenges to achieving adequate patient privacy and confidentiality. Even though we are not able to provide 100% privacy and confidentiality, however, we should be able to improve the situation that exists today. Small steps toward this goal are important and worthwhile.

Dr. James Adams: On the larger issue of privacy and confidentiality, if those goals were the priority in the ED, we would build a physical structure adequate to the demand of the patient in order to enable patient privacy and confidentiality protection. Of course, the caregivers have to be conscientious people, but there are real limits to what a caregiver can do. In my career, I've seen physicians debride and pack extensive sacral decubitus ulcers and residents perform rectal examinations in the hallways.

PR: Let's move on to the second case. Frankly, if I knew this patient had pancreatic cancer before he arrested, I wouldn't be concerned with whether I knew his DNR status. I have watched people die from pancreatic cancer, and the end point of death in this instance is a blessing, not a curse. I would define my mission for this patient in terms of minimizing future suffering as well as responding to the present circumstance.

MC: In the setting of knowing that a patient has a terminal illness, it can be very important to explain

to the wife that a successful resuscitation of someone with a terminal illness is very unlikely. This conversation can provide the wife with a certain amount of relief, and help in giving the wife permission to let the patient go.

JA: I appreciate the emphasis on communicating with the wife. I would emphasize that none of us really want to ask the wife what to do. This puts the family in a terrible situation. I think the conversation is your husband has died, and we're trying to bring him back—would that be his wishes in this circumstance?

PR: Why don't we go on to the third case, in which a family member insists upon sedation for the placement of a nasogastric tube. It is common for different people with various agendas to make demands about what should be done for a patient. The most difficult case is not one like this in which the patient is able to communicate with you, and tell you what he thinks and what his wishes and desires are, but rather the case of the patient who changes his preferences depending on which family member happens to be in the room.

JA: The ethical response is really about what is best for the patient's interests. If the patient needed a little lorazepam for insertion of a nasogastric tube, I would give it. If not needed, I wouldn't give it. Sometimes the family is part of the solution and sometimes the family is part of the problem, and that definitely complicates our lives. Many times I've received letters of complaints from family members even though the patient expressed nothing but appreciation for our efforts.

JJ: Our approach to listening and interacting with the patient's family members is as important as our actions themselves. I would certainly respectfully listen to the family members, and try to explain my reasons for doing whatever my decision was. Usually, I would ask family members to step out while I examine the patient in privacy. I would inquire what the patient's actual wishes are, and then carry on with those while attempting to maintain a respectful relationship to the patient's family members.

JS: Whether or not the patient received 1 mg of lorazepam before the procedure isn't a crucial medical decision that is either going to harm or help the

199

patient in any appreciable way. I was very adamant about not giving the lorazepam, because I didn't feel that it would provide the patient with any benefit, and therefore, wasn't medically appropriate.

PR: The critical point that you are raising has less to do with this case and the lorazepam, and more to do with life-saving procedures or diagnostic tools that clinicians don't feel comfortable proceeding without. At some point you either need to get the patient to commit or simply tell the daughter, "Listen, you can't ask me to jeopardize your father's life because you think it is a good thing to do; I'm not going to do it." When you reduce an argument with a difficult family member to absurdity, you can often convince them of the error of their thought process. I would start by saying to the family, for example, "You can ask me to do a brain transplant, but I'm going to refuse as no amount of money will allow me to perform it safely." From this position, clinicians can often work backwards towards a more reasonable solution.

SG: Ultimately, our primary purpose is to serve the healthcare needs of the patient. Although it is important to placate families, it can't be done to the detriment of our patients, much less endangering our patients' lives. For example, if a patient develops respiratory distress and suffers an adverse event from unnecessary sedation, neither a court of law nor your own conscience would excuse you.

JA: Many families are pushy because they need very much to be in control. A show of confidence and authority, in the context of compassionate care, is often exactly what pushy families need.

PR: I once had a patient with Crohn's disease who presented with a bowel obstruction and desperately needed a nasogastric tube. In response to telling him that he needed the nasogastric tube he said, "I can't tolerate your putting it down, and I can't tolerate having it in. I know I need it, and I'm more than willing to have the surgery, but I simply can't stand the nasogastric tube." Instead of sedating him, I gave him ketamine. Creative solutions and a willingness to change normal practice patterns, in order to provide patients with the comfort care they need, can be extremely important for certain patents.

MC: I think on rare occasions, it requires involvement of the hospital ethics committee, to mediate between the family and the treating medical team. This is particularly helpful when there exists a tension between the family's goals and those of the medical team.

PR: In summary, while we are all willing to provide privacy and respect patient's and families' needs for comfort and confidentiality, by virtue of why the patient is in the ED in the first place dictates how well we can achieve an emergency evaluation and treatment. Privacy, therefore, must be a goal secondary to the primary responsibility of the medical care of the patient. Both economically and logistically, the busier the ED, the less likely will it be possible to provide privacy and luxury to patients, although there are always ways that the individual team members can attempt to protect the privacy needs of the patient.

Section III: Review of the literature

The stories above demonstrate the challenges faced daily by emergency physicians charged with respecting patient privacy and confidentiality while balancing the primary goals of providing high-quality and efficient patient care in the ED. As a society, we understand that control over both one's physical environment and personal information are integral to the protection of an individual's dignity, and thus make efforts to safeguard these values in our day-to-day interactions.[1,2] As healthcare providers, we have the difficult task of upholding our patients' right to dignity while at the same time undermining the fundamental elements of privacy when we obtain even the most basic history and perform a physical examination. In this chapter, we will reflect on how issues of privacy and confidentiality relate to the unique environment of the ED, as well as what we can do as emergency physicians to limit breaches of privacy within the walls of our EDs.

Privacy, confidentiality, and trust

In the strictest sense, the concepts of privacy and confidentiality are separate. While the term **privacy** refers generally to protection of personal space, identity, information, and autonomy, the term **confidentiality** more narrowly pertains to the protection of personal information. The English word "confidentiality" originates from the Latin *confidere*, which is the infinitive of the verb, "to trust."[1] In the ED, as in any clinical environment, it is essential for the physician to establish a trusting relationship with the patient in order to provide quality care; this trust will allow the physician to learn details of a patient's personal and medical history that will aid in diagnosis and treatment, as well as ensure that patients are willing to accept diagnostic plans and treatment recommendations proposed by the emergency physician.

A professional code and legal mandate

The importance of confidentiality within the physician–patient relationship is recognized within the statutes of our profession as well as the laws of our country and states.[2] The Hippocratic Oath, long accepted by medical institutions as an outline for the founding ethical principles upon which physicians should practice, states:

All that may come to my knowledge in the exercise of my profession or in daily commerce with men, which ought not to be spread abroad, I will keep secret and will never reveal.[1]

Beyond fostering quality patient care, protecting privacy and confidentiality in the healthcare setting is, in general, a legal requirement for physicians. Perhaps the most well-recognized example of this is the recently enacted federal Health Information Portability and Accountability Act (HIPAA). This law has many provisions that aim to address the security and privacy of health data, by ensuring that patients are aware of and involved in the sharing of their protected health information between institutions and healthcare providers. Violations of these requirements can result in offending practitioners and institutions being punished by monetary fines or imprisonment. There are also special state and federal laws that separate out and even more strictly protect certain types of medical information considered to be particularly sensitive, including HIV status, genetic test results, and mental health records.[1]

Privacy and confidentiality in the ED

While socially, legally, and professionally recognized as important, patient privacy is routinely overlooked in the routine flow of the ED.[3] We often must interview and examine patients in cubicles separated by curtains, and not in private rooms with solid walls and closed doors. We physically circulate through the ED with cell phones discussing urgent matters with consultants. In academic institutions, we often conduct patient sign-out rounds in a semi-public manner, which can result in the passive transmission of patient information to a myriad of individuals not directly involved in providing patient care. Furthermore, in truly emergent situations like a severe trauma or the seriously ill medical patient, expedited procurement of medical history and sharing of important information between family, other medical providers, and the ED physician may become essential. This can necessitate overlooking generally respected privacy rules, and in turn, can result in unintended breaches of confidentiality.

As demands on emergency physicians to provide efficient patient care increase, the protection of patient confidentiality and privacy may be further undermined. While patients undoubtedly desire high-quality, efficient care, they also have an interest in ensuring that their personal information will be kept private, and that their personal space and autonomy will be respected. It is imperative that we recognize the difference between a truly emergent situation, which calls for expedited sharing of information at the expense of privacy and confidentiality, and when, instead, this is occurring out of convenience to the emergency physician. In maintaining the proper balance, we demonstrate respect for our patients' dignity, autonomy, and wellbeing, ultimately facilitating relationships that allow for open communication and trust.[2]

Our physical space

Most EDs have been built with two important goals in mind: maximize efficiency and ensure patient safety. While understandable, it is unfortunate that patient privacy becomes less of a focus, resulting in common ED features like curtain-separated rooms that allow for size flexibility and easy accessibility, but do little to limit sound transmittal between patient rooms. ED waiting rooms and triage areas encounter a similar problem, as triage personnel must be able to both assess incoming patients and keep a close eye on the door and waiting room, so that critically ill patients will be identified quickly and appropriately triaged.[2] Lastly, as overcrowding continues to stretch

201

the physical space of the ED, we are forced to interview, examine, and treat patients in hallway beds and chairs, which afford even less privacy than curtain-walled rooms.[3]

While these less-than-ideal situations may be a reality for most emergency providers, we can still make reasonable efforts to maintain patient privacy and confidentiality in our daily practice. For "hallway patients," we can attempt to initially see patients in rooms for a history and physical examination, and then rotate patients out of rooms and into hallway space once they are stabilized and awaiting test results and disposition. We can work to limit hallway space next to provider workspaces, as this design can result in the passive transmission of information about other patients in the ED to those located in the hallway. In addition, we can make every effort to monitor the level of our voice while speaking to patients within earshot of others, including curtained rooms.

Emergency physician desensitization to privacy

As emergency physicians we see and hear things about people that most others do not. We are used to dealing with personal struggle and tragedy as a daily part of our job. Not much fazes us, and this desensitization to the experience of privacy for our patients enables us to do our jobs. Imagine, as Dr. Rosen has suggested, if we experienced equal embarrassment to that of the patient for each rectal examination that we performed, or to the humiliation a patient might feel when being undressed during a trauma. Because we become so comfortable operating in an environment where we are privy to a flood of personal information, we are apt to be overly casual in the treatment of that data—especially when doing so allows us to expedite or improve a patient's medical care. What we do not recognize is that when patients experience this phenomenon, they experience it in a different way. Often instead of recognizing that we are trying to improve their individual care by being efficient, the environment and manner in which we practice sends an unfortunate message that we are not concerned about protecting their privacy. This experience by patients undermines the trust that we hope to establish as physicians and thus results in suboptimal care. We must, therefore, remind ourselves to treat patients as we would prefer to be treated and stay vigilant in our efforts to protect patient autonomy, personal privacy, and confidentiality. We must ensure that we make every reasonable effort to keep patient information private and avoid temptation to maximize efficiency by sacrificing confidentiality. For example, we must take care to step out of patient rooms when answering cell phones to speak with consultants and either wait or have nurses step out of patient rooms when we discuss care of other patients located elsewhere in the department.

Observers in the ED

Beyond the usual ebb and flow of medical providers through the ED, there are often additional individuals shadowing providers or otherwise rotating through the ED who may or may not be involved in direct patient care (see also Chapter 16). These individuals include administrators involved in quality assurance activities, nursing and medical students learning to conduct patient histories or physicals, resident and attending physicians from other countries attempting to establish emergency systems, as well as product representatives and actors pursuing medical roles. Training regarding the importance of maintaining patient privacy and confidentiality should be mandatory for anyone who spends significant time in the ED. In addition, patients should be presented with the reasonable option to decline having individuals not involved in their care follow their course of care.

Law enforcement in the ED

Security issues are commonplace in the ED. While some departments have internal security staff, many community sites rely on local law enforcement for all security issues. In addition, law enforcement officials accompany individuals in police custody who need a medical evaluation. While the presence of law enforcement is necessary and often helpful, conflict can arise when patient information is inadvertently relayed to officers. Law enforcement officials are, by occupation, agents of the state, and have no duty to protect the privacy of their detainees, especially against inquiry by other police representatives. On the contrary, they may be required by their own professional codes to report all information they uncover that may be useful in creating a legal case against a person in custody.

Although the simple solution would be to have law enforcement agents physically absent or out of earshot during conversations with and about detainee patients, this is not always possible, especially when the safety of ED healthcare providers or other patients in the department is in question. The emergency physician must make reasonable efforts to respect patient privacy in these situations, asking officers to leave the room for interviews and physical examinations and being sure to discuss test results in private whenever possible. Of course, if a patient needs additional treatment or urgent testing while the patient is in custody, this information will have to be communicated either to the officers or to the healthcare professional at the facility where the patient is to be detained.

Beyond passive acquisition of knowledge while stationed with patients, occasionally officers will ask probing questions of providers regarding results of laboratory or radiographic studies. At times, a physician may feel intimidated or legally obligated to provide this information. In the absence of a court order, the ED physician is under no legal requirement to provide patient information to police, and all usual efforts to maintain patient confidentiality should be upheld.

Mandatory reporting

Occasionally physicians encounter circumstances where they are legally required to breach patient confidentiality (see also Chapter 25). For centuries, medical professionals have been obligated to report instances of certain contagious infectious diseases like tuberculosis or measles to health officials, such as the local department of public health, with the understanding that tracking these cases may prevent further outbreaks of disease.[2] There are laws mandating that any gunshot wound, injury with another "deadly weapon," or dog bite injury must be reported to the local authorities. There are also laws in some US states mandating that physicians report medical conditions such as seizures that may impair a patient's ability to safely operate a motor vehicle.[2] In certain US states patients involved in alcohol-related motor vehicle accidents must be reported to the police.[4] While mandatory reporting laws aim to offer protection for the public at large, they clearly have the potential to lead physicians into morally confusing territory as they require a breach of patient confiden-

tiality and thereby steer physicians away from doing what is in the direct best interest of the individual patient. By enacting such laws, our society has accepted that in certain circumstances the benefit to the public so outweighs the potential harm to the individual that physicians must step out of their usual roles as custodians for their individual patients' health and wellbeing.

While mandatory reporting laws are designed to protect the general public from a dangerous individual or communicable disease, prevent or solve crimes, or to collect epidemiologic data, some of these laws are also enacted with the intent to protect the individual patient from harm.[1,4] For example, suspected child abuse or neglect must be reported to law enforcement officials. It is the expectation, and in fact all US state laws require, that the clinician must act in the best interest of the minor, and file a report. In a similar vein, mandatory reporting laws exist in some US states to report intimate partner violence, and in most states, the abuse of elders. The proposed benefit of such policies is increased identification and prosecution of batterers; however, concerns have been raised about the unintended consequences of such mandated reporting, including possibly increasing retaliatory violence, as well as compromising patient–doctor confidentiality and loss of patient autonomy.[4,5]

Rodriguez et al. conducted a cross-sectional survey of female ED patients and find that almost half of the respondents were opposed to mandatory reporting[6]; these data further complicate the discussion around taking the patient's choice away to have the physician "act in their best interest." The authors of this study argue that further investigations should be conducted to understand the complex issues involved, especially whether mandatory reporting laws for domestic violence actually help these patients or increase their risk of harm.[6] Other strong arguments have been made against mandating reporting in general as there exists the potential to deter patients from seeking medical attention or sharing important parts of their medical history, as doing so may put them at risk for scrutiny by legal and public health authorities. Furthermore, outcomes of mandatory reporting could also potentially result in significant loss of quality of life for the patients involved when they are subsequently barred from driving, incarcerated, or removed from their current living situation.[4]

Regardless of one's personal views on the validity of mandatory reporting laws, we would recommend that emergency physicians become aware of the particular statutes in place in their state of practice. Partially because laws vary from state to state in the United States, significant confusion exists among emergency medicine providers about their legal duty to report.[7-9]

Family members in the ED

It is not uncommon that a patient will be accompanied by a family member or spouse. In the most simple of situations, this family member is the legal guardian or healthcare proxy of the patient, or the patient is competent and well enough to give you permission to openly share medical information with that individual. This ideal circumstance often does not happen, however, leaving the physician to determine what information should be shared with family members as well as to what extent the family member should be present during the physician's assessment and treatment of the patient. Each of these situations will be undoubtedly unique and will require the emergency physician to thoughtfully assess the situation, and to determine a course of action guided by the principles already outlined in this chapter, with the goal being to balance good patient care with maintaining patient privacy and confidentiality.

A particular problem arises in communicating over the phone with a patient's family members. There are two ways in which this generally happens: either the emergency physician initiates a phone call to an individual identified as a healthcare proxy in order to obtain permission to treat/perform procedures, or a family member calls to obtain a status update on their relative. While it is clearly impossible to absolutely determine the identity of an individual whom the physician has never met over the phone, in the first circumstance the physician is reaching out to an identified individual at a listed phone number, which reduces the risk of breaching the patient's confidentiality. In the second circumstance, physicians should be careful to limit information provided over the phone unless reasonably certain of the caller's identity, and they have received permission from the patient to speak with this family member about the patient's condition.[10] It is best to allow the patient themselves to speak with the person on the phone so

that they can monitor the amount and type of information they divulge. Particular caution must be used when treating patients who may have been a victim of violence, as disclosing information about the status of these individuals over the phone has the potential to put not only the patient, but others in the ED, at risk for further violence.

Another common scenario arises when the adolescent minor presents to the ED with a parent. Often the adolescent will request confidentiality regarding certain concerns, test results, and treatments given, particularly for sexually transmitted infections, issues surrounding pregnancy, drug- or alcohol-related complaints, or mental health complaints. This information should be kept confidential as much as is possible in order to build trust between the adolescent and both the individual provider and the healthcare system in general.[11] This necessity is recognized by several national organizations including the American Medical Association, the American College of Obstetricians and Gynecologists and the American Academy of Pediatrics.[11] It is important that the physician lets the adolescent patient know that he or she will have to disclose information to the parent without permission by the patient if there is concern for the patient causing harm to him or herself or to another person. Additionally, every effort should be made within reason to facilitate discussions between the adolescent and the parent regarding situations that will require treatment and follow-up, for example a positive pregnancy test in a young female who is still living at home and is financially dependent on her parents. It should also be emphasized that while you as an emergency physician can uphold confidentiality by not sharing information with the patient's parents, it is possible that they may become privy to that same information inadvertently, particularly in the circumstance where the patient is a minor included on his or her parent's medical insurance plan.[11]

Section IV: Recommendations

• Healthcare providers must recognize the inherent obstacles and work to the best of their ability to provide high-quality and efficient care while being sensitive to the privacy needs of patients.
• While there may be exceptions, such as in cases of mandatory reporting requirements, medical

professionals are tasked with keeping sacred the principles of privacy and confidentiality, thereby preserving the therapeutic relationship between patient and provider.

• In situations where clinicians are in conflict about the best course of action, it would seem advisable to seek counsel of a hospital legal representative or ethics service, whenever available. As Geiderman and colleagues state, "circumstances requiring a breach of confidentiality are rare, and circumstances justifying the invasion of physical privacy are even rarer."[1]

References

1. Geiderman JM, Moskop JC, Derse AR. (2006) Privacy and confidentiality in emergency medicine: obligations and challenges. *Emerg Med Clin North Am.* 24, 633–56.
2. Moskop LC, Marco CA, Larkin GL, et al. (2005) From Hippocrates to HIPAA: Privacy and confidentiality in emergency medicine, Part I: Conceptual, moral, and legal foundations. *Ann Emerg Med.* 45, 53–9.
3. Mlinek EJ, Pierce J. (1997) Confidentiality and privacy breaches in a university hospital emergency department. *Acad Emerg Med.* 4, 1142–6.
4. Gupta M. (2007) Mandatory reporting laws and the emergency perspective. *Ann Emerg Med.* 40, 369–76.
5. Gielen AC, O'Campo PJ, Campbell JC, et al. (2000) Women's opinions about domestic violence screening and mandatory reporting. *Am J Prev Med.* 19, 279–85.
6. Rodriguez MA, McLoughlin E, Nah G, et al. (2001) Mandatory reporting of domestic violence injuries to the police: what do emergency department patients think? *JAMA.* 286, 580–3.
7. McManus J, Margaret ND, Hedges JR, et al. (2005) A survey of Oregon emergency physicians to assess mandatory reporting knowledge and reporting patterns regarding intoxicated drivers in the state of Oregon. *Acad Emerg Med.* 12, 896–9.
8. Houry D, Utz A, DeWitt C, et al. (1999) Colorado physicians' knowledge of and attitudes toward mandatory reporting laws. *Ann Emerg Med.* 34, s71–s2.
9. Turnipseed SD, Vierra D, DeCarlo D, et al. (2008) Reporting patterns for "lapses of consciousness" by California Emergency Physicians. *J Emerg Med.* 35, 15–21.
10. Moskop JC, Marco CA, Larkin GL, et al. (2005) From Hippocrates to HIPAA: Privacy and confidentiality in emergency medicine, Part II: Challenges in the emergency department. *Ann Emerg Med.* 45, 60–7.
11. Baren JM. (2006) Ethical dilemmas in the care of minors in the emergency department. *Emerg Med Clin North Am.* 24, 619–31.

Emergency medicine outside the emergency department

Short-term international medical initiatives

Matthew B. Allen,[1] Christine Dyott,[2] John Jesus[3]

[1]*Research Assistant, Department of Emergency Medicine, Brigham and Women's Hospital, Boston, MA, USA*
[2]*Clinical Research Assistant, Department of Emergency Medicine, Beth Israel Deaconess Medical Center, Boston, MA, USA*
[3]*Chief Resident, Department of Emergency Medicine, Beth Israel Deaconess Medical Center, Boston, MA, and Clinical Instructor, Department of Emergency Medicine, Christiana Care Health System, Newark, DE, USA*

Section I: Case presentation

A 70-year-old woman presented to a makeshift mobile tent clinic where she waited in line for 2 hours among 400 other people to be seen by the visiting medical team. For most of these patients, this was to be the first time in their lives to receive any medical care. The makeshift clinic was staffed by one nurse practitioner, two emergency medicine residents, two fourth year medical students on a tropical medicine elective, two nurses, two nurse educators, and two translators.

Through a translator, the patient communicated that she had experienced approximately 1 month of painless hematuria. There were no known provoking or exacerbating factors. She had no other complaints, and had a negative review of systems. She subsisted by working with her family and village inhabitants to fish and farm along the coast of a local lake. She did note that many of her family and friends also had painless hematuria. The vital signs were: temperature 35.9 °C; heart rate 85 beats per minute; blood pressure 185/90 mmHg; respiratory rate 18 breaths per minute; and oxygen saturation of 100% on room air. The physical examination was remarkable only for immobile, hard, supraclavicular lymphadenopathy. A sample of the patient's urine was obtained for analysis, and eggs were identified consistent with Schisto-soma haematobium. After the resident treated her with praziquantel, the nurse educators spent time teaching her how to avoid future schistosomiasis infections, in addition to stressing the importance of using mosquito nets to avoid malaria, how and why condoms are used, and the methods of using locally grown products to achieve better nutrition.

Section II: Discussion

Dr. Richard Wolfe: What do you think of this presenting scenario, and what would be the optimal way to treat this patient if you weren't in a field clinic in Ghana?

Dr. Peter Rosen: The problems that I have with this case are both medical and ethical in nature. I don't have a particular expertise in tropical disease. I am sure, however, that this woman is not going to get adequate follow-up, and I am sure that this is an incomplete workup. If this were a patient in an ED, I wouldn't stop with identifying *Schistosoma* parasites given the patient's concerning lymphadenopathy. Furthermore, because I have long worked in academic sophisticated tertiary care centers, I fear that I am no longer capable or comfortable with symptomatic treatment without adequate follow-up, without

Ethical Problems in Emergency Medicine: A Discussion-Based Review, First Edition. John Jesus, Shamai A. Grossman, Arthur R. Derse, James G. Adams, Richard Wolfe, and Peter Rosen.

adequate knowledge, and without adequate consultant support. I think medically, to simply treat the hematuria is a sham of providing medical care.

RW: Was there a conscious decision to diagnose and treat only the bladder infection? If so, did you avoid further diagnostic procedures and interventions because they simply weren't available, or because they weren't on your differential diagnosis?

Dr. John Jesus: Everybody noted the lymphadenopathy, and everyone was concerned about metastatic cancer. Almost everyone we met had never seen a physician nor received any medical care prior to our arrival. The closest hospital that might have been able to address the more concerning physical signs and symptoms was multiple days travel away. Generally, this was beyond the means of the people we met, who often depended on the results of their daily labor for food and shelter.

While we considered the possibility of cancer and discussed it at length, we thought it was beyond our capability to address in the field, as well as beyond the patient's means to make the several-day trip to the nearest hospital. We did communicate to the patient that the supraclavicular lymphadenopathy was not normal, that we worried about her health, and that if she had the opportunity, she should go to the capital to receive further diagnostic testing and potential treatments. Even as we communicated this point, however, we acknowledged the very low probability that she would actually be able to follow-up and comply with our recommendations.

RW: The situation appears grim, a field clinic in rural Ghana, a temporizing intervention, and no long-term follow-up for care. Given the challenges of working in these conditions, what benefit could the traveling medical team hope to impart to the population they were treating? Moreover, were there any benefits to be garnered by the providers?

Dr. Shamai Grossman: As emergency physicians, we are trained to care for a vast variety of illness. Though we cannot know everything, we generally have ability to gain access to resources for the information with which we are not yet familiar. In 2010, even in the remote areas of rural Ghana, we can bring a laptop, a handheld computer, or physical textbooks. That said, short-term medical initiatives are replete with

frustration, including the inability to provide the same level of care we are used to providing. Given that frustration, one has to decide if it is worth that frustration in order to be able to provide a minimal level of care when patients in these areas have absolutely nothing else? I would venture to say: "Yes." Some level of reasonable care is better than no medical care. Rather than look at the situation as a frustrating experience, we should approach short-term medical initiatives as an opportunity to use the abilities and skills of emergency physicians to help provide patients in these areas with medical care and improve their health; even if our efforts begin on a small scale, those efforts are clearly better than doing nothing.

RW: In my experience participating in short-term medical initiatives, I have witnessed surgeons literally amputating a limb on the street corner, without first thinking about postoperative follow-up care, or having much of a game plan to address postoperative complications or rehabilitation needs within a country that doesn't make accommodations for disabled persons. Given this situation, I can understand and see a benefit to short-term care to alleviate pain, to address various simple problems. I assume that most of the medical problems seen however, are more chronic in nature. Infectious diseases such as HIV [human immunodeficiency virus] and tuberculosis, for example, require long courses of treatment for months to years. Is this sort of care even possible if foreign medical assistance is present for only 1–2 weeks? Finally, although there are advantages to the provider in terms of education and perhaps emotional fulfillment, short-term medical initiatives also place the providers at risk by exposure to infectious diseases, security concerns, and more. Is the balance of risks and benefits favorable?

PR: I have strong negative feelings about temporary medical services. Our ability to respond with humanitarian aid as well as medical aid, even in a disaster situation is very incomplete. Though I didn't travel to Haiti to assist in the response, I would assume that a lot of the well-intentioned, generous donations of personnel, equipment, and expertise went to waste either because the Haitians wouldn't permit the resources to be used in a useful way, or there wasn't an organized system of delivery. I acknowledge that many well-intentioned and idealistic students acquire a useful educational perspective when caring for patients in the developing world. Despite these benefits, however, working in circumstances that are not organized towards specific achievable goals that will positively affect patients is insufficient and wrong. There are always things that can be accomplished by motivated clinicians, a point I freely acknowledge. Emergency physicians have a special kind of expertise geared toward immediate action and stabilization of acute deteriorations. Their expertise, however, is not very geared towards ongoing and long-term care.

I think that to promise something medical professionals in that environment are unable to provide, namely medical care for any and all conditions, is a mistake. If your medical team can align itself with an organization that is able to establish a more consistent commitment to the provision of care and a permanent facility, then I think the initiative is much more capable of accomplishing its goals. To drop a couple of medical students into a developing country without those resources, however, is promising something that can't be delivered, and is really not doing anything worthwhile.

JJ: These short-term trips do alleviate suffering in the short-term, though I acknowledge that they are not sufficient. Rather than state that initiatives like this are worthless, however, I would argue that the appropriate perspective is to change the initial approach, so that it includes more and more sustainable goals. We should not throw up our hands and say "It's not possible to accomplish sustainable care now, and therefore it's wrong." We do need to start somewhere, and we do so with small projects at first, while acknowledging that we need to do much more.

Secondly, unless a patient's surgical condition is absolutely emergent, it is ethically problematic to operate knowing that the surgeon will not be present to handle postoperative wound management and complications. Similarly, I would include chronic care medicine in a category of interventions we should generally avoid, if we are not prepared to follow the patient over time. Attempting to treat diseases like HIV or tuberculosis in the international setting without ongoing follow-up over a short amount of time only succeeds in promoting non-compliance and bacterial or viral resistance.

PR: Though I recognize that emergency surgery to save a life is more compelling than elective surgical procedures when follow-up care is not possible, I would argue that those efforts don't truly save lives if the surgeons aren't available to address postop care. I think there is more to surgery than the technical operation. If you are not prepared to address all aspects of being a surgeon, then it seems to me that the kinder intervention would be to give the patient some morphine, and let him or her die gracefully, and quickly. I applaud the idealism, energy, and willingness of young people to make the world a better place, but I think that it has to be done within the perspective of making a lasting contribution. It has been my observation that short-term medical initiatives have little guidance, have little leadership, have few educational components, and provide only transient waves of personal fulfillment. I would prefer to see that energy and idealism expressed as a commitment to a program that will make a permanent difference.

JJ: Sustainability is the crux to the long-term ethical justification of any international medical initiatives. I fear that people who are interested in contributing to these efforts abroad, however, will look at sustainability and say, "You know, we don't have the resources or time to engage in international efforts with this approach." I would like to strike a balance between not belittling those current efforts abroad, albeit transient and superficial, and refocusing the efforts towards sustainable interventions. These goals need not last forever, require long periods of commitment, or vast sums of money. Achievable goals of sustainability might include increasing the frequency of these trips, so that the villagers can be seen on a more frequent basis than once in a lifetime. They might also train local healthcare professionals with skills that they could use beyond the presence of foreign medical assistance. Though these efforts are also superficial and inadequate, they are at least a start in the right direction. There are ways that you can increase the duration of the impact beyond foreign assistance, which is a gesture towards sustainability. It is not by any means sufficient, but these small adjustments in perspective and approach can make a significant difference over time.

RW: Where do you think the ethical burden of engaging in international medical initiatives lies? Does it lie with the people who are organizing it and establishing the operational structure in which the participants operate, or does it lie with the medical professionals on the ground, often young and inexperienced, and sometimes innocently, but sometimes arrogantly assuming they are capable of more than they actually are?

SG: It is both the responsibility of the organization and the provider involved in the medical initiative. Ostensibly, organizations should have prior experience in performing medical initiatives. Consequently, the operational goals and objectives should be clear, and the organization of the initiatives should maximize benefit and minimize harm to all parties involved. On the other hand, individuals who volunteer for this type of experience should be equipped with the knowledge and experience to provide a service that will result in some benefit to the patients each of them treats. Regardless of any individual level of education, all individuals should be aware of this principle.

This discussion highlights a deeper ethical question regarding our case: although, we have residents, we have students, and we have a nurse practitioner, the team has no fully trained physician: is it ever appropriate in any scenario to give care when we don't have all the appropriate training tools? I believe this is only appropriate when there is clearly no other choice.

JJ: This case occurred while I was in medical school, and I thought about the ethical justifiability of my own actions given that we had no trained physician on the medical initiative for some time. I would point out a few facts: First, on this initiative was a trained nurse practitioner who had been working within the community for over 10 years. In the United States, as well as in the international setting, nurse practitioners are often the only possible source of care in rural and underserved areas where there are no other options for acute primary care needs. Secondly, the ethics of international medical initiatives without the physician support also depend on defining the scope of the interventions administered. The traditional position on this issue is encapsulated in the following idea, "Some care is better than no care."

In these settings where the need is great, there is a great deal of pressure not to limit the number of people who can help. At the same time, I would argue that anybody who goes there and does anything in

terms of medical interventions, needs to act within the scope of one's own knowledge and training. A good analogy lies with Good Samaritan laws in the United States that protect individuals from legal repercussions when they act to help someone without personal gain, when they act within their scope of knowledge and training. As a result, emergency physicians should not perform a bowel resection because they lack the training to reasonably expect the patient to receive benefit from the procedure. While I don't think that titles like "nurse" and "physician" are necessarily required, I do think that we have to act with humility and within our own limits of knowledge and training.

PR: I don't have any particular problem with students and residents learning from experienced personnel, be they nurses, paramedics, or other health professionals. I do question the ethical justification of operations that are not well organized, and that fail to provide education or reasonably appropriate care. The medical initiatives that work well are those that have the organization and the sense to say, "these are the goals of this particular mission, this is what we can accomplish." Medical initiatives will provide better care, education, and greater sustainability when they have better organization. This concept ought to apply to residencies and medical schools that permit their trainees and students to join short-term international medical initiatives. Residents are somewhat different, because they are already physicians and frequently licensed, even if they are still training and finishing their residency. Furthermore, they are far more capable of facilitating a reasonable degree of medical practice than their medical student counterparts.

JJ: Right now, there is much disorganization among groups involved in short-term medical initiatives. Our approach to changing the focus from short-sighted, short-term goals toward those goals that prolong medical care beyond the presence of foreign medical assistance is as important as recognizing that what care exists today is inadequate. If we take a sledgehammer and beat medical teams over the head with the idea that sustainability is the only way to perform ethical international medical initiatives, I believe our words will be met with a great deal of resistance, resentment and may result in fewer people attempting to join short-term international medical initiatives.

I think a softer, more respectful approach that acknowledges the good work medical teams engaging in these activities already do, while simultaneously aiming to educate practitioners, students, and residents about how to readjust their focus as to emphasize sustainability and reasonable care, is far more likely to result in change of behaviors.

RW: After my experience in Haiti, I believe a large ethical burden lies with the organizations that support and deploy medical initiatives to austere environments. A set of guidelines or code of ethics might help prevent educated, well-intentioned providers from making questionably ethical healthcare decisions. These organizations rely too heavily upon the volunteer services of the providers already taxed with performing a difficult task. Supporting organizations must be able to define the limits and scope of the interventions and services provided, and must be able to provide oversight to ensure the quality of the care provided.

SG: I agree that any organization whose purpose or goal is to assist impoverished nations has an obligation to have clear and direct objectives and protocols. Some of the resultant objectives or protocols will address ethical concerns and others, medical concerns. The salient point, though, is the need for planning, organization, and forethought.

PR: I feel great sympathy for the discrepancy between what we feel is ideal, and what exists in reality today. I, too, would hate to see the energy and idealism of young medical professionals who undertake these missions go to waste. Though I fear that we may become overly bureaucratized and impede medical initiatives in the future, I also believe that we can prevent cavalier providers from making poor choices in a setting with few to no regulations or oversight. There are good organizations that have accomplished a great deal in many places having faced many challenges. Part of what we haven't done well in our educational programs, however, is to educate people with what they need in order to be effective. Just because you're an emergency trained physician doesn't make you automatically a humanitarian. We frequently don't have the language skills, the diplomatic and political skills, the knowledge of local conditions, and we don't have the security skills to always be able to protect ourselves. It is incumbent upon our

residency programs and medical schools to do all they can to protect our young people, and allow them to use their energy and ideals without putting them in harm's way.

Section III: Review of the literature

In recent decades, interest and participation in global health initiatives has increased dramatically. By 2004, 22.3% of American medical students had completed an international educational experience.[1] By 2008, 47% of accredited MD-granting medical schools had established initiatives, centers, institutes, or offices of global health.[2] Emergency medicine in particular has rapidly expanded as a field of international importance. With over 30 nations now having developed and recognized the specialty, interest in global health research and international collaboration are on the rise.[3–8] The trend toward increased participation and funding of short-term international medical initiatives is not without controversy, however, as some have highlighted the ethical hazards of these initiatives, and questioned whether the risk/benefit ratio is imbalanced in favor of visiting volunteers at the expense of local populations.[9–11] Major ethical concerns include patient vulnerability, barriers to linguistic and cultural understanding, resource allocation in austere conditions, the possibility of harm in the absence of follow-up care, lack of sustainability, and the variable expertise of visiting personnel. Yet the process of developing a practical ethics framework to address these issues is in its infancy.[12] We aim to take these ethical concerns seriously by examining them in the literature and suggesting steps toward resolving them. The ethical integrity of short-term international medical initiatives rests on the principles of bioethics, as well as the cooperation, humility, and nuanced understanding necessary to apply them.

The principles of respect for persons, beneficence, non-maleficence, and justice, serve as the basis for US federal regulations governing the treatment of human subjects, as well as the basis for internationally recognized documents including the Belmont Report, the Declaration of Helsinki, and the Council for International Ethical Guidelines for Biomedical Research Involving Human Subjects. Their force thus extends beyond the context of local delivery of healthcare—they are "a set of moral norms that bind all [morally serious] persons in all places."[13] Some have argued that these principles are profoundly limited in their ability to guide ethical decision-making in concrete situations, particularly in international settings.[14,15] Yet, their aim is not to provide concrete directives, but rather a practical framework facilitating evaluation and discussion. DeCamp notes that the vague quality of ethical principles and benchmarks is actually necessary for proper flexibility in collaborating with local communities.[16] The nuances of how abstract principles apply to different circumstances, and fit into unique cultural understandings, is indeed a source of much debate and an important concern in global health.

Vulnerability

In ethical discussions relating to research, the concept of vulnerability describes populations greatly susceptible to abuse, and imposes the obligation to protect them from ethical misconduct. Many of the same considerations outlined in the Belmont Report with respect to research are also relevant to medical care delivered during short-term international medical initiatives. It states that vulnerable groups such as racial minorities, the economically disadvantaged, the very sick, and the institutionalized are characterized by their availability and their "frequently compromised capacity for free consent."[17] In the case of international medical initiatives, diminished capacity for free consent derives from individuals' lack of alternatives for care, minimal knowledge of medical interventions, and extreme poverty. Pinto notes, "Patients may fear to question the authority of a physician, seek a second opinion or refuse an invasive procedure due to a lack of options or a lack of knowledge about alternatives."[18] Based on these concerns, the notion that local populations' willingness to receive care is an indication of the ethical and medical merits of an initiative is misguided.[18,19] Research in the international setting is subject to review to ensure both the validity of the research, and the ethical integrity of research methods including protections against mistreatment of vulnerable participants.[20] At present, no such mechanism of review and oversight exists for short-term international medical initiatives to ensure ethical practices.

The concept of vulnerability may extend beyond the characteristics of the populations receiving care to the circumstances under which they receive it. In the field of public health, ethical frameworks have suggested that questioning the effectiveness of interventions is essential to ensure their ethical integrity, particularly when working with vulnerable populations. Kass writes, "As a rule of thumb, the greater the burdens posed by a program—for example, in terms of cost, constraints on liberty, or targeting particular, already vulnerable segments of the population—the stronger the evidence must be to demonstrate that the program will achieve its goals."[21] Given the austerity of conditions and resource constraints faced by short-term international medical initiatives, systematically acquired data demonstrating effectiveness is difficult to attain.

Recently, there has been increased attention to the need for such information to support more sophisticated assessment of the costs and benefits to communities.[2,15,16] Because the effectiveness of international initiatives is rarely quantified, negative outcomes and other costs may be invisible, and exceed speculation regarding their frequency and severity. Regulations mandating close monitoring and documentation have mitigated this aspect of vulnerability in international research, but for short-term international medical initiatives it remains a significant ethical concern. In the absence of quantitative data, qualitative interviews, written evaluations, close community partnerships, and follow-up assessments on return visits, have been used to monitor effectiveness and support improvements in care.[10,22,23]

Language and culture

Communication and cultural understanding are central elements of effective delivery of medical care. Even within the United States, communication breakdowns and cultural differences are ubiquitous in clinical settings. Indeed, there are over 46 million people in the United States who do not speak English as their primary language; this population is less likely to receive needed care, is less likely to be compliant with treatment regimens, is at greater risk of suffering medical errors, and has been the subject of recent calls for research to more rigorously understand how language affects care.[24] These considerations are often of greater importance and complexity in international settings, where the potential for linguistic and cultural misunderstanding is high. For example, in Ghana, a common destination of short-term medical initiatives, there are 79 spoken languages in an area approximately the size of Oregon.[25] In recent years there has been increased focus on planning for effective methods of communication before arrival, as well as exploratory visits to establish relationships and share information during the planning stages.[11,22] Cultural and linguistic incompetence creates significant risk for patients as miscommunication or misunderstanding can lead to harm. In addition, linguistic barriers undermine clinicians' ability to communicate the risks and benefits of proposed treatments, making informed consent impossible without an interpreter.[26]

Beyond the basic task of communicating linguistically, demonstrating awareness of a culture's beliefs and practices is a key aspect of beneficence in international settings. Cultural understanding fosters an environment of mutual trust and respect, and may translate to better compliance and greater effectiveness of medical treatment.[27–31] The importance of local perception of the project and its staff underlines the need for conscientious behavior more generally. Crump and Sugarman note how this issue applies to the issue of tourism, stating, "Although taking advantage of tourism opportunities in the host country can be personally rewarding, it can be hugely expensive in local terms, and may take the trainees away from the responsibilities they do have, as well as causing local staff to doubt the seriousness of trainees' commitments . . . and the appropriate use of funds."[2] In addition, they note there is reason to believe that many local concerns along these lines may go unexpressed due to cultural propriety, but are nonetheless corrosive to mutual trust and respect.

Even with skilled translators and culturally aware volunteers, it is impossible to eliminate all potential for misunderstanding, as these challenges are inherent to the delivery of medical care in the international setting. The ethical responsibility of both planners and participants is thus to allay these barriers to ethical care to the greatest extent possible.

Lack of adequate time and resources

Short-term international medical initiatives often take place in austere settings where supplies and resources are scarce. Though generally considered in the context of disaster response and the ED, triage is also an important tool during short-term medical initiatives. In fact, the circumstances of international healthcare often fall under the broad definition of "disaster" as a situation in which needs outpace resources. The principle of justice obligates medical personnel to consider medical utility and probability of success in deciding how to allocate scarce resources. It is therefore ethically necessary for volunteers to arrive with an established system of how to quickly identify patients based on their medical needs and the likelihood that they might benefit from available treatments.[13] Because local populations may have extremely infrequent access to care, arrival of an international medical team can draw enormous crowds with problems of varying acuity.[11] The large number of potential patients compared with the relatively small number of medical personnel means some people who come for treatment are not seen at all.

This difficult reality underlines that a "first come, first served" strategy, though simplest to implement, is unfit to distribute resources ethically. There are many existing approaches to triage, and common among them is the utilitarian aim of doing the most good for the most people. The process of assessing and categorizing patients in this way satisfies the principle of justice, in that clinicians who employ it "treat similar cases similarly and equals equally."[32] Understood in this way, the principle of justice validates the care given even though it may be considered extremely limited compared to capabilities in the more developed world.

Though discussions surrounding triage and resource allocation generally take place in relation to the decisions providers make in the clinical setting, institutions and organizations also play an important role in anticipating the needs of the population and determining the goals that offer the most utility in the given circumstances. Established goals can encourage providers to spend their time and apply resources in service of a collectively agreed upon set of concerns. In recent years there has been greater focus on planning trips not only for the sake of establishing good relationships with the host personnel, but also for the purpose of "clarifying the needs and objectives of host communities and countries . . . to cultivate mutually beneficial partnerships . . . and to collaboratively pursue resolution of identified health challenges."[22] Such partnerships can also ultimately ensure that potential costs to the hosts are minimized, lest the initiative place further stress on already limited local resources.[33]

215

Chronic care and elective surgery

Disparities in medical resources are particularly noticeable and ethically relevant in relation to chronic care and elective surgical procedures. In the setting of a short-term international medical initiative, there are many conditions that visiting providers would treat without hesitation in their own country. Yet, in an austere setting, the lack of long-term continuity of care may shift the risk/benefit ratio in favor of withholding those treatments even if they happen to be available. For example, tuberculosis and HIV infection require complex care and meticulous patient compliance over long periods of time. In situations conducive to poor compliance or only intermittent drug therapy, efforts to treat threaten to produce resistant organisms that endanger not only the individual, but also the greater community.[34,35] Similar concerns apply to performing surgical procedures during a short-term international medical initiative: "You have a moral obligation as a surgeon to ensure that your patients receive appropriate post-operative care. . . . It is unethical to perform complicated reconstructive operations only to have them fall apart because patients do not receive appropriate ongoing attention after you have gone."[36] Given the high probability of complications in suboptimal surgical settings and the discontinuous access to care, elective surgery under these conditions presents particularly high risks of doing harm to patients.[37,38] Even life-saving procedures may be inappropriate given the likelihood of poor outcomes and the commitment of significant resources. Though there is a natural impulse to intervene in an acute situation, particularly when one has the training and equipment necessary, a life-saving procedure with a given likelihood of success in the developed world may have little chance of success in substandard conditions. Providers must adopt a spirit of humility to recognize the potential limits to what they can accomplish in the short term and under the given circumstances. Surgical procedures and chronic care require continuity of treatment that is possible only through larger, more sustainable endeavors.

Sustainability

Historically, the success of short-term international medical initiatives had been measured in terms of the number of people who received treatment.[39] More recently, there has been increasing attention to the disparities in access to care that persist after an initiative has left its host country.[10,16,22,23] As discussed above, the discontinuity of care inherent to the short-term involvement of international medical teams introduces risk to an already vulnerable population and limits the extent of the benefit that can be provided. The principle of beneficence therefore requires that initiatives take steps toward providing sustainable benefit to the communities they aim to serve.

In the interest of sustainability, many have emphasized that the role of volunteers should include teaching and training community members to provide necessary services in the absence of foreign medical assistance.[11,22,23] Training local staff can provide extended benefit even on a small scale and without the use of extensive resources. Initiatives have also adopted teaching local providers as a larger-scale goal to great effect. For instance, Operation Smile, which sponsors short-term surgical missions to treat facial deformities, offers training programs for local surgeons, anesthesiologists, and nurses. This initiative has reduced dependence on foreign volunteers and empowers local healthcare professionals; in 2008–2009, local medical volunteers performed 62% of the program's surgeries, and some initiatives are now entirely staffed by local personnel.[40]

Many have identified cooperation with local communities as essential to improving the sustainability of international initiatives to improve health.[10,22,23] Non-governmental organizations (NGOs) can support these efforts by facilitating integration of short-term initiatives into the community infrastructure. The Children's Health International Medical Project of Seattle (CHIMPS) operates with an NGO to optimize the benefits it provides both when its volunteers are present and after they have left.[10] On a larger, multinational scale, the Ghana Postgraduate Obstetrics/Gynecology program involves collaboration between the American and royal colleges of obstetrics and gynecologists, two Ghanaian medical schools, and the Ghana government in order to improve access to trained obstetricians and gynecologists.[41] Results have been promising with regard to sustainability: as of November 2006, 37 out of 38 specialists who completed the program continued to serve communities in Ghana.[42]

While the above initiatives involve working within the context of a preexisting healthcare infrastructure, recent efforts have aimed at establishing continuous access to care and improved health standards in particularly austere settings. The Shoulder to Shoulder Model emphasizes multiple visits to the same site, extensive community involvement, and attention to public health issues such as water, sanitation, hygiene, and health education. In addition, their personnel reflect the organization's commitment to sustainability. While traditional volunteer efforts have been comprised primarily of medical care providers with the aim of treating existing medical conditions, about a quarter of Shoulder to Shoulder teams are non-medical personnel such as engineers, anthropologists, geographers, administrators, and teachers. This diversity of expertise facilitates broader community engagement to address more distal determinants of health.[23]

Delivery of care by non-licensed or inexperienced personnel

The purpose of medical licensure is to grant an individual authority to practice medicine within a given area, and to protect patients by ensuring that medical personnel are qualified and competent.[43] Though it has been common for decades, the practice of using untrained volunteers and medical trainees to deliver care in the international setting has come under scrutiny in recent years.[11,15,33] International humanitarian volunteers may have various levels of medical education or none at all, and yet they participate in the process of delivering medical care. Moreover, their involvement is often without supervision, oversight, or accountability. Pinto writes, "As in other settings, students must balance their learning needs with the right of the patient to appropriate care. In global health work this can be a serious issue, with vulnerable patients, a lack of oversight, and a low likelihood of negative ramifications for students who abuse their position."[15] The opportunity to be deeply involved in patient care is undoubtedly exciting, and offers significant educational benefit to trainees, but it also introduces significant risk to patients. Though physicians-in-training are often encouraged to challenge the limits of their abilities in the setting of teaching hospitals, this highly conditioned proclivity is inappropriate in the setting of international medical initiatives without the close supervision and guidance of fully-licensed physicians.[38]

The Good Samaritan laws protects only physicians who act as a "reasonable and prudent" person would under the circumstances.[44] Similarly international physicians should therefore attempt only interventions that are within the scope of their training, as even licensed physicians must respect the limits of their expertise according to the principle of non-maleficence.[45,46] The frequently expressed notion that "some care is better than no care" can be factually erroneous and ethically hazardous.[47] Many have argued that austere conditions do not permit lapses in attention to patient safety.[36-38] On the contrary, it is important that interventions be as safe and effective as possible to minimize resource-intensive complications and support favorable outcomes. This ideal requires that both trainees and fully licensed physicians exhibit humility and practice within the scope of their training.

Sponsoring institutions have their own ethical considerations in the process of selecting personnel. To the extent possible, short-term medical initiatives to the developing world should incorporate personnel who are both licensed and trained in the particular skills necessary to deliver the care that is relevant to a community. In the interest of both patient safety and the educational objectives of the initiative, the team should also be capable of supervising and mentoring trainees.[11,14,15] Close partnership between local personnel and sponsoring institutions is imperative to ensure that visiting teams include providers qualified to address the community's specific needs and achieve the goals of the initiative.[16,22,23]

Introducing an additional layer of complexity, the conditions and diseases requiring treatment in developing nations are often rare in European and North American populations. This means that even fully-trained clinicians might not be effective in recognizing and addressing the community's needs if they are not experienced in providing care to that population. For example, millions of women worldwide have a vesicovaginal fistula as a result of prolonged obstructive labor, but this condition is quite rare in developed nations. Wall et al. discuss in detail the reasons that normal surgical training, though extensive, leaves surgeons ill-equipped to correct this type of fistula.[36] The problem extends to diagnosis and medical management as well, since even licensed physicians might be inexperienced in working within the constraints of limited laboratory testing.[2] Pinto and Upshur note, "Medical training in a developed world context does not translate to competence in all settings. Rather one should recognize that being in a different setting puts one at a disadvantage, especially in clinical medicine."[15] Initiatives in the preparatory phase should aim to mitigate these disadvantages by attaining thorough knowledge of the working conditions and selecting and training personnel appropriately.

Conclusion

In recent decades, an increasing number of ambitious, well-intentioned individuals have focused their efforts on service to people in the developing world. The time has come to move beyond good intentions. Though austere conditions and logistical complexity often lead to irreducibly suboptimal care, this does not call for abandonment of the short-term international medical initiative paradigm, nor does it justify an attitude of complacency toward diminished standards. Those who aim to serve the developing world should accept disparities only with reluctant necessity, always working to raise the standard of health that is attainable in a given context. Future work should further explore the potential of cooperative partnerships to establish sustainable access to care and mitigate disparities in the long term. With appropriate attention to the nuances of providing ethical care, short-term international medical initiatives may contribute to the development of self-sustaining, long-term improvements to standards of health in the developing world.

Section IV: Recommendations

• Good intentions do not guarantee the ethical integrity of short-term international medical initiatives. Ethical action requires conscientious planning, organization, and behavior based on the principles of biomedical ethics.
• Initiatives should aim to assess their effectiveness in providing benefits to local populations. In the absence of quantitative data, initiatives ought to monitor their impact by other means, including qualitative interviews, written evaluations, close community partnerships, or follow-up assessments.

• Organizations should establish plans for effective methods of communication before arrival.
• Volunteers should be informed about local beliefs and practices to foster an environment of mutual trust and respect.
• Depending on available resources and infrastructure, interventions requiring significant follow-up care or with poor prospects for success may be inappropriate. Providers should consider whether to provide surgical and medical treatments based on assessment of long-term risks and benefits to individuals and communities.
• All initiatives should undertake activities aimed toward sustainability. This may involve training community members to provide basic services, training local physicians and nurses, or working with communities to address distal determinants of public health.
• To the extent possible, volunteers should be trained and licensed to perform the interventions they undertake in the international setting.
• Teams should be capable of supervising less experienced trainees to support effective education and safe patient care.

References

1. Drain P, Primack A, Hunt D, et al. (2007) Global health in medical education: a call for more training and opportunities. *Acad Med.* 82(3), 226–30.
2. Crump J, Sugarman J. (2008) Ethical considerations of short-term experiences by trainees in global health. *JAMA.* 300(12), 1456–8.
3. Levine C, Becker J, Lippert S, et al. (2008) International emergency medicine: A review of the literature from 2007. *Acad Emerg Med.* 15(9), 860–5.
4. Walker D, Tolentino V, Teach S. (2007) Trends and challenges in international pediatric emergency medicine. *Curr Opin Pediatr.* 19, 247–52.
5. Ban K, Pini R, Sanchez L, et al. (2007) The Tuscan emergency medicine initiative. *Ann Emerg Med.* 50, 726–32.
6. Alagappan K, Schafermeyer R, Holliman J, et al. (2007) International emergency medicine and the role for academic emergency medicine. *Acad Emerg Med.* 14, 451–6.
7. Smith J, Shokoohi H, Holliman J. (2007) The search for common ground: Developing emergency medicine in Iran. *Acad Emerg Med.* 14, 457–62.

8. Koplan J, Baggett R. (2008) The Emory global health institute: Developing partnerships to improve health through research, training, and service. *Acad Med.* 83(2), 128–33.

9. Montgomery LM. (1993) Short-term medical missions: Enhancing or eroding health? *Missiology Int Rev.* 21(3), 333–41.

10. Suchdev P, Ahrens K, Click E, et al. (2007) A model for sustainable short-term international medical trips. *Ambul Pediatr.* 7(4), 317–20.

11. Jesus JE. (2010) Ethical challenges and considerations of short-term international medical initiatives: an excursion to Ghana as a case study. *Ann Emerg Med.* 55(1), 17–22.

12. DeCamp M. (2007) Scrutinizing global short-term medical outreach. *Hastings Cent Rep.* 37(6), 21–3.

13. Beauchamp T, Childress J. (2009) *Principles of Biomedical Ethics*, 6th ed. New York, NY: Oxford University Press.

14. Takala T. (2001) What is wrong with global bioethics? On the limitations of the four principles approach. *Camb Q Healthc Ethics.* 10, 72–7.

15. Pinto A, Upshur R. (2009) Global health ethics for students. *Dev World Bioeth.* 9(1), 1–10.

16. DeCamp M. (2011) Ethical review of global short-term medical volunteerism. *HEC Forum.* 23, 91–103.

17. US National Commission for the Protection of Human Subjects of Biomedical and Behavioral Research. (1979) *The Belmont Report: Ethical Guidelines for the Protection of Human Subjects of Research.* Publication No. (OS) 78–0012. Washington, DC: US Government Printing Office.

18. Orton D. (2010) Is third world health care different? *Ann Emerg Med.* 56(3), 308.

19. Jesus JE. (2010) In reply. *Ann Emerg Med.* 56(3), 308–9.

20. Basic HHS Policy for Protection of Human Research Subjects, 45 C.F.R. §46.101 (2009).

21. Kass N. (2001) An ethics framework for public health. *Am J Public Health.* 91, 1776–82.

22. Powell D, Gilliss C, Hewitt H, et al. (2010) Application of a partnership model for transformative and sustainable international development. *Public Health Nurs.* 27(1), 54–70.

23. Heck J, Bazemore A, Diller P. (2007) The shoulder to shoulder model—channeling medical volunteerism toward sustainable health change. *Fam Med.* 39(9), 644–50.

24. Jacobs E, Chen A, Karliner L, et al. (2006) The need for more research on language barriers in health care: A proposed research agenda. *Milbank Q.* 84(1), 111–33.

25. Gordon R. (2005) Languages of Ghana. In: *Ethnologue: Languages of the World*, 15th ed. Dallas, TX: SIL International. Available at: www.ethnologue.com/. Accessed September 10, 2008.

26. Padela A, Imran R, Punekar B. (2009) Emergency medical practice: Advancing cultural competence and reducing health care disparities. *Acad Emerg Med.* 16, 69–75.

27. Arras J. (1990) Noncompliance in AIDS Research. *Hastings Cent Rep.* 20(5), 24–32.

28. Nguyen G, LaVeist TA, Harris ML, et al. (2009) Patient trust-in-physician and race are predictors of adherence to medical management in inflammatory bowel disease. *Inflamm Bowel Dis.* 15, 1233–9.

29. Crigger N, Holcomb L. (2007) Practical strategies for providing culturally sensitive, ethical care in developing nations. *J Transcult Nurs.* 18(1), 70–6.

30. Rentmeester CA. (2008) Case study. Trust, translation and HAART [commentary]. *Hastings Cent Rep.* 38(6), 13–14.

31. Miller J, Leininger M, Leuning C, et al. (2008) Transcultural nursing society position statement on human rights. *J Transcult Nurs.* 19(1), 5–7.

32. Childress J. (2003) Triage in response to bioterrorist attack. In: Moreno J. (ed.) *In the Wake of Terror: Medicine and Morality in a Time of Crisis.* Cambridge: MIT Press, pp. 72–93.

33. Crump J, Sugarman J, Working Group on Ethics Guidelines for Global Health Training (WEIGHT). (2010) Global health training: Ethics and best practice guidelines for training experiences in global health. *Am J Trop Med Hyg.* 83(6), 1178–82.

34. Blumberg H, Burman W, Chaisson R, et al. (2003) American Thoracic Society/Centers for Disease Control and Prevention/Infectious Diseases Society of America: Treatment of Tuberculosis. *Am J Respir Crit Care Med* 167, 603–620.

35. Shin S, Furin J, Bayona J, et al. (2004) Community-based treatment of multidrug-resistant tuberculosis in Lima, Peru: 7 years of experience. *Soc Sci Med* 59, 1529–1539.

36. Wall L, Arrowsmith S, Lassey A, et al. (2006) Humanitarian ventures or "fistula tourism?" The ethical perils of pelvic surgery in the developing world. *Int Urogynecol J Pelvic Floor Dysfunct.* 17(6), 559–62.

37. Raja AJ, Levin AV. (2003) Challenges of teaching surgery: ethical framework. *World J Surg.* 27(8), 948–51.

38. Ramsey K, Weijer C. (2007) Ethics of surgical training in developing countries. *World J Surg.* 31, 2067–9.

39. Dupuis C. (2004) Humanitarian missions in the third world: A polite dissent. *Plast Reconstr Surg.* 113, 433–5.

40. Ott B, Olsen R. (2011) Ethical issues of medical missions: The clinicians' view. *HEC Forum.* 23, 105–13.

41. Klufio C, Kwawukume E, Danso K, et al. (2003) Ghana postgraduate obstetrics/gynecology collaborative residency training program: Success story and model for Africa. *Am J Obstet Gynecol.* 189, 692–6.

42. Anderson F, Mutchnick I, Kwawukume E, et al. (2007) Who will be there when women deliver? Assuring retention of obstetric providers. *Obstet Gynecol.* 110, 1012–16.

43. Federation of State Medical Boards. (2008) *State of the States: Physician Regulation.* Dallas, TX: Federation of State Medical Boards. Available at: www.fsmb.org/pdf/States_2008.pdf. Accessed April 21, 2008.

44. American Medical Association. (2008) *Good Samaritan, Charitable Care Statutes, and Specific Provisions Related to Disaster Relief Efforts.* Chicago, IL: American Medical Association. Available at: www.ama-assn.org/ama1/pub/upload/mm-/395/goodsamaritansurvey_rev20082708.pdf. Accessed July 13, 2011.

45. Bernstein M. (2004) Ethical dilemmas encountered while operating and teaching in a developing country. *Can J Surg.* 47(3), 170–2.

46. Ramsey K. (2008) International surgical electives: Reflections in ethics. *Arch Surg.* 143(1), 10–11.

47. Leow J, Kingham TP, Casey K, et al. (2010) Global surgery: Thoughts on an emerging surgical subspecialty for students and residents. *J Surg Educ.* 67, 143–8.

21

Disaster triage

Matthew B. Allen,[1] *John Jesus*[2]

[1]*Research Assistant, Department of Emergency Medicine, Brigham and Women's Hospital, Boston, MA, USA*
[2]*Chief Resident, Department of Emergency Medicine, Beth Israel Deaconess Medical Center, Boston, MA, and Clinical Instructor, Department of Emergency Medicine, Christiana Care Health System, Newark, DE, USA*

Section I: Case presentation

An earthquake in a moderately developed country destroyed a city of 400 000 people, with no functional hospitals left standing. The closest intensive care unit (ICU) is 300 km away over mostly destroyed roads. Air evacuation is not yet available (48 hours after the event). Most medical staff in the city are dead, injured, or have relocated with their families. There are two foreign military field hospitals in the city, with others expected to arrive in the coming days.

A 22-year-old man is rescued after 46 hours under debris. His 3-year-old daughter is found alive and well, but his wife and mother are dead, and no known relatives are found. He exhibits a moderate crush injury of the lower limbs, with extensive degloving of both legs. The initial examination shows a pale, slightly confused, tachypneic (24 breaths per minute) man with a blood pressure 100/70 mmHg, and a heart rate 110 beats per minute with a regular rhythm. The man is taken by stretcher to the nearby field hospital emergency department (ED) where an arterial blood gas on room air shows PO_2 72 mmHg, PCO_2 28 mmHg, pH 7.28, base excess −8, hematocrit 48%, Na^+ 134 mEq/L, and K^+ 6.1 mEq/L.

The available options are to stabilize the patient and evacuate him to a distant hospital ICU when (and if) feasible; admit the patient to a field hospital ICU, and provide unlimited, unconditional, best available care; admit the patient locally, but provide only limited or conditional care; do not admit the patient to a field hospital, but rather transfer the patient to a local care facility if and when it becomes available; and finally do not admit the patient to a field hospital, and discharge the patient to a refugee camp or the street with very limited comfort care only.

The patient was finally admitted to the field hospital's ICU with an a priori decision documented in the chart, and conveyed to the patient and to the staff, that he would be given 2–3 days of maximal therapy. If his condition worsened he would not be intubated. No renal replacement therapy was available, and therefore it wouldn't be offered.

Section II: Discussion

Dr. Peter Rosen: Is there a difference in the ethical philosophy with which patients are managed in disaster situations? I read a paper recently from Italy that suggests that Hippocratic ethics don't apply in disaster situations because we ignore the advice to do our utmost for individual patients. Do you believe that we cannot afford the "luxury" of Hippocratic ethics in a disaster setting?

Ethical Problems in Emergency Medicine: A Discussion-Based Review, First Edition. John Jesus, Shamai A. Grossman, Arthur R. Derse, James G. Adams, Richard Wolfe, and Peter Rosen.
© 2012 John Wiley & Sons, Ltd. Published 2012 by John Wiley & Sons, Ltd.

Dr. Pinchas Halperin: If Hippocratic ethics calls on us to do our utmost for every patient, and do so with unlimited regard for cost, consequences, and who else is also in need of care at the same time, then yes, I believe we cannot afford the luxury of Hippocratic ethics. There is no question that the ethics of individual patient management in disasters are different, and that we are deluding ourselves if we don't accept that truth.

PR: Do you believe that Hippocratic ethics mandates a degree of care for individual patients that would result in suboptimal care for other patients? In other words, if a physician acts without acknowledging the need to ration resources in lieu of maximally treating one single patient, are the principles and spirit of Hippocratic ethics being followed?

Dr. James Adams: Aristotle's virtue suggests the importance of justice or fairness across all patients. Hippocrates didn't talk about that as much as Aristotle and other philosophers, but the concept of justice requires us to talk about allocation of resources. Hippocrates is concerned with doing the best for the patient in front of us, but doesn't speak to the management of multiple patients with scarce resources. Hippocratic ethics gets overwhelmed in the setting of a disaster, and therefore we need a different model by which to operate.

PR: The reality is that even when we are working under Hippocratic ethics, there is no institution that has infinite resources, and there are many situations in every-day emergency medicine where the kind of care that you render will vary depending on resource availability. For example if you are practicing emergency medicine in a community that has no cardiac catheterization laboratory, you can't offer the same services that you can in an urban environment where there may be multiple hospitals that may have immediate percutaneous angioplasty capability. Do you think we need a modification of Hippocratic ethics for these situations as well as for disaster situations?

Dr. Shamai Grossman: In the practice of medicine we practice to the best of our abilities, though the best of our ability will always be dependent on the resources we have available. If we think that we have maximal resources and a maximal amount of time to utilize them, then we should wake up from our pleas-

ant dream, as that situation does not exist. Wherever we find ourselves, no matter what we do, we're obligated to take the best possible care of our patients. The best possible care of our patients is determined by the circumstances in which we find ourselves, which may or may not change from one moment to the next. The basic principles and obligations are the same: resources change, ethics do not.

PH: I would like to present the micro versus macro perspectives of the situation, if you will. The case presented was an actual case I was called to evaluate in Turkey. I ran a highly sophisticated ICU that we brought with us in the midst of total destruction. Within the field hospital, we could take care of this patient. However, outside of the hospital there was nothing. If we were to send this patient outside the ICU, he would have been dead by the next day. We were then faced with a difficult decision: Do you make use of the resources you have because you have them, or do you also look at how you manage resources based on where the patient comes from and where he will return? I have heard that this was a significant issue for colleagues who went to Haiti. They had fairly good resources within their medical facility, but their patients had few or no medical resources before or after visiting their facility.

PR: Moreover, your team did not have infinite resources within their facility. One has to make a judgment about which patient should even be triaged into the facility in the first place.

PH: I purposefully mentioned that the patient had a 3-year-old child. One could argue that in the setting of a devastating natural disaster, triage decisions regarding the father have a direct effect on two persons. If the father dies, the baby will likely die within a few days as well, as there will be no one to care for the child. Should this affect one's decision-making? Should the father "count" as two lives? I'm not sure I know, but the variables are complicated and not easily discounted.

PR: That introduces the concept of whether utilitarian philosophy is to be utilized to judge the number of patients and relatives who benefit from the care provided. A simpler decision however, has to be made with what are you doing to your resources when you use them for a patient who has a lower probability of surviving than perhaps 20 other patients who are less injured. This situation is similar to battlefield triage considerations, where the goal of treatment is not to address the health needs of the most wounded casualty, but rather to treat the less wounded casualties in as rapid a fashion as possible in order to restore them to battle condition.

JA: At the time of a disaster, it is critically important to assess the quality of your information about current and future needs. An important question to consider is, "What casualties are yet ahead?" We would hate to underutilize our resources and allow a salvageable patient to die, only to later realize that we had the necessary resources if we had known the anticipated would never arrive. Yet, information can also be incomplete. We knew, for example, in this case that the 3-year-old would be orphaned, but for many patients we wouldn't know the future implications of their death. We may believe we have adequate understanding of the situation in hindsight, but may frequently make mistakes in the chaos of a disaster situation. It is easy to criticize decisions with the benefit of hindsight, but prospectively it is very hard to know, very hard and difficult to put in place ground rules or an obvious clear course of action.

PR: Petrini has suggested that one of the newer ethical theories in European medical ethics is the concept that we as individuals owe something to the community as part of what he calls solidarity.[1] He explains that we might accept a lower level of care on the basis that we are doing something good for someone else. I find this an interesting idea, which I hope would be true, but I have a hard time conceiving of it being realistic in terms of people who were being asked to accept less care for the benefit of strangers or those whom they dislike.

PH: The cost of solidarity is unacceptable. Consider having five people with certain skills that may be necessary to save many lives. For example, caring for people who can operate water systems is very important, as it will save thousands down the line. From a utilitarian approach it makes sense to care for them before others. Taking care of people based on considerations other than utilitarianism, represents a slippery slope at the bottom of which lies unethical decisions based on arbitrary needs of solidarity, for

example, rather than on decisions that actually save lives.

Do we need to produce a theoretical construct, or do we, in fact, need to produce site-specific, time-specific principles to guide caregivers, in order to ensure that everybody is applying the same principles to their work rather than applying personal and cultural values?

SG: I would argue that any utilitarian approach can lead one down a slippery slope. Who decides who is more valuable to the population? Is utilitarianism ever an appropriate triage tool? This begs the question once more: Do disaster ethics require a different ethics? I would again argue that they should not.

JA: There has been a huge amount of discussion about allocation decisions. We're prone to human emotion and bias, but everybody knows that allocation decisions frequently break down at the bedside, and that human sympathies win out. This issue will need to be addressed for a coordinated consistent disaster response. Carrying out rationing at the bedside is enormously difficult for us, because we're accultured into a Hippocratic philosophy and ethic. Those rationing decisions are morally hazardous as well. I'm not sure how to make this work, but in planning for this sort of situation, the first thing we can ask for is awareness on the part of the caregiver.

PH: If you were the commanding officer of the unit, having just landed in Haiti or in Pakistan with a limited amount of blood sufficient for 50 operations, should you instruct your staff to use only a certain number of units on any one patient though not using more may mean their death? In other words, should you preserve this valuable resource for 10 other patients?

JA: That is exactly what you have to do. Preexisting rules have to be put into place to decrease the phenomenon of deciding at the bedside how to allocate resources.

PH: I don't think it's fair or appropriate to leave such a decision to a caregiver who is personally involved in the management of any individual patient. Because some emotional attachment is inevitable, it behooves the disaster commander (or appointed representative with authority) to make these decisions a priori. At the very least, the disaster commander is able to have a detached perspective, and can prevent decisions from occurring that are based upon irrational thought processes.

PR: These decisions can't be left to the physician on the scene, but rather must happen in advance through an organized group structure. This is not only because it will ensure greater rationality of allocation decisions, but also because it will spare physicians the emotional burden of making such determinations on their own in the setting of caring for individual patients.

Dr. John Jesus: Though I agree with the importance of preestablished protocols and guidelines prior to arrival to a disaster scene, I would also raise a note of caution regarding implementation of a pure utilitarian approach. Attempting to produce the greatest net benefit can lead to negative consequences for some that may not be ethically justifiable.

In addition, one key difference between triage in disaster areas and triage in modern EDs is that in the ED, we try to address the most urgent medical needs. Though patients will often wait for several hours to see a physician, eventually all the patients needs will be met. Disaster triage, on the other hand, purposefully excludes the medical needs of those patients who cannot be saved with available resources. These patients are triaged as expectant, and resources will be directed elsewhere. This can be a severely stressful situation for clinicians triaging disaster victims, and I would like to emphasize the importance of emotional preparation prior to arrival.

PH: I propose a different method of approaching disaster response. Within this approach, we must make a two-step decision regarding the rationing of resources. The first decision is whether a certain person is let into the medical facility at all. This decision is made quickly, over a few seconds to minutes. Once the person is allowed to enter the medical facility, a second triage decision is necessary. For example, we need to decide how much blood we're going to give them if they go on bleeding, or how much of a certain medication that is in short supply. This decision, on the other hand, is made much more deliberately.

PR: It's useful to get into the mindset that ideal care is not necessary for survival. Patients will survive and receive some benefit from an adjusted standard of care that becomes necessary within the situational stress of a disaster. The reality in disaster situations like the one in Haiti is that efficient amputations that require little resources will still have a significant impact on the lives of patients in a country unable to provide ongoing care and resources for handicapped persons. Survival is unlikely for a bilateral lower extremity amputee. As a result, I believe physicians need emotional preparation not only for the sake of being more efficient and humane in a disaster situation, but also for the sake of their own emotional wellbeing. Having a method of debriefing avoids buildup of resentment and bitterness towards the situation and one's colleagues.

PH: Another issue of importance is that the participants in disaster response are often young and inexperienced. While their intentions are to assist in the response, their participation leans more heavily toward gaining experience rather than on the benefits of the services they are able to provide. Though I would argue that it is essential to educate these inexperienced personnel about the principles of disaster response and ethics, it infrequently occurs.

PR: Ideally, appropriate preparation for disaster response would include the formulation of teams that would pair inexperienced team members with those with greater skills and expertise. This would allow for the opportunity for idealistic young physicians and nurses to participate and gain valuable experience in the care administered, an important intervention for future disaster responses. This ideal situation cannot happen, however, without prior preparation and without a proper command structure. Everybody who has ever been involved in a disaster can remember the absolute chaos that occurs when there is no disaster team in charge. Such efforts are well intentioned but uncoordinated, and frequently result in counterproductivity.

PR: Is there a way to educate disaster victims about the fact that ideal circumstances are impossible, and that a different perspective on medical practice is necessary to respond effectively? As you probably noticed during Haiti, not only were people criticized for arriving unprepared, but they were immediately criticized for the type of care they were able to administer. This may not have occurred inside Haiti, but it was certainly true in the international press.

PH: I have never encountered a situation during which disaster victims ever complained about the care they received, or demanded a higher standard of care. More often than not, disasters in need of an international response occur in poorer countries, where the victims are not intimately aware that they are receiving a standard of care different from what physicians would ordinarily be able to provide in their countries or anywhere else for that matter.

JA: Unfortunately, criticism is to be expected. When I was in the military and we were deployed, the first rule upon arrival was that somebody had to dig the latrines. The second rule was to set up the tents and send one-third of your personnel to sleep, because somebody has to be available at night and next day. Everyone wants to get on the ground and immediately engage in the disaster, but we have to think about the bigger perspective. That said, when a desperate population observes disaster response personnel going to set up the food and digging latrines, I can understand if they think, "Why aren't they helping?" I'm not sure that there's any way to participate in disaster response without facing criticism. Furthermore, you have to do the right thing despite possible criticism.

PH: Strict adherence to those principles, however, can be taken to an extreme. There are times when sending one-third of your team to eat and sleep is clearly the correct course of action. There are other situations when the team ought to postpone their rest and meals for a few hours even though that approach doesn't follow strict disaster response teaching. When we traveled to Turkey for a disaster response mission, for example, we were operational 48 hours before a couple of other teams mainly because they adhered to the rules of disaster response—some degree of flexibility is important.

JJ: Public perception of disaster response is important to continue the flow of supplies and support for aid initiatives. Also, medical professionals tend to favor triage principles that maximize the number of lives saved, whereas the public generally favors the approach that gives priority to the sickest patients, which is not appropriate in a disaster scenario. It strikes me as relevant and advantageous to proactively publicize the basis of disaster triage and resource allocation principles in operation. The goal of such transparency is to justify any departure from public preference, and help assuage public criticism.[2]

PR: It is important to have a public relations area set up, and to have administrators deal with the media so that medical professionals can focus on delivering care. Such an approach helps control the flow of information.

PH: In addition to setting up a public relations team, it is equally important to educate our press colleagues ahead of time and make them part of your team. Giving them a background understanding of disaster triage will contextualize any deviation from the standard of care provided in modern healthcare facilities. In my experience, integrating the press has been useful in gaining support for our initiatives.

PR: Yet another issue that comes up frequently in disaster situations is the flow of patients whose medical problems are unrelated to the disaster. Many non-disaster patients, however, may have greater acuity than many disaster victims. How should non-disaster patients be prioritized? Should disaster-related medical problems take precedence?

PH: The distinction you are referring to is typically described as "disaster-related" and "routine" care. True of most disaster scenarios, however, is the loss of operational local medical infrastructure. As a result, disaster-related injuries or patients with routine care needs are all victims of the disaster. The patient suffering from ketoacidosis because of a loss of insulin supplies, for example, should not be placed in a separate category from the person with a crushed leg from falling concrete blocks. In fact, after the first few days of disaster response, medical teams on the ground are primarily concerned with replacing the work of the local medical infrastructure and taking care of "routine cases" because people have nowhere else to go. I see no ethical difference, and certainly no basis for allocating resources based on such a distinction.

PR: Do you feel disaster ethics is still a topic of concern in medical ethics, or do you feel that the series of disasters that have occurred over a short time span have demonstrated that we have a good handle on these issues?

JA: This is still a big problem. We saw in the response to Hurricane Katrina that clinicians working in hospitals with limited resources had very difficult choices to make, and they had to make them on their own. Situations like these highlight the importance of preplanning and consideration of possible scenarios and the appropriate actions that accompany them.

PH: It is certainly important to have prepared, clear-cut definitions of what principles should be utilized in particular situations. Without training, individual clinicians will be left to make their own decisions without considering important variables or weighing the potential consequences appropriately.

PR: You cannot manage a disaster with individual effort. It requires a well-trained team with an effective command structure in order to efficiently achieve disaster response objectives.

Section III: Review of the literature

Triage is a central strategy of disaster relief efforts, yet recent events suggest the task of establishing priorities and planning for difficult decisions remains underdeveloped.[3] Disaster triage is an uncomfortable topic within contemporary bioethics and disaster management, introducing complexities that push the limits of accepted ethical ideals. The Hippocratic Oath and traditional principles of clinical bioethics have been notably difficult to apply to triage in disaster scenarios.[4] Establishing priorities when needs exceed resources requires thoughtful consideration of the motivations underlying disaster relief efforts. Insofar as it unfolds within the irrational contingency of destruction and suffering, triage is inherently tragic.[5] All systems and ethical frameworks of triage are therefore subject to criticism and debate that are frequently based on concerns of the competing philosophies of utilitarianism and egalitarianism.[6] We aim to clarify these positions and examine their influence on contemporary ethical discussions surrounding disaster triage. Disaster relief takes place at the intersection of clinical care, public health, disaster management, and humanitarian relief, and ethical frameworks for understanding disaster triage reflect this uniquely simultaneous commitment to the interests of individuals and populations.[1,7] Discussion of the principles for resource allocation therefore extends beyond the decision-making of individual clinicians and leads to an understanding of triage as a large-scale system of priorities aimed at achieving particular ethical ideals.[8,9] Exploring the difficult ethical issues surrounding disaster triage will hopefully serve as a

basis for broader discussion and understanding of relevant societal values. The ethical content of disaster relief strategies is not for ethicists alone to decide, as it must reflect the values of the people it aims to serve.

Triage: origins and concepts

Origins of triage

The earliest known use of triage was during the Napoleonic Wars, when the French military surgeon Baron Dominique-Jean Larrey instituted a system of identifying and treating the soldiers whose needs were most urgent. In reflecting on the Russian campaign, he summarized his approach: "Those who are dangerously wounded should receive the first attention, without regard to rank or distinction. They who are injured in a less degree may wait until their brethren in arms, who are badly mutilated, have been operated on and dressed, otherwise the latter would not survive many hours; rarely, until the succeeding day."[10] Early British systems of triage, on the other hand, aimed to optimize overall outcomes with maximum efficiency.[4] These conceptions of triage reflected the sensibilities of their respective historical and cultural contexts. Larrey's egalitarian approach emerged in the years following the French Revolution, echoing its motto, "Liberty, equality, fraternity!"[6] The British focus on efficient pursuit of the greatest overall benefit appears to have been similarly conditioned by contemporary intellectual trends; it embodied the principle of utility articulated by Jeremy Bentham and developed by John Stuart Mill.[11] Triage therefore appeared not as a unified and coherent set of principles, but rather as a general strategy whose conceptual content was subject to the influence of societal norms and values.

Egalitarianism

The concept of egalitarianism resonates with the tradition of political liberalism, and is based on the conception of the self as a free and self-determining entity. According to egalitarian lines of thought, the self is capable of setting ends for itself and thus distinguishing itself from other individuals. This capacity for self-determination is the basis of individuals' equal standings in society and is an important aspect of liberal political theory and practice. Hartman notes, "This concept of social equality is a cornerstone of American law for promoting fairness in judgment about classification of similarly situated persons, and for reducing arbitrariness in the exercise of that judgment."[12] Affirmations of basic equality also rest on Aristotle's principle of formal justice, "treat like cases as like," and inform the principle of justice in contemporary biomedical ethics.[13,14] The Ethics Committee of the Society of Academic Emergency Medicine identifies justice as a virtue fundamental to the practice of emergency medicine: "[Justice] is required to ensure that medical decisions are made with reason and honesty . . . EPs [emergency physicians], confronted by medical and management decisions, must ensure fairness and consistency in patient care."[15] In general, egalitarian conceptions of triage involve commitment to helping those patients whose conditions are most critical, even if this strategy limits potential benefit to other patients.[6,11]

Utilitarianism

Utilitarian determinations of the good are based on the aggregate happiness of a population within a given scope of concern. A population is made up of persons, which utilitarianism conceptualizes as "sites of utility where activities such as having pleasure or pain, happiness, and desire-fulfillment take place."[16] Bentham and Mill therefore understand subjective experiences as largely irrelevant so long as the overall distribution of happiness is favorable. Mill is explicit about this hierarchy, stating, "I must again repeat what the assailants of utilitarianism seldom have the justice to acknowledge, that the happiness which forms the utilitarian standard of what is right in conduct is not the agent's own happiness but that of all concerned."[17] Based on these priorities, many consider utilitarianism the most straightforward ethical justification for the practice of triage. Indeed, triage is frequently characterized as an attempt to "do the most good for the most people."[2,18] From a utilitarian perspective, the practice of prioritizing patients is thought to be valid because it produces the greatest overall benefit through efficient allocation of resources. Utilitarianism's attention to populations rather than individuals has led many to affirm its principles as central to the field of public health.[19–21] It is important to note, however, that the magnitude of the aggregate benefit is independent of its distribution within a population; the scope of concern may include the concerns of many but actual benefits could be restricted to a few. The characterization of utilitarianism as "doing the most good for the most people" is therefore deeply misleading because it implies that sharing benefits between many individuals has intrinsic utility or value. Because priority lies with the summation of positive and negative outcomes, triage by utilitarian values may dictate that some individuals suffer avoidable morbidity or mortality if these sacrifices appear necessary to achieve the optimal outcome overall.[2]

Triage and the concept of disaster

The American College of Emergency Physicians offers the following definition of disaster: "A medical disaster occurs when the destructive elements of natural or man-made forces overwhelm the ability of a given area or community to meet the demand for health care."[22] A disaster is therefore a situation in which the need for care exceeds available resources. The word "resources" refers not only to supplies of medications and equipment, but also to facilities, mechanisms of transport, and personnel.[8] These definitions allow significant flexibility in applying the concept of disaster to diverse contexts and conditions. The discussion surrounding disaster triage employs primarily an "all-hazards" approach rather than attempting to address specific conditions arising from particular types of precipitating events such as explosions, earthquakes, or hurricanes. Many aspects of the debate apply most directly to large-scale mass casualty incidents in which the gap between resources and need is most significant.[8,23,24] Because disasters undermine the healthcare infrastructure's ability to satisfy societal needs either through destruction of health-related resources or increasing the demand for care, all disasters necessitate some form of triage regardless of the precipitating event. Even brief, self-limited events that do not damage community infrastructure necessitate triage due to subsequent surges in patient flow.[24] Larkin and Arnold note that responsible stewardship of resources is a strong ethical obligation, and the World Medical Association provides the following admonition: "Triage must be carried out systematically, taking into account the medical needs, medical intervention capabilities and available resources."[25,26]

The variables that bear on triage are heavily dependent on the nature of the disaster. Damage to vital infrastructure can lead to significant need for medical care in the days and weeks following the onset of an event. Such circumstances may therefore precipitate public health emergencies requiring attention not only to concerns of individual patients, but also to interests of the community.[1] Disaster relief efforts in large-scale events are thus characterized by two objectives: providing care to individuals, and attending to the wellbeing of the affected population through conscientious resource allocation.[1,4,6,7,11] Though these concerns clearly overlap and stem from the ethical principle of beneficence, they are nonetheless distinct with regard to their guiding principles and judgments.

To highlight this distinction, many have articulated the inability of the Hippocratic Oath to identify a physician's duties in a disaster scenario.[1,4,5,27] Veatch states, "All disaster triage is a violation of the Hippocratic Oath."[4] As interpreted in modern medical ethics, the Hippocratic Oath describes a physician's duty to promote the wellbeing of the patient. In fact, this is not simply one duty among others—it is the physician's **sole** duty. This duty to patients is sometimes referred to as "fidelity," and it fosters patients' trust and confidence in their physicians.[11,14] Moskop argues that because it compels physicians to provide or withhold treatment based on established criteria, triage of any form threatens the formation of relationships of trust between doctor and patient. In addition, changing disaster conditions may require shifting of priorities and resources in the midst of care. When performed in service of the principle of utility to the detriment of an individual patient, such changes in care are in violation of a physician's duty as interpreted in the Hippocratic Oath and expressed in the tradition of egalitarianism.[4] The duality of a physician's role in disaster scenarios demonstrates underlying tension between the utilitarian aim to alleviate the suffering of a population, and the egalitarian conception of individuals as ends in themselves.

This conflict is also readily apparent in the differences between "everyday triage" in hospital settings and disaster triage. In the former, it is usually possible to meet all patients' needs. Everyday triage in the hospital setting determines the order in which patients will receive treatment, but does not typically limit their access to care.[28] The implications of disaster triage are more profound in that they often dictate which individuals will not receive any care. Several thinkers note that discussions regarding the ethical foundations of triage are frequently based on triage in a hospital setting, where access to resources supports respect and attention to the needs of individual patients.[1,29] Petrini therefore raises an important concern regarding the limitations of utilitarianism: "A utilitarian approach may not be a fully adequate framework for planning and executing disaster responses because the history and practice of triage also incurs an egalitarian ethics that focuses on assisting those in greatest need: that is, on the needs of particular individuals."[1] There has been significant attention to the tensions between public health and individual rights, and many have identified a need for balance between considerations of patients and communities.[30-33] The duality explored here reveals that the widespread notion of triage as intrinsically utilitarian is a significant oversimplification.[6] In addition, the tensions that emerge for the physician in a disaster scenario indicate that both utilitarian and egalitarian lines of thinking offer compelling principles relevant to disaster triage.

Many have recognized that uncompromising commitment to either extreme is problematic, and that most ethicists employ a mixture of principles in analyzing triage.[1,6,33,34] In his work *Triage and Justice*, Winslow applies Rawls' political philosophy to the ethics of triage in an effort to achieve proper balance between egalitarian and utilitarian principles.[33,35] Rawls articulates a theory of justice resting on principles of fairness in the distribution of social goods. He does not advocate strict equality, but nonetheless affirms that individuals have equal rights to certain liberties and opportunities in society.[36] Even a cursory glance at Rawls' work reveals a deep-seated interest in balancing concern for individuals' experience and the wellbeing of communities. Central to his theory is the idea that social, political, and economic goods should be distributed so as to optimize benefits to society's most disadvantaged individuals. This "difference principle" has been used to provide ethical justification for approaches to triage that blend utilitarian and egalitarian ideals.[6,11,33] An alternative approach to focusing attention on the most vulnerable members of society is the concept of solidarity, which is based on "a feeling of togetherness that implies a commitment to the most disadvantaged."[6] Though it appears similar to the Rawlsian understanding of distributive justice in sentiment, it is relatively vague and less developed as a set of principles capable of motivating policy and allocation decisions.

Application of Rawlsian political philosophy to matters of healthcare has been the subject of significant debate and further discussion.[33,35,37,38] One source of criticism is Rawls' own claim that his philosophy addresses questions of macroallocation of societal goods. The traditional understanding of triage and medical resource allocation is one of small-scale decision-making unfolding at the level of individuals.[35] This view is inconsistent with many contemporary understandings of triage as a key aspect of public policy that extends from microallocation to broader considerations on the societal level.[1,8,23] The difference principle can therefore be coherently applied to assess appropriateness of triage strategies on the level of government policy and institutional guidelines, particularly in large-scale disaster events.

To apply the difference principle, one must define the worst possible outcome within a given set of possibilities. Winslow argues that rational agents would agree that in considering how to distribute finite medical resources, the worst possible outcome for an individual is death. Strategies of triage and resource allocation should therefore address the needs of those who are at greatest risk for mortality, but who also have a reasonable chance of benefiting from available treatments.[33] This notion of triage resonates with the ideals of the Sphere project, which aims to establish standards for disaster relief. It maintains that the primary motivation of disaster relief efforts is "to alleviate human suffering amongst those least able to withstand the stress caused by disaster."[39] Applying these principles requires understanding of the ethical dimension of variables shaping a disaster scenario.

Ethical considerations of disaster triage

Urgency and narratives of care

Disaster triage operates based on urgency of need. Assessments of need direct caregivers to withhold resources from those with trivial medical complaints as well as those who have little chance of benefiting from available care.[11,26,40] The refusal to care for those without reasonable hope of recovery is widely accepted as ethically necessary in disaster scenarios. The World Medical Association notes, "It is unethical for a physician to persist, at all costs, at maintaining the life of a patient beyond hope, thereby wasting to no avail scarce resources needed elsewhere."[26] Triage algorithms such as the simple triage and rapid treat-

ment system, or "START" are designed to support timely assessment of victims' needs and assignment of categories to facilitate patient management.[40] START is thought to be the most prevalent system of disaster triage, and other systems aimed at prioritizing treatment include SAVE, MASS, and SALT.[8,41] Kennedy et al. note that no single algorithm is necessarily ideal for disaster relief under a particular set of circumstances.[40] This fact underlines the importance of effective planning and communication of agreed upon protocols. Common to most disaster triage strategies is the practice of categorizing some victims as "expectant."[40,41] Victims whose needs clearly extend beyond what can be provided are considered unlikely to survive even with available medical assistance, and are thus given no priority in the hierarchy of resource allocation. Categorizing individuals as expectant is based not only the victim's condition, but also on how their needs fit into the given context, "the specific circumstances of time and place."[11]

Urgency is therefore a dynamic concept that depends not only on a patient's condition, but also on the evolving capabilities of the disaster response.[34,40] In order to incorporate the relevant variables in determining the likelihood that a patient will benefit from medical attention, it is often useful to consider "narratives of care." Such an approach fosters thinking beyond initial interventions to anticipate what further resources might be necessary to achieve a positive outcome. On presentation, an individual might require fluids and basic wound care. Though many think of triage as a "snapshot" decision of whether to provide this care at a moment in time, the approach is severely limited because it ignores future costs that may be significant and exceed local capabilities. The likelihood that an individual will require surgery, dialysis, or extended use of antibiotics is relevant to considerations of whether they should receive any care whatsoever.[42] Indeed, without the ability to address the patient's needs over time, initial investment of resources may go to waste by simply delaying mortality that is inevitable under the circumstances.

After the devastating earthquake in Haiti, physicians repeatedly encountered the difficult question of whether to provide care to those who had suffered crush injuries. Given the high likelihood of developing rhabdomyolysis and subsequent renal impairment in a setting without dialysis capabilities, there was little chance that these individuals would survive even with treatment.[42] Further complicating the decision is the question of how circumstances might change over time. Care that is unavailable today might be available tomorrow, and vice versa. Such uncertainty underlies many nuances of disaster management and decision-making.[43] Utilitarian approaches in general require prediction of the consequences of an action, which is frequently undermined by the rapidly changing circumstances and poor situational awareness characteristic of a disaster scenario.[11]

In large-scale disasters, the "circumstances of time and place" extend far beyond individual EDs, hospitals, and even local healthcare networks. Such situations require that considerations of need and available resources encompass regional interests, and also be motivated by situational awareness.[44] Bostick and Subbarao argue for a macro conception of triage to promote justice and effectiveness in large-scale disaster events.[8,9] They note, "The public health preparedness community must reconceptualize disaster triage as a population-based system process."[8] Though Iserson and Moskop distinguish the concept of triage from rationing and allocation, others do not employ this distinction, particularly when considering triage as a multi-tiered process in the setting of a large-scale disaster.[8,9,28,44] Burkle et al. identify use of health emergency operations centers (HEOCs) as a key aspect of the incident command system framework capable of coordinating efforts at different scales of disaster response.[44] Such an approach recognizes the ethical significance of broader considerations of disaster management and the role of HEOCs in promoting fairness and effectiveness in macroallocation decision-making.[45]

The cost and likelihood of victims' achieving good outcomes depends not only on disaster-related circumstances, but also on conditions that preceded the event. For example, analyses following earthquakes find highly positive correlations between age and mortality.[46,47] Such data suggest this population is vulnerable, and that attempts to address its medical needs once a disaster has occurred might be resource-intensive and ineffective. A more cost-efficient approach might involve disaster preparedness initiatives to mitigate this population's risk of poor outcomes and need for disaster care.

Preexisting medical conditions and disabilities also raise important questions about allocation of scarce resources, since comorbidities lead to complex and costly narratives of care with lower probabilities of success. Significant evidence linking baseline level of health to socioeconomic status raises the question of whether disaster triage offers unequal benefit to those with reliable access to medical care.[48] The interconnectedness of medical and economic variables suggests that even when based on "medical criteria," triage cannot avoid incorporating socioeconomic considerations. Bell notes, "The 'victims' in general macroallocation contexts frequently are casualties of antecedent inequalities, that is, their lower socioeconomic status . . . "[49] Though clearly unacceptable from an egalitarian point of view, these disparities in disaster response arguably do not represent a radical departure from the systemic inequalities that already exist within the healthcare infrastructure. Disaster planning and response are committed to social justice in being attentive to particularly vulnerable populations.[50] Yet because disaster relief is usually short term and unfolds within a given context, it is reasonable to question the extent to which it is capable of radically surpassing the underlying conditions that undermine equitable distribution of medical wellbeing.[51]

In the years since Hurricane Katrina, there has been increased attention to incorporating the elderly, the chronically ill, and people with disabilities into disaster preparedness plans to reduce their risk of poor outcomes and limit dependence on disaster relief services for basic care. Such approaches may prove useful in avoiding situations that lead to unequal treatment, morbidity and mortality, and significant consumption of resources.[51–54]

Questions of societal value
Though strict egalitarianism dictates that individuals have equal standing within society, and should therefore be treated equally, disasters frequently challenge the importance of equity in allocating resources. Arguments for equity often exclude considerations of disaster scenarios as dynamic events, and instead focus on distribution of goods at a moment in time.[6,45] In most cases, the scope and impact of disasters evolve and develop after their onset. Indeed, research has suggested that particularly in events affecting infrastructure, mortality peaks in the days and weeks after the original event.[47] Because certain individuals may contribute to disaster recovery through their particular knowledge and skills, there are strong utilitarian motivations for both protecting them and ensuring

they are healthy enough to perform tasks vital to the health of the community. For example, treating the minor injuries and ailments of utility workers to ensure the supply of water and electricity provides enormous "downstream" benefit by preventing a public health crisis.[55] Similar strategies exist to ensure that healthcare personnel have received proper vaccinations during an influenza pandemic to maintain the healthcare infrastructure and thereby attain maximum benefit from prophylactic resources.[56,57]

Such a strategy need not challenge directly the notion that everyone is equal, since the argument is not that these individuals are intrinsically more deserving of treatment, survival, or prophylaxis. Rather, the basis for this strategy is that without securing the underlying determinants of public health, the population as a whole will suffer.[55,57] Some have argued that incorporating such questions of societal value into triage inevitably leads to unjust distribution of resources, since those judged to contribute the most to society are often the most educated and integrated into society's existing structures of influence.[49,58] While it is certainly true that disadvantaged groups are unlikely to be prioritized as having societal value, they are also the most likely to suffer unacceptable outcomes due to lack of water, electricity, and security after a major disaster.[59,60] Given their significant vulnerability in a public health crisis, preventing further deterioration of infrastructure and other determinants of health at the expense of equity clearly serves the interests of those who are "least able to withstand stress caused by disaster."[26]

Analogous situations arise when considering how to prioritize parents with young or otherwise dependent children. It has become particularly clear in the wake of Hurricane Katrina that mothers and children are a vulnerable subset of the population with unique needs and therefore require special considerations.[61,62] From a utilitarian perspective, the interests of parents should be of higher priority because their fates are closely linked with the survival of others. Although this idea makes obvious mathematical sense, strict egalitarians would argue that this approach violates a basic principle of fairness, since there is no reason a parent's life is of intrinsically greater value than that of someone without children. Indeed, an egalitarian might ask, "Why should another individual be less entitled to care based on a personal choice or inability to have children?"

To prioritize the life of a parent is to abandon the ideal of equality. Both the egalitarian and utilitarian views are coherent and logical, and it is not immediately clear how to resolve the dilemma. One way to reconcile these views is to apply concepts of distributive justice, and consider the question of how to protect those who are most disadvantaged in a given situation.[6,33] Deviating from the ideal of equality by giving the parent priority might be justifiable because the resulting disparity is in service of a profoundly vulnerable population. In a society attentive to distributive justice, one can argue that the ideal of equality would still be operative in a certain sense, since as a child everyone would have enjoyed the same protections as those employed in the present scenario.[63] Of course, if the nonparents in this scenario were at significant risk for mortality, then they would themselves qualify as vulnerable, and therefore be entitled to adequate care within a distributive justice framework.

Further considerations include whether more abstract ideas of "benefit" should ever be used to guide triage decisions. Examples include prioritizing critical care of the only remaining child in a family, the brothers and sisters having been killed in the disaster. Perhaps a spiritual leader of the community who is in critical condition might be saved, but requires an inordinate amount of resources, and his or her survival is far from certain. Though they push the limits of "responsible stewardship of resources," considerations of symbolic value seem ethically valid if they align properly with societal priorities. Strong societal priorities can bend outcomes of utilitarian thinking in unexpected ways. For example, Olsen suggests that "extremely risk-averse" utilitarians might opt for a distribution of benefits that includes a safety net to ensure they do not end up in an unacceptable position as individuals, which would resemble distributive justice.[58] It becomes particularly obvious in these considerations that in order to appear reasonable and just, ethical standards for disaster triage must stem from societal values. There have been many arguments in favor of transparency of the ethical principles guiding triage practices as well as community involvement in determining them.[2,8,44,64] Ethicists cannot assume they know a society's values a priori. Childress offers a good example, suggesting those who conceive of triage in a purely utilitarian fashion might overlook important social concerns that do not fit into that ethical framework:

> Society may have a stake in protecting the patient–physician relationship and the delivery of health care from the economic language of investment and return. It may value the relationship of "personal care" even when it is not productive. If the physician looks through the patient to society and tries to realize society's goals, the relationship of personal care and trust would be radically altered.[65]

Although the discussion of resource allocation has primarily involved physicians and others in the healthcare field, there is no obvious reason these groups should have unique authority in answering ethical questions. In fact, several have pointed out good reasons to question physicians' judgments on questions of macroallocation given their deep involvement in microallocation settings where clinical bioethics are sufficient.[1,4,18] The conversations necessary to further develop the ethics of disaster triage must therefore include diverse cultural and ideological viewpoints representative of the community as a whole.

The tragedy of triage

"An acceptable theory of justice must conform with our strong intuitions about what is fair and just in particular cases," Elster suggests.[66] While it is certainly true that a theory of justice must resonate with peoples' values and make intuitive sense as a conceptual framework, this in no way guarantees that its application will appear fair or just in particular cases. As Hume notes, in matters of life and death, "The strict laws of justice are suspended and give place to the stronger motives of necessity and self-preservation."[67] Insofar as disasters themselves are without reason, applying a theory of justice in this context cannot overcome the underlying senselessness of threats to individual wellbeing. Both the physician and the dying victim might feel at the moment of their encounter that disaster triage is deeply flawed to permit such suffering to continue untreated. Even a clear intellectual understanding of the ethical requirement to withhold care from the dying may crumble under such circumstances, leading to inappropriate care and failures of stewardship. Some have discussed the struggle between systems of disaster triage and empathy as an enormous emotional and psychological burden capable of generating significant stress and cognitive dissonance.[5] DeWaal describes this experience in strong but appropriate terms:

> On entering the profession, the doctor has taken the Hippocratic Oath and is committed to the best interests and rights of the individual patient. Triage, though, compels the healer to decline to treat the badly wounded soldier . . . The humanitarian physician must look into the eyes of a man or woman in the most desperate need of his or her expertise, and withhold that help. It is an act of cruelty.[5]

Such a narrative highlights the importance of preparing disaster relief personnel for the unique stresses of carrying out disaster triage, and working outside the scope of clinical bioethics.

One of the unfortunate aspects of disaster triage is that despite its perceived importance in determining patient outcomes, there has been essentially no scientific evaluation of its effectiveness.[8,40,68–70] The absence of systematically acquired data demonstrating the impact of disaster triage strategies is understandable given the significant barriers to conducting research in disaster situations, but it is nonetheless disconcerting from an ethical standpoint.[71–73] Several studies have assessed the interrater reliability, ease of use, and accuracy of some triage systems, but without data supporting causal inference between algorithms and outcomes in disaster settings, these results have been of little use in trying to improve the quality of disaster triage methods.[41,70,74–77] Despite the limitations in evaluating effectiveness of triage methods, evidence does suggest that triage affects mortality after a disaster. Analysis of data from several terrorist attacks indicates a positive linear correlation of over-triage and critical mortality.[78] Researchers should view the barriers to attaining effectiveness data as impediments to achieving more ethical practices. Without dedicated attempts to study the actual impact of current methods, uncomfortable doubts will persist and the path forward will remain obscure.[79]

Conclusion

Disasters expand needs beyond available resources; thus they necessitate difficult choices and invite reflection on the basic principles that motivate disaster response. Beneficence toward both individuals and populations positions disaster relief at the intersection of clinical medicine, public health, disaster management, and humanitarian relief, introducing nuanced tensions between distinct sets of priorities. Triage in the disaster setting is therefore properly understood not only as a tool to support clinical decision-making, but also as a framework for achieving a collectively agreed upon balance between the interests of the one and the many. Considered in terms of Aristotle's definition of virtue as a golden mean between deficiency and excess, disaster triage is a means of attaining virtue. Although its ideals are in some cases as old as medicine itself, actual systems of disaster triage have emerged only recently. Triage strategies in disaster settings are therefore in need of validation on multiple levels. Future work must assess the effectiveness of different approaches to support evidence-based practices. Equally important is the ongoing conversation about the social values and priorities that orient triage strategies and provide them with ethical content. When equipped with triage systems evaluated by these standards, physicians may serve society's interests and ideals even when circumstances undermine its stability.

Section IV: Recommendations

• Consider the resources available. Note that the word "resources" refers not only to medications and medical supplies, but also staff, facilities, equipment, ability to transport patients, etc. Triage involves assessments of what you can reasonably expect to accomplish for patients, which is largely shaped by the resources available to you in relation to peoples' needs.

• Coordinate between multiple levels of disaster response to foster sound situational awareness and cooperative micro- and macroallocation decisions in pursuit of collectively agreed goals.

• Consider the nature of the disaster, particularly the type of damage it might cause to the healthcare infrastructure, what medical problems are likely to be prevalent in the aftermath, how it might change or develop to affect need and resource availability, and how it might impede patient transport and arrival of external support.

• Understand the population's medical and public health needs independent of the disaster scenario, as

these variables will likely condition the disaster response as well. Be mindful of the needs of vulnerable populations, since they are likely to bear an unequal burden of the poor outcomes after a major disaster.

• Adopt a collectively agreed algorithm for triaging patients based on quickly attainable information. Adapt the algorithm to the particular scenario as necessary. In general, disaster triage strategies withhold treatment from those unlikely to benefit and from those whose complaints are minor.

• When deciding whether to provide treatment, consider the patient's potential future needs such as surgery, dialysis, wound care, and antibiotics, and assess the likelihood that they will be available. Responsible stewardship includes attentiveness to narratives of care and withholding care when no path to a good outcome is evident.

• Prepare for unique emotional and psychological burdens arising from the dissonance between the drive to relieve suffering and the ethical obligations to withhold care from individuals you likely would have treated under other conditions.

• Consider prioritizing treatment and prophylaxis of healthcare workers, utility workers, and others whose skills will be of use in the disaster relief effort. Doing so will limit the scope of the disaster, ease the burden on limited resources, and maximize benefit to the community from available treatments.

• Further research is necessary to learn about how specific triage strategies compare with one another in improving outcomes in disaster scenarios.

• Make efforts to ensure transparency of ethical principles guiding triage decisions, and proactively involve the community in discussion of its concerns, values, and priorities relating to disaster relief.

References

1. Petrini C. (2010) Triage in public health emergencies: ethical issues. *Intern Emerg Med.* 5, 137–44.
2. Sztajnkrycer MD, Madsen BE, Báez AA. (2006) Unstable ethical plateaus and disaster triage. *Emerg Med Clin North Am.* 24, 749–68.
3. Fink S. (2009) The deadly choices at memorial. *New York Times Magazine*, August 25.
4. Veatch RM. (2005) Disaster preparedness and triage: Justice and the common good. *Mt Sinai J Med.* 72(4), 236–41.

5. DeWaal A. (2010) The humanitarians' tragedy: escapable and inescapable cruelties. *Disasters*. 34(S2), S130–S7.

6. Baker R, Strosberg M. (1992) Triage and equality: An historical reassessment of utilitarian analyses of triage. *Kennedy Inst Ethics J*. 2(2), 103–23.

7. Lin JY, Anderson-Shaw L. (2009) Rationing of resources: Ethical issues in disasters and epidemic situations. *Prehospital Disast Med*. 24(3), 215–21.

8. Bostick NA, Subbarao I, Burkle FM, et al. (2008) Disaster triage systems for large-scale catastrophic events. *Disaster Med Public Health Prep*. 2(S1), S35–S9.

9. Subbarao I, Bostick NA, Burkle FM, et al. (2009) Re-envisioning mass critical care triage as a systemic multitiered process. *Chest*. 135(4), 1108.

10. Larrey DJ. (1814) *Memoirs of Military Surgery, and Campaigns of the French Armies*, vol. 2 (trans: Hall RW). Baltimore, MD: Classics of Medicine Library.

11. Moskop JC, Iverson KV. (2007) Triage in medicine, Part II: Underlying values and principles. *Ann Emerg Med*. 49, 282–7.

12. Hartman RG. (2003) Tripartite triage concerns: Issues for law and ethics. *Crit Care Med*. 31(5S), S358–S61.

13. Aristotle. (2000) *Nichomachean Ethics* (Crisp R, ed.). Cambridge: Cambridge University Press.

14. Beauchamp T, Childress J. (2009) *Principles of Biomedical Ethics*, 6th ed. New York, NY: Oxford University Press.

15. Larkin GL, Iserson K, Kassutto Z, et al. (2009) Virtue in emergency medicine. *Ann Emerg Med*. 16(1), 51–5.

16. Alexander JM. (2003) Capability egalitarianism and moral selfhood. *Ethical Perspectives*. 10(1), 3–21.

17. Mill JS. (2001) *Utilitarianism*, 2nd ed. (Sher G, ed.). Indianapolis, IN: Hackett Publishing Company.

18. Repine TB, Lisagor P, Cohen DJ. (2005) The dynamics and ethics of triage: rationing in hard times. *Mil Med*. 170, 505–9.

19. Dawson A, Verweij M. (2006) Introduction: ethics, prevention, and public health. In: Dawson A, Verweij M (eds) *Ethics, Prevention and Public Health*. Oxford: Oxford University Press.

20. Bayer R, Fairchild ALR. (2004) The genesis of public health ethics. *Bioethics*. 18, 473–92.

21. Beaglehole R. (2004) Public health in the new era: improving health through collective action. *Lancet*. 328, 2084–6.

22. American College of Emergency Physicians. (2000) *ACEP Policy Statement: Disaster Medical Services*. Dallas, TX: 22. American College of Emergency Physicians. Available at: www.acep.org/workarea/downloadasset.aspx?id=33620. Accessed December 21, 2011.

23. Burkle FM. (2002) Mass casualty management of a large-scale bioterrorist event: an epidemiological approach that shapes triage decisions. *Emerg Med Clin North Am*. 20, 409–36.

24. Kipnis K. (2010) Overwhelming casualties: Medical ethics in a time of terror. *Account Res*. 10(1), 57–68.

25. Larkin GL, Arnold J. (2003) Ethical considerations in emergency planning, preparedness, and response to acts of terrorism. *Prehosp Disaster Med*. 16, 53–7.

26. World Medical Association. (1994) *Statement on Medical Ethics in the Event of Disasters*. Available at: www.wma.net/en/30publications/10policies/d7/. Accessed August 8, 2011.

27. Gert HJ. (2005) How are emergencies different from other medical situations? *Mt Sinai J Med*. 72, 216–20.

28. Iserson KV, Moskop JC. (2007) Triage in medicine, Part I: Concept, history, and types. *Ann Emerg Med*. 49, 275–81.

29. Wynia MK. (2007) Ethics and public health emergencies: restrictions on liberty. *Am J Bioethics*. 7, 1–5.

30. Roberts MJ, Reich MR. (2002) Ethical analysis in public health. *Lancet*. 359, 1055–9.

31. Gostin LO. (2008) Public health and civil liberties in conflict. In: Gostin LO (ed.) *Public Health Law. Power, Duty, Restraint*. Berkeley, CA: University of California Press.

32. Pellegrino ED, Thomasma DC. (2004) The good of the patients and the good of society: striking a moral balance. In: Boylan M (ed.) *Public Health Policy and Ethics*. Dordrecht: Kluwer Academic Publisher.

33. Winslow GR. (1982) *Triage and Justice*. Berkeley, CA: University of California Press.

34. Caro JJ, Coleman N, Knebel A, et al. (2011) Unaltered ethical standards for individual physicians in the face of drastically reduced resources resulting from an improvised nuclear device event. *J Clin Ethics*. 22(1), 33–41.

35. Shevory TC. (1986) Applying rawls to medical cases: An investigation into the usages of analytical philosophy. *J Health Polit Policy Law*. 10(4), 749–64.

36. Rawls J. (1971) *A Theory of Justice*. Oxford: Oxford University Press.

37. Daniels N. (1974) Rights to health care and distributive justice: Programmatic worries. *J Med Philos*. 4, 179–80.

38. Daniels N. (1981) Health care needs and distributive justice. *Philos Public Aff*. 10, 164.

39. Sphere Project. (2004) *Humanitarian Charter and Minimum Standards in Disaster Response*. Oxford: Oxfam Publishing.

40. Kennedy K, Aghababian RV, Gans L, et al. (1996) Triage: Techniques and applications in decisionmaking. *Ann Emerg Med*. 28(2), 136–44.

41. Garner A, Lee A, Harrison K, et al. (2001) Comparative analysis of multiple-casualty incident triage algorithms. *Ann Emerg Med*. 38(5), 541–8.

42. Merin O, Ash N, Levy Gad, et al. (2010) The Israeli field hospital in Haiti—Ethical dilemmas in early disaster response. *N Engl J Med.* 362(e38), 1–3.

43. McCaughrin WC, Mattammal M. (2003) Perfect storm: organizational management of patient care under natural disaster conditions. *J Healthc Manag.* 48(5),295–308.

44. Burkle FM, Hsu EB, Loehr M, et al. (2007) Definition and functions of health unified command and emergency operations centers for large-scale bioevent disasters within the existing ICS. *Disaster Med Public Health Prep.* 1, 135–41.

45. Rubinson L, Hick JL, Hanfling DG, et al. (2008) Summary of suggestions from the task force for critical care summit, January 26–27, 2007. *Chest.* 133, 1–7.

46. Tanida N. (1996) What happened to elderly people in the great Hanshin earthquake. *BMJ.* 313, 1133–5.

47. Liang NJ, Shih YT, Shih FY, et al. (2001) Disaster epidemiology and medical response in the Chi-Chi earthquake in Taiwan. *Ann Emerg Med.* 38, 549–55.

48. Daniels N, Kennedy BP, Kawachi I. (1999) Why justice is good for our health: The social determinants of health inequalities. *Daedalus.* 128(4), 215–53.

49. Bell N. (1981) Triage in medical practices: An unacceptable model? *Soc Sci Med.* 15F, 151–6.

50. Lo B, Katz MH. (2005) Clinical decision making during public health emergencies: ethical considerations. *Ann Intern Med.* 143, 493–8.

51. Blumenshine P, Reingold A, Egerter S, et al. (2008) Pandemic influenza planning in the United States from a health disparities perspective. *Emerg Infect Dis.* 14(5), 709–15.

52. Andrulis DP, Siddiqui NJ, Gantner JL. (2007) Preparing racially and ethnically diverse communities for public health emergencies. *Health Aff.* 26(5), 1269–79.

53. Dyer CB, Regev M, Burnett J, et al. (2008) SWiFT: A rapid triage tool for vulnerable older adults in disaster situations. *Disaster Med Public Health Prep.* 2(S1), S45–S50.

54. Desalvo KB, Kertesz S. (2007) Creating a more resilient safety net for persons with chronic disease: Beyond the "medical home." *Soc Gen Intern Med.* 22, 1377–9.

55. Kass NE, Otto J, O'brien D, et al. (2008) Ethics and severe pandemic influenza: maintaining essential functions through a fair and considered response. *Biosecur Bioterror.* 6(3), 227–36.

56. Verweij M. (2009) Moral principles for allocating scarce medical resources in an influenza pandemic. *J Bioethic Inquiry.* 6(2), 159–69.

57. Vawter DE, Garrett JE, Gervais KG, et al. (2011) Attending to Social Vulnerability When Rationing Pandemic Resources. *J Clin Ethics.* 22(1), 42–53.

58. Olsen JA. (1997) Theories of justice and their implications for priority setting in health care. *J Health Econ.* 16, 625–39.

59. Zoraster RM. (2010) Vulnerable populations: Hurricane Katrina as a case study. *Prehosp Disaster Med.* 25(1), 74–8.

60. Davis JR, Wilson S, Brock-Martin A, et al. (2010) The impact of disasters on populations with health and health care disparities. *Disaster Med Public Health Prep.* 4(1), 30–8.

61. Callaghan WM, Rasmussen SA, Jamieson DJ, et al. (2007) Health concerns of women and infants in times of natural disasters: Lessons learned from Hurricane Katrina. *Matern Child Health J.* 11, 307–11.

62. Pfeiffer J, Avery MD, Benbenek M, et al. (2008) Maternal and newborn care during disasters: Thinking outside the hospital paradigm. *Nurs Clin North Am.* 43, 449–67.

63. Daniels N. (1988) *Am I My Parents' Keeper? An Essay on Justice Between the Young and the Old.* New York, NY: Oxford University Press.

64. Powell T. (2008) Allocation of ventilators in a public health disaster. *Disaster Med Public Health Prep.* 2(1), 20–6.

65. Childress J. (1970) Who shall live when not all can live? *Soundings.* 53, 340–50.

66. Elster J. (1992) *Local Justice: How Institutions Allocate Scarce Goods and Necessary Burdens.* New York, NY: Russell Sage Foundation.

67. Hume, D. (1999) *An Enquiry Concerning the Principles of Morals* (Beauchamp T, ed.). Chicago, IL: Open Court.

68. Jenkins JL, McCarthy ML, Sauer LM, et al. (2008) Mass-casualty triage: time for an evidence-based approach. *Prehosp Disaster Med.* 23, 3–8.

69. Auf der Heide E. (2006) The importance of evidence-based disaster planning. *Ann Emerg Med.* 47, 34–49.

70. Cone DC, MacMillan DS. (2005) Mass-casualty triage systems: A hint of science. *Acad Emerg Med.* 12(8), 739–41.

71. Collogan LK, Tuma F, Dolan-Sewell R, et al. (2004) Ethical issues pertaining to research in the aftermath of disaster. *J Trauma Stress.* 17(5), 363–72.

72. Levine C. (2004) The concept of vulnerability in disaster research. *J Trauma Stress.* 17(5), 395–402.

73. Kass N. (2001) An ethics framework for public health. *Am J Public Health.* 91, 1776–82.

74. Risavi BL, Salen PN, Heller MB, et al. (2001) A two-hour intervention using START improves prehospital triage of mass-casualty incidents. *Prehosp Emerg Care.* 5, 197–9.

75. Sacco WJ, Navin DM, Fiedler KE, et al. (2005) Precise formulation and evidence-based application of resource-constrained triage. *Acad Emerg Med.* 12, 759–70.

76. Kahn CA, Schultz CH, Miller KT, et al. (2009) Does START triage work? An outcomes assessment after a disaster. *Ann Emerg Med.* 54(3), 424–40.

77. Sanddal TL, Loyacono T, Sanndal ND. (2004) Effect of JumpSTART training on immediate and short-term pediatric triage performance. *Pediatr Emerg Care.* 20, 749–53.

78. Frykberg ER. (2002) Medical management of disasters and mass casualties from terrorist bombings: how can we cope? *J Trauma.* 53, 208.

79. Burstein JL. (2009) Mostly dead: Can science help with disaster triage? *Ann Emerg Med.* 54(3), 431.

22

The emergency physician as a bystander outside the hospital

Zev Wiener,[1] *Shamai A. Grossman*[2]

[1]*Medical Student, Harvard Medical School, Boston, MA, USA*
[2]*Vice Chair for Resource Utilization, and Director, Cardiac Emergency Center, Division of Emergency Medicine, Beth Israel Deaconess Medical Center, and Assistant Professor of Medicine, Harvard Medical School, Boston, MA, USA*

Section I: Case presentation

A 56-year-old otherwise healthy woman boards an airplane for a 12.5-hour flight from Tokyo to New York. About 7 hours into the flight the patient develops crushing chest pain radiating to her left arm with associated diaphoresis and dyspnea and seconds later sustains a cardiac arrest. The pilot announces overhead, "Is there a physician on board?" and an emergency medicine resident and a pathologist from the former Soviet Union respond. They discover that the airplane (a non-US-based carrier) keeps no medical equipment on board. The closest landing field is in a small town in Alaska, while Anchorage, the closest medical center with a 24-hour catheterization laboratory is 30 minutes away. The emergency physician's wife, concerned that her husband will be sued, and that resuscitation will be futile in any event, sets out to comfort the family. Nevertheless, her husband and the pathologist begin cardiopulmonary resuscitation (CPR), including mouth-to-mouth resuscitation. They insist that the airplane land at the closest airstrip, and that the pilot contact air traffic control to notify the nearest medical facility and arrange for an emergency medical crew to meet the airplane. Despite the dangers of a field landing, the pilot skillfully lands the plane approximately 5 minutes later. A team of paramedics board the plane and declare the patient dead on arrival.

Section II: Discussion

Dr. Peter Rosen: One of the strangest and most unfortunate consequences of malpractice fear in the United States has been the unwillingness of physicians to act as clinicians outside of their hospitals or office practices. Many states have rules that allow a physician to be exempt from litigation if the help is provided without charge. Some countries other than the United States have made physician response a legal responsibility. The notion that a physician can only apply professional expertise in optimal circumstances is not consistent with what I understand to be the practice of medicine. First, we should consider that giving the individual on an airplane the best possible care can put the rest of the passengers and crew at risk. How should this affect our decision-making?

Dr Richard Wolfe: I agree that physicians have a responsibility to provide care to people in need. It is not ethically justifiable to ignore a patient when your assistance is required, because of fear of litigation. In our case, while assisting the pilot and crew in making a decision about where to land the plane, one has to take responsibility for the safety of everyone on board, a risk/benefit assessment. In this case, a clinician has three possible options. First, one could decide to stop resuscitation because the patient is beyond saving. The ultimate decision to land and where, is

Ethical Problems in Emergency Medicine: A Discussion-Based Review, First Edition. John Jesus, Shamai A. Grossman, Arthur R. Derse, James G. Adams, Richard Wolfe, and Peter Rosen.
© 2012 John Wiley & Sons, Ltd. Published 2012 by John Wiley & Sons, Ltd.

always up to the pilot, and no physician can do anything but offer advice. No pilot will accept that advice, if he or she deems the landing to be unsafe. Second, one could go to the nearest available airport, though landing at an airport or an airstrip ill equipped for commercial airlines might place the passengers in danger. Finally, landing in Anchorage is a third option that facilitates a safer landing, and provides the patient with access to medical resources.

PR: Most American carriers now provide sophisticated first-aid equipment on all flights. In the absence of sophisticated equipment, what are the probabilities of providing effective life support, and when do you think it's medically reasonable to pronounce this patient dead?

Dr. Shamai Grossman: US carriers are significantly different from carriers outside the United States. First, every US carrier is currently mandated by law to carry basic life-saving equipment including an external defibrillator, as well as a full array of resuscitation medication, oxygen, intubation equipment, and more. I believe that we're obligated to try to do something for this patient. If you have no equipment, you can perform basic CPR. If that's all you can do, it's all you can do. Nevertheless, I acknowledge that a couple minutes of CPR is probably not going to be effective if the patient does not receive defibrillation or resuscitation medications.

RW: There are case reports of people surviving prolonged resuscitation efforts, up to and beyond 1 hour. I'm not sure how much of that was done with the benefit of oxygen, or if those patients benefited from intermittent episodes of return of spontaneous circulation. Nevertheless, there are reports of people who do survive long periods of cardiopulmonary arrest, and return after prolonged resuscitation with good neurologic function.

PR: Prolonged CPR is going to be virtually impossible on an airplane. I think that the other issue is that there are precedents for not providing either prolonged CPR, or withholding resuscitation efforts altogether. In the Seattle system, for example, they have not provided CPR to patients known to be in asystole for over 30 years.

SG: Even if the patient were able to be saved, appropriate personnel may not be available to help them on an airplane.

PR: The qualifications of those who respond to the call for a doctor on a flight are highly variable. There are many physicians who are trained in unrelated fields, or who don't have any training, yet are eager to get involved, to have everyone witness them acting as a physician. There are also those physicians who refuse to volunteer for fear of being sued. Do you have any recommendations on how to interact with the flight crews, and how to interact with the other physicians in an effort to address this?

Dr. James Adams: It's really tough to validate who's licensed and who's not. Doctors often don't carry their licenses, and in many cases I've seen nurses and paramedics step forward to help. I wonder if there is a generational difference regarding which physicians are most likely to step forward. The physicians I know would step up and wouldn't hesitate to provide what ever care they could. However, I've heard stories of younger physicians too afraid and hesitant to do anything but silently sit in their seat. I hope that isn't a widespread phenomenon.

RW: I think we can agree that anyone who would remain seated, in essence refusing to volunteer, misunderstands what the role of a physician is in society; in some ways I find that a breach of one's ethical duty as a physician.

SG: Most US airlines, if not all, are connected to a medical control system that helps the flight crew and any physicians on board care for the patient. Moreover, if you are a volunteer physician, you're obligated to show a license or somehow prove you're qualified to provide patient care. Though this requirement might assist in filtering out people who are not physicians, a pathologist may be the only licensed physician on the plane. Once you've been able to verify someone's qualifications, it becomes the discretion of the pilot or the head flight attendant to decide who is actually going to treat the patient. There are now actually eight states in the United States that mandate a response to people in peril. I suspect this is in response to a growing trend of physicians who are more inclined to stay silent, and not put themselves at putative risk for subsequent malpractice litigation.

RW: All physicians should act regardless of what the state mandates. It's our duty. The possibility of a lawsuit shouldn't influence a physician's decision.

Dr. John Jesus: Although we all believe physicians have an ethical obligation to act, it's important to explore how that obligation differs from legal responsibilities. As previously explained, for example, eight states have a positive duty to assist people who need assistance. That leaves 42 states that don't have a positive duty to act. Additionally, the case includes a resident physician. A physician's lack of extensive experience is not, in any way, an excuse for failure to assist an ill person. Insofar as Good Samaritan statutes require us to act within our own skill set and knowledge base, a young inexperienced resident may find himself in a difficult situation. On airplanes, the salient point is to be transparent about that knowledge base and that skill set, and to maintain actions within the scope of expertise.

RW: I agree that you need to be clear and open about what your skill set is. By the same token however, you are a physician, and regardless of your level of training, you should be able to contribute what you can.

PR: The licensed resident physician must understand that when he steps outside of his residency, he has the same privileges and responsibilities as a fully trained physician. I think we must teach residents that it's okay to use their skills outside the hospital and comfort zone.

JJ: Not all medical students are required to do ACLS (advanced cardiac life support) or PALS (pediatric advanced life support) courses upon graduation. Insofar as they consider themselves to be physicians, and there is an ethical responsibility to stabilize patients outside of a hospital setting, I think its incumbent upon medical schools to provide that training to their students.

PR: No matter how little training you received in medical school, you're still likely to possess more practical knowledge than the average lay person. Furthermore, there is an ethical responsibility one takes on by virtue of finishing medical school. Could medical schools do a better job with the curriculum of emergency medicine? We've been arguing the need for practical skills training for over 35 years.

RW: In the instances when I have found myself trying to help someone on a plane with several other physicians, each person relays his or her background and expertise, and the group usually defers to the person with the most expertise. It is important not to defer to someone who does not have an appropriate skill set.

PR: The conflicts I have had have not been with other physicians, but rather have been with the flight crew. I've been in several situations on airplanes, in which I've been asked to help, and have been prevented from approaching the patient because of various passengers or flight crew personnel with some paramedic training who attempt to take over the patient's care. I've had the same problem when I've stopped to help people in motor vehicle accidents. I've even been told to go on my way, despite having the expertise.

RW: If, after you've made it clear what your skills are, and you're ordered away by the people who ultimately have responsibility for the patient's care, then this may be one of those times when it is appropriate to defer to their judgment.

PR: Another issue to consider is the question of when to stop resuscitation. The reality is that we simply don't have good markers of who should have resuscitation attempted or stopped.

SG: A patient with multiple comorbidities is far less likely to survive a cardiac arrest than a young or otherwise healthy patient. For instance, a patient who has an ejection fraction of 10% or a severe cardiomyopathy, would be far less likely to survive a cardiac arrest than the patient who has a healthy heart. When to stop resuscitation also depends on the etiology of the arrest. In this case, the patient is likely having a large myocardial infection with myocardial irritability. The patient will likely not survive unless that patient is quickly reperfused. The key to giving this patient a chance for survival is to administer a thrombolytic drug, or perform a percutaneous intervention. Without those interventions, the likelihood of patient survival is vanishingly small. One clearly has to take into account these variables in deciding to what extent resuscitation should be prolonged or attempted at all.

PR: In most circumstances, physicians who find themselves on an airplane with a pulseless patient, will not have the privilege of knowing any patient-specific information. The best advice I can give clinicians in this situation is simply to try. If your efforts don't work, then stop.

SG: Included in the variables a physician must consider as he attempts to care for an ill patient, is how those decisions will affect the physician and the rest of the passengers on the plane.

PR: The reality is that when we practice emergency medicine we're not doing something that is particularly safe. All of us run risks of acquiring disease from our patents. We don't know that this patient did not die of meningitis, for example, or some other communicable disease, and I think that part of being a physician is to accept that risk. It isn't always convenient, it isn't always safe, and it isn't always fun.

JA: Despite the difficulty and the serious concerns doctors can feel in a situation like this, we still have to rise to the highest standards, and do what we feel is right and do so to the best of our abilities.

JJ: Caring for patients on an airplane is not an extremely rare circumstance. The rate of these medical incidents is also likely to increase over time as the elderly population continues to grow and the globalization process accelerates. To some extent, we can predict the kinds of medical problems that are likely to occur. A few examples include insulin-dependent diabetics who fail to maintain their schedules of eating and checking their glucose levels, patients who are prone to clotting and developing a deep venous thrombosis or a pulmonary embolus, and patients with chronic respiratory or cardiac disorders who are vulnerable to the atmospheric changes in the cabin of a plane.

Section III: Review of the literature

The question of a bystander's responsibility to intervene in a stranger's plight has been probed for centuries by the ethical Judeo-Christian tradition.[1] (Of note, this dilemma does not appear to feature as prominently in the ancient Eastern traditions, see Tang, for example.[1]) The Hebrew Bible begins with the story of Cain and Abel, in which Cain's rhetorical question, "Am I my brother's keeper?" is implicitly answered in the affirmative (Genesis 4:9). Subsequently, the Hebrew Bible explicitly commands, "Do not stand idly by the blood of your neighbor" (Leviticus 19:16). The Babylonian Talmud codifies a legal obligation to perform life-saving efforts on behalf of a stranger, even if such an effort requires expenditure of funds on the part of the intervener (BT Sanhedrin, 73a; see Rabbeinu Asher, Sanhedrin 8:2). The parable of the Good Samaritan is well known to students of Christianity, and has been applied by modern legal systems to protect intervening bystanders from legal liability (Luke 10:25–37). While these ancient sources have all focused on the obligation of a civilian, the unique obligation—or lack thereof—of the physician bystander has not been well explored.

Ethical considerations

If a civilian witnesses a fellow human drowning in a river, and can easily provide a life preserver at no apparent risk of harm—physical, financial, or otherwise—is there an obligation to do so? Similarly, if a truck driver observes a major accident on a remote road and has easy cell phone access, is there an obligation to notify the paramedics? Whether one relies on common intuition, Kantian categorical imperatives, utilitarian pragmatism, or Biblical law, most would agree that failure to participate in such situations is morally reprehensible. A civilian is ethically obligated to do whatever is safely within his or her capacity to assist in the rescue of a fellow human being.

If one accepts the civilian's ethical obligation to intervene, what of the responsibility of the off-duty emergency physician? Although emergency medicine relies heavily upon the use of technology and resources available only in staffed emergency departments (EDs), emergency physicians possess a wealth of knowledge and skills that could be of critical assistance, even in the field. Consequently, what is the scope of the emergency physician's obligation to intervene outside of the hospital? One could envision three possible responses:

- First, an off-duty emergency physician is no different **in practice** from any civilian. A civilian is obligated to "do as much as he can," which usually means dialing 911 in medical emergencies. Therefore, an off-duty emergency physician is similarly only obligated to perform minimal interventions, such as dialing 911.
- Second, an off-duty emergency physician is no different, **in principle**, from any civilian; the two merely differ with regards to the scope of what they are able to perform. An off-duty emergency physician is bound by the same civilian imperative to "do as much as he

can," but, while a layperson's "as much as he can" is limited to dialing 911, an emergency physician's "as much as he can" extends to taking pulses, performing chest compressions, mask breathing, etc. Fundamentally, however, there is no qualitative distinction between the essential nature of their obligations to intervene.

• Third, an off-duty emergency physician carries a higher degree of moral obligation. This is not the case of simply a "civilian who happens to know more"; rather, the physician maintains a categorically distinct identity with concomitantly novel responsibilities. This approach differs from the second option, in that it allows for a broader distinction between the civilian and the physician. Accordingly, perhaps an off-duty emergency physician may be obligated to intervene in situations in which an ordinary civilian would not, such as situations with higher degrees of risk or inconvenience.

Beyond the characterization of the essential nature of the physician's obligation to intervene, numerous other specific ethical considerations underlie this question. For example, *primum non nocere*—"first, do no harm".[2] How does intervention outside of the hospital fit into this principle? On the one hand, an off-duty emergency physician without appropriate equipment or training for field work may do more harm than if he or she merely desisted from intervention. Accordingly, non-intervention might be the ethically "safe" policy. On the other hand, however, one might argue that remaining silent in the face of an obvious threat actually constitutes a form of "doing harm." In other words, can acts of omission ever be as blameworthy as acts of commission?

Furthermore, one must consider the possible distinction between life-threatening and non-life-threatening conditions. For example, if an off-duty physician observes someone suffering from a gouty flare which is causing severe pain but no threat to life, perhaps the obligation to intervene is diminished relative to the obligation to intervene in a life-threatening myocardial infarction. This issue may depend on which of the aforementioned approaches one chooses to adopt.

One must also consider the appropriate balance between immediate obligations and long-term benefits. Even if one maintains that an emergency physician has an obligation to incur some degree of risk in intervening outside of the hospital, if the risks are too

great, perhaps it is not only **unnecessary** to intervene, but even **unethical**. If a physician's intervention risks a malpractice lawsuit or the contraction of hepatitis C, the physician's lost years of service might ultimately result in fewer patients being helped. Is it appropriate to weigh the long-term benefits to patients against the immediate necessity of the victim, or does the present need always take precedence?

Finally, even if a physician does assume a higher standard of ethical responsibility, perhaps this standard applies only towards one's patients, as opposed to society as a whole. Such a distinction would naturally necessitate a precise definition of exactly who qualifies as a "patient." These are just a few of the many general ethical considerations that must be borne in mind when approaching this complex question.

Ethical arguments supporting intervention

Once we have accepted the premise that ethical principles would likely obligate a non-medical civilian to intervene to the best of one's abilities (i.e., dialing 911) when there is no obvious threat to self, a doctor should seemingly hold no less of an obligation. At the very least, an off-duty emergency physician should be obligated to intervene by dialing 911. But perhaps the off-duty physician's moral obligation is considerably greater than that of a layperson. In choosing to become a physician, one has elected a profession that has dangers and responsibilities, akin to a career of a police officer or firefighter, which obligates one to a higher ethical standard, and which may even involve the potential risk of contraction of a disease, litigation, or personal harm. The question of exactly how much risk a physician must assume may certainly be debated extensively, and is an entire subject unto itself. Nevertheless, without specifying exact guidelines, the choice to become a physician entails that one serve society even when off-duty, and even in the face of a certain degree of risk, beyond that which a layperson would be expected to assume, is involved.

This argument must acknowledge the unique status of medicine as a profession. Medicine is not simply a "9 to 5" occupation, but rather, an essential definition of one's identity that transcends time and location. The source of this distinction, however, must be elucidated. Perhaps this responsibility is inherent in becoming a physician simply by virtue of its near universal acceptance: Because most doctors perceive themselves as holding a higher degree of ethical responsibility, irrespective of the reason, all doctors are similarly bound to this level of responsibility. The weakness of this argument, however, is that it leaves open the possibility that any individual physician may personally elect **not** to subscribe to the general consensus. Indeed, some physicians who enter the medical profession may not be aware of the ethical responsibility that their choice entails, and never consensually accept this responsibility.

A similar yet distinct source for the higher ethical imperative of the off-duty physician may stem from the specific codes of conduct that have been formalized and instituted by physicians over time.[3] The Hippocratic Oath (modernized in 1964 by Louis Lasagna), for example, affirms, "I will remember that I remain a member of society, with special obligations to all my fellow human beings, those sound of mind and body as well as the infirm."[4] The *International Code of Medical Ethics* of the World Medical Association (2006) contends that "a physician shall give emergency care as a humanitarian duty unless he/she is assured that others are willing and able to give such care."[5] The code of ethics of the Canadian Medical Association (2004) requires a physician to "provide whatever appropriate assistance [he] can to any person with an urgent need for medical care."[6] Lastly, the principles of ethics of the American Medical Association state "A physician shall, in the provision of appropriate patient care, except in emergencies, be free to choose whom to serve."[7] These societal recommendations, however, may also not fully suffice. Not all medical students take the Hippocratic Oath on graduation or are aware of these standards. And even among those who are aware of these standards, the non-specific formulations of many of the responsibilities certainly remain open to diverse interpretations.

One might also posit that the higher ethical standard of physicians stems from the unique value and quality of their knowledge. By virtue of their broad training backgrounds, physicians of all specialties are better suited to diagnose and manage emergent illnesses than untrained civilians. Their unique ability to assist may confer a de facto ethical obligation to intervene, regardless of whether or not an individual physician has personally volunteered to do so. Moreover, the universal and organic nature of their knowledge, which deals with problems of disease that transcend all barriers of culture, race, or geography, may further oblige a physician to a higher degree of service to humanity.

Beyond the nature of medical knowledge, arguments of societal reciprocity may also support a physician's obligation to intervene. All privileges come with responsibilities. The police officer's unique privilege to carry a loaded weapon comes with a concomitant responsibility to risk his or her life to protect others who are in danger. Similarly, a physician's unique privilege to acquire the exclusive knowledge of healing and to be privy to people's most intimate secrets and problems comes with the responsibility to serve society to the best of one's abilities, even if doing so poses some risk to one's own personal or professional wellbeing. A final point in support of a positive duty to act may be an application of basic Kantian principles: Because I would want another person with medical knowledge to assist me if I were in need, I am ethically obligated to do the same, even if it is beyond the technical call of duty. Whatever the source of this ethical obligation, a tenable position emerges, which maintains that off-duty emergency physicians are obligated to intervene, even if the intervention poses some degree of risk.

Ethical arguments against intervention

The arguments against an ethical obligation to intervene may reject either of the two aforementioned assumptions. First, one could reject the uniqueness of the medical profession, stating that medicine is fundamentally not different from any other vocation. Just as a lawyer, musician, or plumber who is off-duty bears no ethical obligation to voluntarily help a stranger in need of his or her specific services, so too a physician holds no such obligation. Although the consequences of a physician's failure to intervene may indeed be far graver than those of the other listed professions, this difference is technical rather than fundamental, and ultimately has no bearing on the categorical principle that workmen who are off-duty are not bound to serve with their expertise. Indeed, a physician who does not intervene has technically not violated his or her mandate to "do no harm," and has not made the patient any worse off than if the physician had never chanced upon the scene in the first place.

Alternatively, even if one accepts that physicians are held to a higher ethical standard than other professions, one could still maintain that countervailing ethical responsibilities supersede the value of intervention. As noted before, intervention outside of the hospital virtually always entails some degree of risk, be it the risk of contraction of an illness (e.g., intervening on a patient whose human immunodeficiency virus (HIV), hepatitis, or tuberculosis status is unknown), the risk of violence (perhaps the patient's intentions are malicious, or the event has occurred in an unsafe neighborhood), or the risk of litigation. Physicians are not trained to work in such environments, and therefore may be unable to accurately assess the risk involved in a particular situation. Moreover, physicians are not police officers or firefighters, for whom the assumption of high risk is germane to their profession. Incurring such risks is not only non-obligatory, but perhaps equally unethical, as voluntarily risking one's health or career may ultimately limit the physician's ability to help many more patients in future years.

One could further argue that the unique responsibility of physicians to treat is solely towards their "patients." Perhaps the definition of one's "patients" does not extend to strangers outside of the hospital. Only in the hospital, where both parties have consented to medical intervention (the patient has consented to receive treatment, and the physician has consented to practice medicine) does the ethically binding patient–doctor relationship exist. One could argue that if a homeless man of unknown hepatitis status is brought into the ED, he becomes a "patient," and the doctor is not only required to treat the patient, but also to assume certain risks while doing so. But if the physician encounters that same homeless man on the street, the man is not considered a "patient," and the responsibilities inherent in the patient–doctor relationship do not apply.

Finally, the immense stress involved in the daily practice of medicine requires some breaks. The hours of medical training and practice are very demanding, and rates of burnout among physicians are of serious concern to society.[8] Placing physicians under a perpetual obligation of service may ultimately compromise their ability to deliver quality care to their true patients in the long term. Even though the frequency of such bystander situations is extremely low, the fact that a physician must always leave home with a feeling of being "on call" (even if only subconsciously) may have negative psychological effects on the ability to serve in the long run. It may also result in fewer individuals electing to pursue the practice of medicine.

Assessment of arguments

It is difficult to deny the unique ethical station of the medical practitioner, due to both the special value of medical knowledge as well as the reciprocal benefits that exist between him or her and society. Additionally, the irreversible and time-sensitive nature of life-threatening emergencies significantly strengthens the arguments in favor of an ethical obligation to intervene, despite the fact that a stranger may not be one's "patient" and that a perpetual obligation of service may contribute to burnout. In light of these factors, physicians are ethically obligated to intervene to the best of their abilities in life-threatening situations, as long as no major risk to personal safety can be identified. Although risk of litigation does pose a significant concern, such fear is ultimately insufficient grounds to justify non-intervention. The risk of litigation is a non-fatal risk that is less likely to occur, while the risk to a person's life is irreversible and imminent. By similar logic, while intervention in non-life-threatening situations is meritorious, it cannot be deemed ethically obligatory, given that the threat to the patient is reversible and not time sensitive.

The specifics of each situation must be assessed individually. In some situations, for example, prompt summoning of additional medical help may be more valuable than attempts to intervene (as in a pulseless patient who requires prompt defibrillation), while in other situations, immediate intervention may be preferable (as in the application of a tourniquet to a massive hemorrhage). Sometimes, the immediate emergency will supersede all other concerns (as in a physician who witnesses an emergency while travelling to a recreational event), while other times, a physician may have to judiciously overlook an immediate emergency for the sake of a larger good (as in a physician who witnesses a small-scale emergency on the way to responding to a large-scale natural disaster).[3] These distinctions ultimately require prudent judgment on the part of the physician, and, while general guidelines may be offered, every case remains unique.

In light of the argument that a physician's intervention outside of the familiar hospital setting may cause more harm than good, hospitals and training programs should encourage periodic reviews of field emergency medical procedures, and physicians should always consider the suggestions of trained first-responders on scene. In addition, protocols detailing an off-duty physician's role in assisting bystanders, particularly when other first responders are at the scene, should be disseminated.

Legal considerations[9]

"Good Samaritan" statutes encourage prompt emergency care by protecting individuals from civil liability for any negligent acts or omissions committed while providing voluntary emergency care. Since the passage of the first "Good Samaritan" statute in 1959, all US states have enacted some form of this legislation.[10]

Over the years, numerous limitations have been applied to the immunity afforded by "Good Samaritan" legislation. While many jurisdictions protect anyone who administers emergency care, others limit coverage to specified medical personnel, or to physicians alone. "Good Samaritan" statutes often require that the emergency assistance be offered "in good faith" and without expectation of payment.[10] Some courts have stipulated that only interventions performed in an "ordinary reasonably prudent" manner are protected by the statute.[11] Similarly, courts have limited the protection of "Good Samaritan" statutes to acts that do not constitute gross negligence or willful and wanton misconduct. In *Higgins* v. *Detroit Osteopathic Hospital Corp*, for example, the court ruled that a physician's misreading of an X-ray did not constitute gross negligence, and was therefore eligible for statutory immunity.[12] Other limitations to the law include requirements that the situation be deemed an "emergency," that the emergency was not created by the individual who intervenes, and that the assistance be rendered "without objection" of the victim (see, for example, *Flynn* v. *United States* and *Botte* v. *Pomeroy*).[11,13]

"Good Samaritan" laws are designed to encourage intervention by individuals who may otherwise have refrained from doing so. As such, physicians who have preexisting duties to a particular patient may not be covered by these laws. Some courts have ruled that only doctors treating patients in emergencies when they were not on call, or bound by a similarly binding professional obligation, were covered by the statutory protection. Similarly, in *Colby* v. *Schwartz*, the court ruled that emergency physicians who provided treatment in the ED to the victim of an automobile accident as part of their normal duties could not be considered volunteers and were therefore ineligible for statutory immunity.[14]

While "Good Samaritan" legislation traditionally serves to exempt from liability those who choose to intervene, some US states, including Florida, Ohio, Massachusetts, Minnesota, Rhode Island, Vermont, Washington, and Wisconsin, have broadened these laws to include "duty to rescue" obligations—a requirement to provide "reasonable assistance" to strangers in peril.[15] In practice, however, these laws are rarely applied in the United States.[16] Other countries, however, including Portugal, the Netherlands, Finland, Italy, Norway, Russia, Turkey, Denmark, Poland, Germany, Romania, France, Greece, Switzerland, Spain, and Belgium, do enforce a general duty to rescue, imposing fines and in some cases imprisonment for failure to assist.[17] In 1998, the State of Israel, following ancient Talmudic law, passed a modern law that similarly obligates bystanders to offer assistance in emergency situations and provides for restitution of financial losses suffered by bystanders as a result of their intervention.[18]

Existing policies and guidelines

Given the arguments above and the varied but genuine legal consideration involved in bystander care, the American College of Emergency Physicians (ACEP) describes the expectations of a physician bystander as follows:

Because of their unique expertise, emergency physicians have an ethical duty to respond to emergencies in the community and offer assistance. This responsibility is buttressed by local "Good Samaritan" statutes that protect health care professionals from legal liability for good-faith efforts to render first aid. Physicians should not disrupt paramedical personnel who are under base station medical control and direction.[19]

Conclusions

While all people are ethically obligated to assist others in peril, the essential value and the benefits of the practice of medicine place a higher ethical obligation on the off-duty emergency physician to serve society. Therefore, even though field intervention invariably entails some degree of risk to self or career, an emergency physician is obligated to intervene in the assistance of a life-threatening medical situation. One is not, however, required to take undue risks to personal safety, as such risks are both beyond the call of duty and may compromise the physician's ability to assist patients in the future.

Section IV: Recommendations

- Ultimately physicians are defined by their ability to save human life.
- Although strong arguments might be made for physicians to be treated like any other bystander, both their choice of profession and the unique nature of their abilities make it difficult to allow the withholding of essential services in the absence of a significant threat to personal wellbeing.
- Each physician should become familiar with the particular "Good Samaritan" legislation in his or her own locale, in order to best be able to conform to the standards of care and to enable one to receive statutory immunity.
- Physicians should also consider, when appropriate, suggestions from other professionals, and first-responders who may also be on scene.
- Hospitals and training programs should encourage periodic study and review of practical medical interventions in the field, as these interventions may differ significantly from a hospital-based physician's daily activities.

References

1. Tang LY. (1935) *My Country and My People*. New York, NY: John Day Press, p. 177.

2. Smith CM. (2005) Origin and uses of primum non nocere—above all, do no harm! *J Clin Pharmacol*. 45(4), 371–7.

3. Daniels S. (1999) Good samaritan acts. *Emerg Med Clin North Am*. 17(2), 491–504.

4. University of California San Diego. (n.d.) *Hippocratic Oath: Modern Version*. Available at: http://ethics. ucsd.edu/journal/2006/readings/Hippocratic_Oath_ Modern_Version.pdf. Accessed July 5, 2011.

5. World Medical Association. (n.d.) *WMA International Code of Medical Ethics*. Available at: www.wma.net/ en/30publications/10policies/c8. Accessed July 5, 2011.

6. Canadian Medical Association. (n.d.) *CMA Code of Ethics*. Available at: http://www.cma.ca/index.php/ci_ id/53556/la_id/1.htm. Accessed July 5, 2011.

7. American Medical Association. AMA's Code of Medical Ethics (6/01). Available at: www.ama-assn.org/ama/ pub/physician-resources/medical-ethics/code-medical-ethics.page. Accessed July 5, 2011.

8. Waguih WI, Lederer S, Mandili C, et al. (2009) Burnout during residency training: A literature review. *J Grad Med Educ*. 1(2), 236–42.

9. Veilleux DR. (2011) *Construction and Application of "Good Samaritan" Statutes*. 68 A.L.R. 4th 294.

10. Good Samaritan Laws—The Legal Placebo: A Current Analysis, 17 Akron L. Rev. 303 (1983).

11. Botte *v.* Pomeroy, 438 So.2d 544 Fla. App. D4 (1983).

12. Higgins *v.* Detroit Osteopathic Hospital Corp., 154 Mich. App. 752, 398 N.W.2d, 520 (1986).

13. Flynn *v.* United States, 681 F. Supp. 1500 (D Utah, 1988).

14. Colby *v.* Schwartz, 78 Cal. App. 3d 885, 144 Cal. Rptr. 624 (2nd Dist, 1978).

15. Vermont Good Samaritan Act, Duty to Aid the Endangered Act (Good Samaritan Law); Title 12, Chapter 2; SS 519.

16. Rosenbaum T. (2004) *The Myth of Moral Justice: Why Our Legal Systems Fail to Do What's Right*. New York, NY: Harper Collins, p. 247–8.

17. Rosenbaum T. (2004) *The Myth of Moral Justice: Why Our Legal Systems Fail to Do What's Right*. New York, NY: Harper Collins, p. 248.

18. *Laws* 1670, 6 Tammuz 5758 (June 30, 1998), p. 245.

19. American College of Emergency Physicians. (n.d.) *Code of Ethics for Emergency Physicians*. Available at: www.acep.org/content.aspx?id=29144. Accessed July 5, 2011.

23 Military objectives versus patient interests

Kenneth D. Marshall,[1] Kathryn L. Hall-Boyer[2]

[1]Resident Physician, Department of Emergency Medicine, Beth Israel Deaconess Medical Center, Boston, MA, USA
[2]CEP America, Attending Emergency Physician, Memorial Medical Center, Modesto, CA, and Colonel, Army Reserve (Retired), USA

Section I: Case presentation

A 25-year-old male detainee, shot in the right chest, arrives by Medevac helicopter to an Echelon II medical facility staffed with a forward surgical team. A search for weapons was done prior to the patient's arrival. Vital signs are blood pressure 90/50 mmHg, pulse 120 beats per minute, respiratory rate 24 breaths minutes, oxygen saturation 95% on a non-rebreather mask. No additional injuries were apparent. There were penetrating wounds to the right anterior and posterior chest above the nipple line. The breath sounds were diminished on the right. The remaining physical examination was normal. The patient was accompanied by an armed guard and a hospital interpreter was at the bedside. The patient stated, "Save me, save me, I'll tell you everything." A Medevac helicopter was expected to land in 2 more minutes bringing in two soldiers injured in the same firefight as the patient.

Section II: Discussion

Dr. Peter Rosen: I have just finished reading a biography of Mithridates, who was famous for capturing prisoners and testing poisons on them.[1] The attitudes towards medical care and the aid we bestow upon prisoners have been somewhat different in every war

that has ever been fought. In World War II, there were classic examples of field hospitals operating on all troops, whether or not they were enemy combatants. In contrast, there were also horrifying stories of treatment bestowed on the wounded enemy. This issue is one that each society is probably going to have to choose its own direction to follow. The situation resonates with the interaction of emergency medicine and civilian life because we often have to treat the perpetrators and victims of avoidable accidents or violent crimes simultaneously. For instance, drunk driving and gang warfare can raise ethical issues similar to this case. Can the Hippocratic Oath guide us?

Dr. Arthur Derse: The Hippocratic Oath stipulates no differentiation between a nobleman and slave, and obliges a physician to care for the sick no matter the station and no matter the position in society. The strict application of the Hippocratic duty to all patients under all circumstances is a fairly recent phenomenon, stimulated in part by the atrocities that occurred in World War II, when we learned that prisoners were used for ethically unjustifiable experimentation. In addition to the new emphasis on the Hippocratic duty, these events also led to the Nuremburg Code, which placed restrictions on the use of prisoners for experimentation.

PR: Do our military personnel receive any instructions as part of their training about how to interact

Ethical Problems in Emergency Medicine: A Discussion-Based Review, First Edition. John Jesus, Shamai A. Grossman, Arthur R. Derse, James G. Adams, Richard Wolfe, and Peter Rosen.
© 2012 John Wiley & Sons, Ltd. Published 2012 by John Wiley & Sons, Ltd.

with prisoners, and handle their medical needs? I was in the army from 1965 to 1968, and I do not remember the topic ever being raised.

Dr. Kathryn Hall Boyer: Before deployment, every physician soldier must take an online detainee medical care course. The military's teaching carries the same obligations stipulated in the Hippocratic Oath, namely, that all the patients receive the same medical care. Regardless of affiliation, we are obligated to treat all patients by their level of acuity. Military teaching also emphasizes that military physicians should not be involved in prisoner interrogation. Their treatment cannot be contingent on their cooperation or sharing of intelligence which they may or may not have.

PR: The military physician's role has not been the same throughout history, however. In the Austrian Empire, for example, Empress Maria Theresa passed a law that required prisoners to pass a medical examination before they could be tortured. Unlike her son Joseph, with whom she was co-regent, she was opposed to the abolition of torture.[2] Psychologically, it is useful to focus on being professional in your delivery of care, and the fact that there are other injured casualties on the way changes nothing. Military physicians are going to have to deal with shortages of supplies and resources regardless of the makeup of wounded patient affiliation. That said, we can't overlook the psychological stress of having to take care of someone who may have just killed a friend, or experience the multiple casualties of a car bombing when simultaneously attending to the medical needs of the perpetrator. It is important to have considered our own ethical values before we ever find ourselves in this situation. I'm happy to hear that since I've been in the military, there's a more coordinated educational process.

Dr. John Jesus: As every physician graduates from medical school, an oath is taken to care for anyone who comes through the hospital door regardless of station. As I understand it, when a physician joins the military, an oath must be taken to place the mission first, and to follow all legal orders from a commanding officer. This combination of obligations may set up a difficult situation for the military physician. It is also worth noting that military physicians are working under very stressful and potentially chaotic condi-

tions. When Henry Beecher wrote his article in '66 identifying a series of unethical or questionably ethical research studies conducted at premier institutions in the United States, he noticed that many, if not all, questionably ethical or unethical decisions made were made out of thoughtlessness or with a lack of consideration, rather than with a willful disregard for patients' rights. This notion negates the idea that we have to be bad people in order to make bad decisions. The situational stress on the battlefield, I would argue, may exacerbate this situation, and may lead to ethically unjustifiable decisions.

PR: There are many administrative decisions made by the army for the sake of the army rather than for the sake of an individual patient—for example, discharging a patient out of the service rather than treating a previously undisclosed chronic medical condition when a condition is finally discovered, perhaps to avoid the cost burden of managing a chronic disease. On the battlefield, triage has a different goal than in civilian practice. For instance, preferential treatment may be given to the less injured, in order to restore them to combat duty sooner.

KB: There are some differences in a soldier's right to privacy while in the military. Though military physicians undergo Health Insurance Portability and Accountability Act (HIPAA) training, some situations require a patient's commander to know a soldier's medical condition. If a soldier is HIV [human immunodeficiency virus] positive, for example, the commander must be notified, because that soldier can no longer deploy to theaters of operation, and must be transferred to a non-deployable unit. When I was deployed to Afghanistan, battlefield triage operated much like civilian multiple casualty incident triage. The patients labeled "red," or those who had immediate treatable conditions, were addressed first. There were some patients who were too sick or injured to manage with a reasonable expectation for survival within the environment of a battlefield emergency station. They were kept comfortable and labeled "expectant."

KB: Regarding our case, there may be limited resources and space to treat all patients arriving at the medical facility. I would suggest placing the chest tube, while readying oneself for the next group of wounded patients coming into the facility. To push a patient who happens to be an enemy combatant aside to make room for the other patients coming in would be an inappropriate and an unethical decision.

PR: Is there ever an appropriate non-objective utilization of resources? For example, some time ago when I was practicing in a small town in Wyoming, I received a patient with a self-inflicted gunshot wound to the head, and simultaneously four very gravely injured teenagers from an automobile crash. All five of the patients clearly needed blood, and needed it immediately. The blood bank at the rural hospital had two units of O negative blood available; any other blood had to be matched to type-specific call-in donors. I was faced with a man who attempted to commit suicide after killing his wife and her lover after he found the two together, side by side with four teenagers who had a rollover crash from poor weather conditions. Should the circumstances surrounding patients' injuries affect our clinical decision-making?

Dr. Shamai Grossman: The Talmud describes a classic scenario that may be instructive in our discussion of this case. In the story, two people have just enough water to allow one person to survive. Do you split the available resources, knowing that both people will die? Or do you give one person the whole bottle of water, and allow at least one person to survive? The Talmud goes through all sorts of discussions about qualities that might justify choosing one person over the other. Ultimately, the heavy argument may come down to recognizing that a decision that causes both people to die is clearly wrong. We do need to sometimes make those very hard life and death decisions that allow some to survive, knowing others will not. Applying this concept to the emergency department (ED) 1700 years later is still difficult. Situations that involve limited resources enabling the appropriate treatment to some patients, but not others, do exist. Clearly there is going to be some subjectivity when we are faced with two equally injured patients requiring the same resources. It's a situation we never want to have to face, because when we make these decisions we are "playing God." Some situations, however, require that we decide how to allocate resources in a way that we think will do the most good.

PR: In most decisions labeled "ethical dilemmas," information exists that can make the decision more

clear. In the case that I cited involving the patient who attempted to commit suicide and the four injured teenagers, I did not experience any difficulty in making the decision to withhold blood from the patient who attempted to commit suicide, because I didn't believe he would have survived even if he had received blood. I didn't want to waste the resource on someone who probably wouldn't survive when I might have been able to save one of the teenagers. It's human nature to use every piece of data that we can find to help make these difficult choices. The alternative is to do precisely what the Talmud argues: treat everybody with justice and have no one survive. When push comes to shove, during a war we're going to use criteria in our decision-making that is subjective, and perhaps not always ethically defensible. I, for one, would probably not hesitate to use my resources for my troops first. Others might feel that one should treat patients on a first come, first served basis. What would other people do in this situation?

JJ: My honest answer is to admit that I don't know what I would do. This scenario is a very difficult scenario that I have not yet experienced, and I wouldn't presume to know how I would act. That said, I do have a few considerations that may guide military physicians in similar decisions. There are sources of authority that military personnel can use to guide them through military ethical issues, including the Geneva convention. Within the Geneva Convention, it is mandated that **military physicians prioritize treatment to the most severely injured casualties**; it prohibits any threatening or demeaning treatment of prisoners of war, and **requires that military physicians disobey any unlawful orders**. There is an apparent trend toward the separation of military objectives and the obligations of a physician.

Medical ethics, however, generally do not label any one rule or principle as absolute. The principles of medical ethics are prima facie obligations such that each of them should be followed unless an equally important competing principle outweighs it in the pursuit of the greatest balance of right over wrong. We already have certain exceptions for societal interests that take precedence over individual interests. One example is the reporting of sexually transmitted infections and communicable diseases with potential societal impact to the Department of Public Health or the Centers for Disease Control. If we have deemed societal interests to be more important than individual interests in a civilian setting when larger societal interests are at stake, is it necessarily unethical to include military objectives in medical decision-making when we are forced to allocate limited life-saving resources?

PR: I understand your reluctance. The confusion this very question produces is going to recur in medical practice if you haven't spent some time trying to organize your ethical approach to these difficult decisions. It is important to avoid ethical paralysis when a medical decision needs to be made under time constraints. I don't think that there is a right answer to every ethical question. I do think that the more prepared you are to make difficult decisions, whether or not anyone else agrees with your choice, the quicker you'll make them, and the more comfortable you'll feel having made them.

AD: The military has paid more attention to this issue, and is more familiar with the difficulty of the situation of treating a patient whom one does not feel is worthy of treatment. I'm not aware of a specific educational objective focused on instilling in our residents a non-judgmental attitude, and the expectation that sometimes they have to treat patients whom they feel are not worthy of optimal treatment. It is worthwhile for emergency physicians to think about this issue.

PR: Part of our education of residents has to include attitudes towards patients; I've noticed every year, one or more residents becoming depressed by the reality that many patients we care for are not likeable human beings. It leaves the emergency physician often feeling that their chosen career is life wasting; that he has spent many years trying to develop the tools and skills with which to help people, and is rewarded with another alcoholic drug-crazed individual who will not use any of the gifts of health that are being bestowed by the good care of the physician. We have to learn how to withhold judgment, so that we can still care for these difficult patients. There is an educational role that is ongoing with many residents who should understand that their discontent with emergency medicine is predicated on assuming responsibility for what happens after you take care of the patient. Just because I treat an alcoholic who goes from the ED to the nearest bar to get drunk again, does not mean I have failed the patient.

SG: The question is whether we really want to accept those answers as solutions. It is our human nature that we must struggle with our feelings about patient care. I cannot be the judge. I cannot be the jury. All I can be is the physician whom I have been trained to be: that is to treat patients and provide the best care possible to every patient as they come through my door. We must sometimes distance ourselves from patients' personalities and qualities to provide care. That's perhaps the most trying element of the practice of emergency medicine, and makes practicing in the military setting even more trying.

PR: There are a couple of recommendations we can make. The first is, to focus on how the integrity of the profession can mitigate your individual feelings for a patient. For example, I'm willing to treat patients I abhor, and give my utmost to see that they receive the best treatment because I feel I owe it to my profession. I do not want to live in a society in which people are not able to have access to the services of a physician unless they happen to be a member of the right party, or unless they happen to have the right amount of money, or unless they happen to have the right skin color. Avoiding this situation is more important than giving in to my human feelings of dislike for certain patients.

Where possible, accept and acknowledge that you are having these feelings, and see if you can find a colleague who will take over for you. I remember a young man in a trauma bay who came in with a gunshot wound to the abdomen. He had a swastika tattooed on the center of his forehead, and when I came in to start his assessment, he looked at me and he said, "No fucking Jew is going to take care of me." In order to avoid allowing my anger to affect the care I would have given the patient, I passed the case onto the resident and supervised the resuscitation more in the background to avoid confrontation with the patient.

My second observation is that military medicine is different from civilian medicine, whether we want it to be or not. Moreover that is a stress on the military physician who comes from the civilian sector. For example, in World War I, venereal disease was not considered a service-connected disability, and therefore could not be treated by army physicians. But after the advent of penicillin, venereal disease was just another infectious disease to be treated. I think the army changes its attitudes towards disease sometimes in ways that don't seem to have any logic. These decisions often seem to be predicated upon how the service will minimize spending in caring for the patient. It can be very frustrating, and though it hasn't necessarily altered the ethics of the individual physician, it certainly alters the realities under which they are forced to practice.

KB: Today, military personnel continue to receive the medical care they need. There are times, however, when commanders can make it difficult for soldiers or sailors to receive medical care by making it hard to miss duty. In the past, I have known situations in which physicians had to explain to commanders more about soldiers' medical conditions in order for them to understand the extent of their medical needs. In general, one cannot discharge someone from their position very easily, unless they're within the first 6 months of their enlistment. If the army discovers an undisclosed, preexisting condition within the first 6 months of service, the soldier or member of the medical personnel may be discharged immediately as an act of fraudulent enlistment. The military emphasizes that military physicians ought to treat enemy combatant patients humanely, because how we treat them may have an effect on how our captured soldiers are treated. If the word gets out that we take good care of all patients regardless of affiliation, we hope that our soldiers are treated similarly.

PR: I think the best reason for treating all patients regardless of affiliation was articulated by Plato some 2000 years ago in *The Republic*. He says that the reason to be good is not because it will win you success, it's not because there are laws that mandate it, and you don't want to fall afoul of the law; it's because you have to protect your own soul. The reason to take good care of patients is not only in the hope that this kind of behavior will be generalized, but because, if you don't, your soul will suffer.[3,4]

Section III: Review of the literature

This case represents a unique challenge that emergency physicians in military service may face: when

one's moral obligations as a physician conflict, or appear to conflict, with one's military obligations. This review explores the nature of such conflicts, and discusses how an emergency physician can approach them. We first set the stage by explaining from a philosophical point of view how these potential conflicts arise, and then discussing the role-specific obligations of military ethics, as well as medical ethics, and the various attempts to reconcile the two. We then describe specific types of conflicts that emergency medicine physicians in particular may face as they strive to discharge their duties both as physicians and members of the military. In the course of these discussions, we will give recommendations about how physicians in these dual roles can think about approaching such situations.

Different roles, different duties

When military duties conflict with the duties of medicine, it presents a dilemma that can be especially difficult for physicians to resolve. The source of the conflict stems from two unique sources of moral demands: the special moral obligations binding physicians, and the demands and obligations of serving in the military. Military ethics are the principles and duties necessary to guide behavior in a context radically divergent from everyday life. The purpose of the military is to subdue one's enemy by whatever means available, which often means seeking to injure or kill other human beings. In order to maintain moral orientation in this unique milieu, concepts such as honor, loyalty, and submission of one's autonomy to authority become key for the soldier. The ethics of medicine on the other hand gets its impetus from the physician–patient relationship. Patients approach physicians from a position of vulnerability: they entrust physicians with personal information and with control of their medical welfare, and must rely on physicians to act in their best interest. Society likewise depends on the expertise of physicians, and authorizes the training and privileges given to them in exchange for work on behalf of patients. Following the Hippocratic tradition, physicians are thought to have several special duties: they must work primarily for their patients' interests rather than focusing on their own interests. They must attend to the demands of justice in practice. Finally, they must respect the autonomy of their patients. Even in this brief discussion, the possibility of conflict is obvious. Interests of a prisoner or soldier may not coincide with those of the mission or fighting force. In such situations, a physician may be forced to choose between acting in the interests of the patient and the military under which he or she serves.

Before moving on to specific types of ethical conflict, it is worth noting that organizing wartime medical operations differently than they are today might avoid some of these conflicts altogether. Today, battlefield physicians serve under the command of militaries: they are supported by, owe allegiance to, and are bound by the (legal) orders of the military. However, this is a contingent historical fact—wartime medicine could be practiced by neutral third parties only. Such an approach was discussed in the early Geneva conventions 150 years ago, but rejected on practical grounds, yet some physicians advocate for this arrangement today.[5] This different structure would free the physician from an oath or obligation to any military force, thus largely dissolving the conflict between one's duties as a physician and soldier. However, for the foreseeable future, physicians will continue to serve as medical officers in military hierarchies, and so will potentially face the kinds of ethical conflicts to which we now turn.

Physician roles in torture and interrogation

We now move to several scenarios that could present a moral dilemma to the emergency physician serving in a military setting. The set of scenarios discussed are by no means exhaustive, but they are illustrative of the types of difficult decision which an emergency physician serving in the military may face.

The first of these scenarios involves physician involvement in interrogation or torture of prisoners of war, of which history provides numerous examples. Here we deal with three basic related situations: (1) the physician is ordered to use a medical expertise in devising, supervising, or practicing interrogation or torture; (2) the physician suspects torture based on the examination of the patient, or other interaction with someone under the physician's care; and (3) the physician is asked to clear a detainee for participation.

Consider then the situation in which a physician is ordered to participate in torture. The case of military commanders ordering physicians to participate in torture of prisoners sadly had ample precedent, from the notorious behavior of physicians in Nazi Germany to Uruguayan physicians exercising torture during the dictatorship of the 1970s.[6,7] The ethical response to such a case should be straightforward; however wide its practice among modern thinkers, torture is virtually universally condemned as immoral. This moral judgment is reinforced in documents such as the third and fourth Geneva conventions, the World Medical Association Declaration of Tokyo, and the United Nations *Convention Against Torture*. It is expressed and given legal force in the eighth amendment to the US Constitution.[8-10] Thus, any order to perform torture (whether to a layperson, and doubly so to a physician) is immoral, and should not be followed.

Related to this strong moral argument against physician involvement in torture is the duty of physicians to report suspicion of torture or mistreatment of those under their care. Of course, as a corollary to the moral proscription against torture, all persons have a duty to avoid complicity with acts of torture, and thus to take steps to prevent or report it. Moreover, the Geneva conventions and US military training require prisoners of war and detainees be given regular physical examinations by medical personnel, and specifically require physicians to report abuse.[11] Discharging this obligation will generally require great courage and dedication on the part of the military physician, as reporting or trying to prevent what is believed to be abuse may involve substantial personal or professional risks. The example of American physicians failing to report signs of abuse among the prisoners at Abu Ghraib (such as cuts, bruises, bruised genitals, and patients collapsed from exhaustion or abuse) is a sobering reminder that the obstacles to fulfilling this duty are not always overcome.[12] Moreover, the moral vision required to see that one has a duty to report potential abuse or to disobey an order will first depend on whether a physician can identify torture when it is discovered, as whether a given case constitutes torture often may be difficult for a physician to discern.

However, even if it is unclear whether an order, if carried out, would be an instance of torture, such an order would likely at minimum require the physician to be participating in interrogation or punishment. Such participation has caused controversy in recent years in the United States, for instance in the case of American physicians leaving records open to aid interrogators in devising interrogation strategies at

Guantanamo Bay, and more controversially still, American physicians and medics overseeing interrogations at Abu Ghraib.[13-16] These types of situation require more nuanced analysis. It should be noted at the outset that there is a strong presumption against direct physician participation in such activities.

The theoretical argument against participation in interrogation comes from the physician's duties of fidelity: because the doctor–patient relationship is founded on trust, the physician must function as a trustee for the patient's medical welfare. There is agreement by thinkers from diverse theoretical perspectives that by overseeing or otherwise participating in interrogation, the physician no longer prioritizes the patient's wellbeing, and instead gives primacy to societal or institutional obligations.[17,18] Further, even if the physician strives to keep the detainee's interest foremost, the detainee is unlikely to trust the physician who is participating in interrogations, preventing the flow of communication necessary to have a beneficial clinical relationship.

Against this line of thought, other commentators have argued for a role for physicians in interrogations. According to this position, when a physician takes on a role of an interrogator, he or she is acting primarily as combatant rather than physician.[15] The thought here is that the Hippocratic ethic of dedication to patient wellbeing applies only to physicians who are serving clinical functions, so that if physicians use their medical training to fulfill other societal functions, there is no imperative to hold the patient's wellbeing above other values.

However, a strong consensus has developed against this line of thinking. As Bloche and Marks argue, "the proposition that doctors who serve these social purposes don't act as physicians is self-contradictory. Their 'physicianhood'—encompassing technical skill, scientific understanding, a caring ethos, and cultural authority—is the reason they are called on to assume these roles."[15] This counterargument enjoys wide assent. Physicians remain bound by the ethics of medicine even when not serving in primarily extra-clinical capacities. There is substantial agreement that physician involvement in interrogation is acceptable only in quite restricted advisory roles.[19-21] Given these more theoretical considerations, it is unsurprising to find that codes of medical ethics firmly limit physician involvement in interrogation. In 2008, the American Medical Association reinforced its position on this

issue in the member code of ethics, saying "Physicians must neither conduct nor directly participate in an interrogation, because a role as physician-interrogator undermines the physician's role as healer and thereby erodes trust in the individual physician-interrogator and in the medical profession."[22] These considerations of medical ethics generally are reinforced by the special role accorded to healthcare personnel by the laws of war. As codified in the Geneva conventions, medical personnel are distinguished explicitly from those in combatant roles: they are given certain protections, but must fulfill a number of obligations as well.[23] Sidel and Levy give a helpful summary:[24]

• Regarded as "noncombatants," medical personnel are forbidden to engage in or be parties to acts of war.
• The wounded and sick soldier and civilian—friend and foe—must be respected, protected, treated humanely, and cared for by the belligerents.
• The wounded and sick must not be left without medical assistance, and the order of their treatment must be based on the urgency of their medical needs.
• Medical aid must be dispensed solely on medical grounds, "without any adverse distinction founded on sex, race, nationality, religion, political opinions, or any other similar criteria."
• Medical personnel shall exercise no physical or moral coercion against protected persons (civilians), in particular to obtain information from them or from third parties.

Thus, physicians serving medical roles in wartime are forbidden from acting in roles that could be construed as combatant roles, and are also not to exercise "physical or moral coercion" against detainees. Abiding by these conventions of war is near universally regarded as a reciprocal moral obligation among nations, and thus their proscription on physician behavior is another layer of moral argument against physicians playing an active role in interrogations. Consistent with these considerations, the training manual for wartime medicine produced for military healthcare personnel states that: "Healthcare providers charged with the care of internees should not be actively involved in interrogation, advise interrogators how to conduct interrogations, or interpret individual medical records/medical data for the purposes of interrogation or intelligence gathering."[25]

One role in which physicians' expertise may be used, however, is in screening prisoners for participation in interrogation. As mentioned before, detainees held by a warring army have the right to a medical entrance screening examination. As part of this care, physicians may communicate to their commanders whether or nor a detainee is physically capable of undergoing interrogation safely, much as emergency physicians provide input on work restrictions in the civilian sector. That is, the physician may play a protective role, preventing the prisoner from undergoing interrogation if it would be medically dangerous to the prisoner. In this role, the physician is using his or her expertise to work for the detainee's interests, while also providing information useful to the forces under which they serve.

Triage scenarios

Triage is a morally loaded concept in medicine with which emergency medicine physicians are particularly familiar. In the military setting, the moral strains involved in its appropriate application can be more acute. Adapted from the French term meaning "sort into three groups," triage in the medical arena is prioritization according to medical need in the setting of limited resources. As it pertains to emergency situations, triage is the temporal prioritization of patients according to the urgency of their medical needs in order to derive the greatest medical benefit possible from the resources at hand. This driving principle applies whether the resources are being split among the more and less urgent cases in an ED, a mass casualty incident, or in wartime. The specific priorities shift in response to the balance of resources, patients in need of treatment, and acuity of injury.

As in civilian mass casualty incidents, triage of patients under battle conditions sometimes requires a different model than that at relatively resource-rich medical facilities in the industrialized world. As outlined in *Emergency War Surgery*, wartime triage divides patients into three major groups (some of which are further subdivided; the discussion here is excerpted for brevity)[25]:

• **Emergent:** This group of wounded will require attention within minutes to several hours of arriving at the point of care to avoid death or major disability.

• **Non-emergent:** This is the group of patients that, although injured and may require surgery, does not require the attention of the emergent group, and lacks

significant potential for loss of life, limb, or eyesight.

• **Expectant:** This group of wounded, given the situation and resource constraints, would be considered unsalvageable.

The primary difference between this model and that practiced at civilian centers is the addition of the "expectant" category. As explained in the previous edition of the same textbook, "Casualties in the expectant category have wounds that are so extensive that even if they were the sole casualty, and had the benefit of optimal medical resource application, their survival still would be very unlikely."[26] In the resource-rich environment of civilian medical centers, patients meeting these criteria may be treated quite aggressively since this can be done without substantial negative impact on other patients' treatment. When resources are more limited, pursuing aggressive treatment for one patient who is very unlikely to benefit comes at an expense. Other patients with emergent but more likely reversible needs may deteriorate or die for want of the resources dedicated to the irreversibly injured patient. This fact is why situation-responsive models of triage are required.

Military physicians utilize three different models of triage depending on battlefield conditions, as explained in Beam's discussion of battlefield ethics: those of non-austere, austere, and extreme conditions.[27] Triage in non-austere conditions functions like that in civilian centers' everyday operations; treatment priority is dictated by acuity, and full treatment is pursued within the limits of patient autonomy and physician judgment of efficacy. In austere conditions, when resources are more limited, the focus changes to saving as many lives as possible within constraints of available resources. Priority will be a blended determination of acuity and likelihood of survival. In austere conditions, some patients with a very small but non-zero chance of survival will receive aid and comfort, but not resuscitative measures. Finally, Beam points to the possibility of extreme conditions, in which the forces to which the physician belongs are being overrun, and in which the availability of each individual soldier may be determinative of the success of the campaign. In such situations, he argues that physicians may justifiably adopt a triage model in which patients with non-life-threatening injuries who might quickly be returned to the fighting force should be treated first, with all other patients assigned priority according to austere-conditions model. Several aspects of these models of triage may raise ethical qualms for the physician. A general worry will be discussed, followed by two concerns specific to military medicine: the problem of what to do with enemy combatants or civilians, and whether Beam's extreme conditions model is appropriate.

The general concern is, given the Hippocratic ideal of focusing exclusively on the benefit of one's patient, whether a physician may ever withhold resources from one patient to serve the interests of another. Given the wide practice of triage in EDs and in other areas, a consensus clearly exists that this practice is morally sound, but it is helpful to remember why this is so. In the context of emergency or battlefield medicine, in which multiple patients present requiring treatment, the ethical ideal of physician fidelity to the interest of a single patient is inapt. In such situations, the physician or healthcare team has a duty to focus on the medical wellbeing of all the patients, and so fidelity to the interest of individual patients is superseded by fidelity to the goods of medicine and the interest of all patients needing attention.[28] There is nothing, in principle, objectionable to the practice of prioritizing patients in such situations.

However, triage must occur within certain constraints. First, as mentioned, the medical wellbeing of patients must be the primary concern of the healthcare team. Second, priority of treatment should be according to medical need, not morally irrelevant institutional or social concerns.[29,30] This has been a hallmark of battlefield triage since its inception; the originator of triage, Napoleon's chief surgeon Dominique Jean Larrey, developed the triage model that treated soldiers according to medical need, "without regard to rank or distinction."[31] Nonetheless, when military physicians serve under the auspices and command of one of the warring armies, knowing that the soldiers under the same command are striving at great risk to wound or kill the enemy, they may feel compelled to give greater priority to their own wounded, rather than enemy combatants or civilians.

This is the situation in the case that opens this chapter. From a medical perspective, there is no question about the right course of action. According to Beam's classification, this is an austere environment, and the patient's most serious problem is a quickly fatal as well as quickly reversible medical condition.

The only reason not to intervene is the fact that this is an enemy combatant; so the question is, under even austere conditions of war, should enemy combatants have the same priority as a friendly soldier? Historically, the answer was not always thought to be yes. As Swan and Swan note, "traditionally US combat casualty care has been directed towards US casualties first, allies second, civilians third, and the enemy fourth."[32]

This kind of thinking, however, is a moral tragedy. In adopting this approach, the physician abandons the ethical demands of medicine in favor of military objectives. Moreover, the special role reserved for medical units in the ethics and law of war is ignored. This position has been argued by a number of physicians and ethicists, and reinforced by international committees and treaties. In the almost 150 years since the first convention of Geneva, international consensus has consistently reaffirmed that in time of war, a physician must treat patients according to acuity only, ignoring considerations of military or political affiliation, race, nationality, or the like. Such affirmations appear in the first Geneva treaty, the World Medical Association "Declaration of Geneva," and "Regulations in Time of Armed Conflict", and the "Red Cross fundamental rules of international humanitarian law applicable in armed conflicts."[33–36] Moreover, this order of priorities is taught in US military training manuals as the appropriate approach to triage.[21] Thus, in the opening case, the clear moral duty of the physician is to treat the enemy soldier, and this would be the case even if a group of less or equally seriously injured friendly soldiers were also present.

Despite this forceful conclusion, a question remains as to whether battlefield conditions may become so dire that exceptions to this moral imperative exist. Some authors believe, as Beam, Howe, and others argue, that in the most extreme circumstances, exceptions are necessary.[37,38] Others, such as Sidel and Levy, argue that the moral conflict between military goals and the aims of medicine in such cases are irresolvable, and hence demonstrate why physicians should serve in a wholly neutral capacity rather than under the command of a warring army.[24] One such case taken to be a paradigm is discussed by Beecher: in the North African theater of World War II, a very small shipment of the then new wonder drug, penicillin, arrived in the hospitals that were overcrowded with soldiers, some wounded in battle, some also "wounded in brothels" suffering from venereal disease. There was a critical shortage of manpower on the front lines, and soldiers suffering from venereal disease could more easily be returned to battle if treated. As a result, the penicillin was given to the soldiers with venereal disease despite limited availability of the medication. Beecher concludes, "In terms of customary morality, a great injustice was done; in view of the circumstances, I believe that the course chosen was the proper one."[39]

Non-military crisis situations suggest that despite the strong moral force of triage only according to medical need, there are some situations in which extra-medical considerations give moral justification to deviate from typical triage priority. For instance, in natural or human-made disasters or disease outbreaks, it would be justifiable to treat or inoculate healthcare providers first if they could then aid in relief to others. Similarly, if a disaster was to occur at sea, it might be legitimate to treat a subset of crew members whose good health and function are necessary to reach or summon aid. In such situations, non-medical qualities become nonetheless morally relevant, and can be justifiably considered in making triage decisions.[29]

The challenge for the physician is to determine what features meet this criterion of moral relevance. The ideal of military medicine, both as discussed by bioethicists and reified in international law, is to practice medicine from the vantage of neutrality with respect to the particular biases, interests, and claims of the warring parties. Thus, the criterion the physician should use to discern whether there is reason to give weight to extra-medical considerations in making triage decisions is whether a physician without allegiances of nationality, brotherhood, or self-interest would give weight to the extra-medical considerations. According to this approach, "military necessity," "success of the mission," or commands of superiors would not *by themselves* provide sufficient reason for deviating from typical austere-conditions triage.

Rather, the physician will have a number of factors in mind: whether and how much the deviation in question will harm those whose treatment will be changed or delayed as a result, whether the exception in question will truly make a decisive contribution to the campaign that might outweigh the harm caused to the aggrieved, and also whether the campaign is

itself just and aimed at morally worthy versus morally suspect ends. This does not imply that the physician must adopt a "view from nowhere," attempting to make a decision without appeal to settled values or principles. However, the idea is to abstract away from goals of pure material or national self-interest or morally incidental allegiance.

This approach does place a remarkable epistemic burden on the physician, and making the fine theoretical and empirical judgments required for a decision may easily outstrip the physician's intellectual resources in times of true crisis. In such situations, if the physician believes that the command which is being served under is just, and if one trusts the commander's assessment of the need to deviate from typical rules of triage, the orders of command may be used as a guiding heuristic. On the other hand, a physician may also question the moral judgment of command, in which case the orders of command might not be a compelling reason.

Where does this leave Beecher's famous case of penicillin rationing: was the distribution morally correct? The answer is that it depends on details that his account leaves unspecified. He does not say what ultimately happened to the soldiers who did not receive penicillin, and we do not know precisely how thin were the margins of victory, or if a different distribution of medicine would have had a material impact on the war. It takes little imagination to conceive of circumstances under which such use of resources would have been either justifiable or not. Such complex situations make general rules or pronouncements of little value. Here, as in so many circumstances in medicine, the physician must take the limited information that is available, and using moral sense and clinical judgment, strive to make the best decision possible.

Section IV: Recommendations

• Recent studies demonstrate a substandard understanding of the Geneva conventions by medical students, and there is some evidence that even US military medical personnel have not internalized the conventions' requirements.[40,41] Physicians should receive more instruction on the requirements of international law and military physicians should receive even more comprehensive training on this topic.

- The ideal of military medicine as presented in international treaties governing the conduct of war points toward an ethics of neutrality as undergirding military medical practice. Military physicians should acknowledge this and come to terms with their own biases and loyalties, which may interfere with delivering care to those about whom they are ambivalent or whom they consider enemies.
- Military ethics emphasizes the importance of submission to legal authorities, not authority per se.[42] Physicians should understand the difference and be prepared to ignore or reject orders inconsistent with the laws of war.

References

1. Mayor A. (2010) *The Poison King: The Life and Legend of Mithradates Rome's Deadliest Enemy*. Princeton, NJ: Princeton University Press.
2. Kann RA (1980) *A History of the Habsburg Empire, 1526–1918*. Berkeley, CA: University of California Press.
3. Bloom A. (1968) *The Republic of Plato. Translated with Notes and an Interpretive Essay*. New York, NY: Basic Books.
4. Hamilton E, Huntington C. (eds) (1961) *The Collected Dialogues of Plato*. New York, NY: Pantheon. Princeton University Press, p. 71.
5. Howe EG. (2003) Point/counterpoint: A response to Drs. Sidel and Levy. In: Beam TE, Sparacino LR. (eds) *Military Medical Ethics*. Washington, DC: Office of the Surgeon General, Department of the Army, and Borden Institute, pp. 312–20.
6. Lifton RJ. (1986) *The Nazi Doctors: Medical Killing and the Psychology of Genocide*. New York, NY: Basic Books.
7. Bloche MG. (1986) Uruguay's military physicians: Cogs in a system of state terror. *JAMA*. 225, 2788–93.
8. International Committee of the Red Cross (ICRC). (1949) *Geneva Convention Relative to the Treatment of Prisoners of War (Third Geneva Convention)*, 12 August 1949, 75 UNTS 135.
9. World Medical Association. (1975) *Declaration of Tokyo*. Adopted by the World Medical Association, Tokyo, Japan. October 1975.
10. UN General Assembly. (1984) *Convention Against Torture and Other Cruel, Inhuman or Degrading Treatment or Punishment*. United Nations, Treaty Series, vol. 1465, p. 85.
11. Lounsbury DE, Brengman M, Bellamy RF. (2004) *Emergency War Surgery*. Third United States revision of the emergency war surgery NATO Handbook. Washington DC: US Department of Defense, pp. 34.4–34.8.
12. Zernike K. (2004) Only a few spoke up on abuse as many soldiers stayed silent. *New York Times*. May 22, A1.
13. Slevin P, Stephens J. (2004) Detainees' medical files shared: Guantanamo interrogators' access criticized. *Washington Post*. June 10, A1.
14. Lewis NA. (2004) Red Cross finds detainee abuse in Guantanamo. *New York Times*. November 30, A1.
15. Bloche MG, Marks JH. (2005) When doctors go to war. *N Engl J Med*. 352, 3–6.
16. Miles SH. (2004) Abu Ghraib: Its legacy for military medicine. *Lancet*. 364, 725–9.
17. Pellegrino EP. (2003) The moral foundations of the patient-physician relationship: The essence of medical ethics. In: Beam TE, Sparacino LR. (eds) *Military Medical Ethics*. Washington, DC: Office of the Surgeon General, Department of the Army, and Borden Institute, pp. 3–21.
18. Beauchamp TL, Childress JF. (2001) *Principles of Biomedical Ethics*. New York, NY: Oxford University Press, pp. 312–19.
19. Annas, GJ. (2008) Military medical ethics—physician first, last, always. *N Engl J Med*. 359, 1087–90.
20. Stotland NL, Heyman JM. (2008) Correspondence: Military medical ethics. *N Engl J Med*. 359, 2728–9.
21. Levine MA. (2007) Role of physicians in interrogations. *Virtual Mentor*. 9, 709–11.
22. American Medical Association. (2008) *Opinion 2.068 Physician Participation in Interrogation. Code of Medical Ethics 2008–2009 Edition*. Chicago, IL: American Medical Association, pp. 30–1.
23. Vollmar LC. (2003) Military medicine in war: the Geneva Conventions today. In: Beam TE, Sparacino LR. (eds) *Military Medical Ethics*. Washington, DC: Office of the Surgeon General, Department of the Army, and Borden Institute.
24. Sidel VW, Levy BS. (2003) Physician soldier: A moral dilemma? In: Beam TE, Sparacino LR. (eds) *Military Medical Ethics*. Washington, DC: Office of the Surgeon General, Department of the Army, and Borden Institute.
25. Lounsbury DE, Brengman M, Bellamy RF. (2004) *Emergency War Surgery*. Third United States revision of the emergency war surgery NATO Handbook. Washington, DC: US Department of Defense, pp. 3.1–3.17, 34.4.
26. Bowen TE, Bellamy RF. (1988) *Emergency War Surgery*. Second United States revision of the emergency war surgery NATO Handbook. Washington, DC: US Department of Defense, pp. 184–6.
27. Beam TE. (2003) Medical ethics on the battlefield: the crucible of military ethics. In: Beam TE, Sparacino LR.

(eds) *Military Medical Ethics*. Washington, DC: Office of the Surgeon General, Department of the Army, and Borden Institute.

28. Moskop JC, Iserson KV. (2007) Triage in medicine, Part II: Underlying values and principles. *Ann Emerg Med.* 49, 282–7.

29. Beauchamp TL, Childress JF. (2001) *Principles of Biomedical Ethics*. New York, NY: Oxford University Press, pp. 270–2.

30. Baker R, Strosberg M. (1992) Triage and equality: An historical reassessment of utilitarian analyses of triage. *Kennedy Inst Ethics J.* 2, 102–23.

31. Moskop JC, Iserson KV. (2007) Triage in medicine, Part II: Concept, history, and types. *Ann Emerg Med.* 49, 275–81.

32. Swan KG, Swan KG Jr. (1996) Triage: the past revisited. *Mil Med.* 161, 448–52.

33. International Committee of the Red Cross. (1864) Convention for the amelioration of the condition of the wounded in armies in the field. Geneva: 35. International Committee of the Red Cross. Available at: www.icrc.org/ihl.nsf/FULL/120?OpenDocument. Accessed December 23, 2011.

34. World Medical Association. (n.d.) WMA declaration of Geneva. Available at: www.wma.net/en/30publications/10policies/g1/. Accessed December 23, 2011.

35. World Medical Association. (n.d.) WMA regulations in times of armed conflict. Available at: www.wma.net/en/30publications/10policies/a20/. Accessed December 23, 2011.

36. Red Cross fundamental rules of international humanitarian law applicable in armed conflicts. (1978) In: Roberts A, Guelff R. (eds) *Documents on the Laws of War*, 2nd ed. Oxford: Clarendon Press.

37. Madden W, Carter BS. (2003) Physician-soldier: A moral profession. In: Beam TE, Sparacino LR. (eds) *Military Medical Ethics*. Washington, DC: Office of the Surgeon General, Department of the Army, and Borden Institute.

38. Beam TE, Howe EG. (2003) A proposed ethic for military medicine. In: Beam TE, Sparacino LR. (eds) *Military Medical Ethics*. Washington, DC: Office of the Surgeon General, Department of the Army, and Borden Institute.

39. Beecher, H. (1970) *Research and the Individual*. Boston, MA: Little Brown and Company.

40. Boyd JW, Himmelstein DU, Lasser K, et al. (2007) US medical students' knowledge about the military draft, the Geneva Conventions, and military medical ethics. *Int J Health Serv.* 37, 643–50.

41. Carter BS. (1994) Ethical concerns for physicians deployed to Operation Desert Storm. *Mil Med.* 159, 55–9.

42. Kirkland FR. (2003) Honor, combat ethics, and military culture. In: Beam TE, Sparacino LR. (eds) *Military Medical Ethics*. Washington, DC: Office of the Surgeon General, Department of the Army, and Borden Institute.

Public health as emergency medicine

SECTION SIX

Public health as emergency medicine

24 Treatment of potential organ donors

Glen E. Michael,[1] *John Jesus*[2]

[1]*Assistant Professor of Emergency Medicine, University of Virginia, Charlottesville, VA, USA*

[2]*Chief Resident, Department of Emergency Medicine, Beth Israel Deaconess Medical Center, Boston, MA, and Clinical Instructor, Department of Emergency Medicine, Christiana Care Health System, Newark, DE, USA*

Section I: Case presentation

A 22-year-old man was brought to the emergency department (ED) by ambulance after suffering a gunshot wound to the head. The patient was intubated by paramedics in the field, without the need for any sedative or paralytic medications. On arrival he had a Glasgow Coma Scale (GCS) score of 3 with fixed and dilated pupils. The examination and imaging studies showed the bullet crossing the midline, and strongly indicated that the patient's life was not salvageable, and therefore evaluation for brain death was initiated. Meanwhile, the patient became profoundly bradycardic, and a continuous infusion of norepinephrine was started to increase the patient's heart rate and maintain adequate blood pressure. The patient's driver's license indicated that he had previously consented to be included in the state's organ donor registry.

Section II: Discussion

Dr. John Jesus: In 2009, 28 000 transplants were performed while there were over 100 000 people waiting for organs, leaving a 70 000-person gap. Every year that gap continues to grow. This issue has also been heavily addressed in popular culture. Two major motion films, *John Q* and *Seven Pounds*, have high-

lighted organ transplantation and dramatized the topic. Finally, the *Washington Post* published an article on March 15, 2010, detailing a study underway in Pittsburgh, in which federal funds were to be used to rapidly identify patients whom doctors were unable to save, and take steps to preserve their organs so that a transplant team could quickly retrieve them.[1] Given this context, is addressing the care of potential organ donors in the ED an appropriate focus for the emergency physician?

Dr. Glen Michael: Generally, we tend to think of the task of referring patients for potential organ donation as being the job of critical care specialists in the intensive care unit (ICU), but data suggest that this need not be the case. In my recent study, I report that when patients are referred from the ED for potential donation, they are more likely to become successful organ donors than patients referred from the ICU. There are several reasons for this. Patients in the ED are often early in the course of their illness, which means there are fewer complications that could compromise the patient's organs, such as multisystem organ failure, ventilator-associated pneumonias, or sepsis. Interestingly, families are just as likely to consent to donation when the referral is made from the ED as when it is made from the ICU. These findings suggest that the ED is an ideal place to begin thinking about organ donation.

Dr. Arthur Derse: Another important set of questions relates to how a patient's wishes are carried out in the ED based on the wishes of the family. For instance, that *Washington Post* article raised concerns about how organ harvesting can raise suspicion in the family even if a patient had registered themselves as an organ donor.[1] The Uniform Anatomical Gift Act says that no one has the right to revoke an individual's anatomical gift except in cases where the deceased patient is an emancipated minor. Legally speaking, it is acceptable to harvest a patient's organs if that is in accordance with the patient's documented wishes even if this is in conflict with the wishes of the family. Even though the law allows it, few organ procurement organizations and transplant surgeons ever go against the wishes of the family due to concerns about how that would affect subsequent donations. The concern is that if an entire community is upset that organs are retrieved against explicit wishes, that experience might ultimately decrease the number of future donations.

GM: What other conflicts need to be considered regarding potential organ donors?

AD: One important distinction to consider is the difference between brain death and cardiovascular death, and how this can complicate clinical and ethical scenarios. Brain death is the newer concept; for years organs could not be taken from "live patients" because it would violate the "dead donor rule," which basically says that you cannot cause the patient's death through the removal of vital organs. Brain death was developed not only from recognition that patients' brains could be "dead" even while their bodies had residual cardiac activity, but also because of the need to identify patients who were on an irreversible road to death and whose organs could appropriately be harvested.

JJ: That said, there are still religious groups within the United States and Canada who do not recognize brain death, and this further constrains the emergency physician in making rapid organ donation referrals. You raised the distinction between what is legally permissible and what is reasonable, based on the wishes of the family when considering procurement of organs. Another illustrative example along those lines involves the discussion in the literature of "loopholes" in the dead donor rule. For instance, if one were to procure non-essential organs from patients in

persistent vegetative states or from anencephalic babies, you could accomplish organ procurement without causing death and without violating the dead donor rule. Despite the fact that this practice is technically permissible, very few such procedures have actually been done due to concerns voiced by surgeons and society about degrading the patient. This issue of public acceptance is of central importance; as a result, it will prove very difficult to have physicians and surgeons move forward with procuring organs before the family is available to consent to these procedures.

AD: Generally, it is far more effective to have a representative from the organ procurement organization (OPO) approach the family. In the ED, this might not always be possible, and the treating clinician may need to initiate the discussion. In such situations, the timing of this decision is important. The discussion and decision regarding organ donation becomes appropriate only when the family has decided to discontinue treatment. For example, at the Pittsburgh and Allegheny General Hospital, the protocol stipulates that one cannot inquire about the patient's donor status until a decision has been made to stop life-sustaining treatment. Once the family has reached a decision about treatment, then the discussion about organ harvesting is legitimate and valuable. This raises the issue of needing to differentiate between the roles of the treating physician and the role of the organ procurement organization. This differentiation is in the best interests of the physician, the patient, and the family. It is best carried out by separate professionals.

JJ: The previously cited *Washington Post* article refers to organ procurement in the ED as "ghoulish."[1] It is a shocking experience to be informed of the loss of a loved one in the ED, and then be approached by procurement organizations in the ED within minutes of the patient's death. This experience of shock and discomfort with the rapidity of the process may be a significant impediment to the procurement process.

AD: With this concern in mind, it is important to recognize the timing constraints of potential organ procurement after cardiopulmonary death versus brain death. In situations involving cardiac arrest, the surgical teams really do need to procure organs within minutes, whereas brain death scenarios offer more flexibility regarding how quickly the intervention occurs.

GM: Regarding the word "ghoulish," it occurs to me that just because something seems ghoulish, doesn't mean we should abandon the possibility of performing a procedure that has potential utility.

AD: A number of procedures in emergency medicine can appear "ghoulish." Applying electricity to someone's chest probably looked pretty ghoulish initially, but it has now become a common and well-accepted practice.

JJ: It may be helpful to consider the similarities between the word "ghoulish" and the concept of "repugnance." Leon Kass, head of the former President's Council on Bioethics, suggests that a feeling of repugnance is the starting point for questioning whether or not something is morally right. This is a useful concept, but it should not be used as a basis for ethics or law in and of itself. Feelings of discomfort are a cause for reflection, but discomfort alone cannot be the basis for determination of what is ethically and legally permissible.

AD: I have found that many of the barriers to addressing organ transplantation in the ED are more concrete and less philosophical. Is this consistent with your experience?

JJ: Yes, one major barrier I have noticed is a lack of cognizance. Given the high patient volume coupled with limited time and resources, it is natural for residents and physicians to simply fill out a death certificate, call the medical examiner, and move on to the next patient. The lack of a protocol for making referrals is also a barrier to making early referrals from the ED. When a potential organ donor is in the process of dying in the ED, the act of making the referral is an ad hoc effort. A nurse or a technician might suggest it, after which we'll look to the internet for information regarding whom to contact—it's just chaotic. Another logistical impediment to early referral from the ED is that when we do call the organ bank, we are made to answer dozens of questions. Even though this might take just 5 or 10 minutes, it might still be a significant burden for the emergency physician simultaneously caring for an entire department of patients.

GM: I do worry about the growing number of public health interventions being forced upon us as emergency physicians. Referral for transplantation is certainly important to consider in the ED, but it is not without cost in terms of how it affects the balance between emergency medicine's commitment to matters of public health and its commitment to individual patient care.

JJ: The addition of public health measures to our job description as emergency physicians may sometimes diminish our effectiveness in treating patients and negatively affects patient flow. If we could uncouple these roles, and delegate the time required to make a referral away from the clinical staff, we could address many of the problems we've identified. Also, deepening the involvement of OPOs [organ procurement organizations] in the ED would educate OPO representatives about the time and resource constraints particular to the ED. Better understanding of the issues involved could be the basis for an improved system and protocol for referrals. Within an ideal system, the physician could quickly submit a referral, after which the OPO would take responsibility for the more time-intensive information accrual and decision-making.

AD: I think this approach has merit. It also addresses another concern, which is the psychological burden for emergency physicians. It's important to consider the difficulty of being a physician who is doing everything possible to save a patient, who must then shift gears not only to withdraw life-sustaining treatment, but also to initiate a conversation with a distraught family about organ donation. This scenario poses burdens not only to the family, but also to the emergency physician. Another point I'd like to raise involves the determination of brain death. This is complicated by the fact that many institutions require that this determination be made by a neurospecialist, and that it takes time. Such protocols make it difficult to establish brain death in the ED.

GM: I agree, but one interesting implication of overcrowding and increased ED boarding times is that many ICU patients now linger in the ED as boarders for hours on end. As a result, it is becoming more common for brain death to be declared while patients remain in the ED. Moreover, there is a growing movement to pursue "uncontrolled donation after cardiac death" as a way of expanding the pool of potential organ donors. The ED and emergency providers will be on the front lines of these efforts, should they prove feasible. Are there patients who are definitely not candidates for organ donation?

JJ: More often it is the case that medical personnel fail to refer patients to an OPO because of their misconceptions about eligibility for donation. There are instances in which a physician will not refer a patient because the patient has cancer, or some sort of infection. Yet, these conditions are not necessarily contraindications to all organ transplantation. Certain cancers don't affect certain organs, localized infections don't preclude transplanting unaffected organs, and systemic infections like hepatitis B or C do not preclude transplantation of organs to other hepatitis B or hepatitis C patients in life-saving situations. We should be careful not to make conclusions with erroneous information regarding who is and is not eligible. OPO criteria for referral are purposefully broad in order to include as many potential donors as possible. Refer all potential organ donors, and allow the OPO to decide who is and is not suitable. We must also think of organs other than heart, liver, and kidney, since corneas, skin, and bone are almost always useful for transplantation.

AD: This applies to elderly patients as well, who may have some tissues that could be enormously useful to other individuals.

JJ: We've discussed many of the barriers to the referral of potential organ donors from the ED. What are some solutions to these problems?

GM: First I'll touch on a few points of consensus. It is important to maintain differentiation between yourself as the treating physician, and the OPO representative who should be the one to approach the family about the question of organ donation. Next, it is important to simply get the process started. Making that referral to the OPO is the most critical intervention in the organ donation process, and this can be done from the ED. Another more controversial issue we have not yet discussed is "organ life support," wherein treatments are aimed at preserving the patient's organs for donation rather than for the benefit of the patient himself. If you have established that there is brain death and organ procurement is in line with the patient's wishes, the family's wishes, and

the clinical scenario, then I think it is acceptable to preserve organ function by use of pressors, or heparin to try to maintain perfusion to the desired organs. Such organ-sustaining treatment would not be acceptable if it was against the wishes of the patient or the family, nor if it would hasten the patient's death.

JJ: We can take simple steps to educate the public about these issues. Perhaps flyers in the waiting room or in the family counseling room would make inroads toward better educating our patient and family populations.

AD: It might also be helpful for emergency physicians to carry a little card that runs through the steps involved in considering organ transplantation, to ensure clinicians are making the appropriate considerations for the interests of the OPO and the patient.

GM: Our discussion has often highlighted the juxtaposition between the law and what is acceptable to society. Another example of this friction concerns the Uniform Anatomical Gift Act and its subsequent revisions in 2006. The original Act stated that if you are a physician with a patient who is a potential organ donor, you are required to maintain life-sustaining treatments until the OPO can arrive to determine whether the patient is suitable for transplantation. This directive was supposed to trump patients' expressed wishes about life-sustaining treatments, family preferences about such measures, and physician assessment of futility. The directive, however, conflicted with ethical norms, our professional fiduciary responsibilities, and societal opinion. In fact, this particular directive was reversed a year later to allow physicians to act in accordance with patient or family wishes independent of OPO determinations of a patient's suitability for donation.

AD: This issue of societal wishes is important. Clearly there is a societal wish that we do everything we can to increase the numbers of organs donated. In some other countries, for example, people are presumed to be organ donors though each individual has the opportunity to opt out of the status of organ donor. In the United States, we have different concerns regarding the intrusion upon people's bodies, and we have not been willing to move towards a default donor status. In addition, popular conceptions of organ procurement are shaped by the media and by popular culture. Even fictional gruesome stories highlighting illegal organ procurement and presenting a negative picture of organ transplantation on the whole can shape people's beliefs and undermine their good faith.

JJ: To summarize, from a logistical perspective, there are many barriers to using the ED as a place for processing organ transplantation. Firstly, determination of brain death is a lengthy process. Furthermore, reconciling the family to both patient death and organ transplantation is time consuming and often beyond the ability of the ED physician simultaneously responsible for a full complement of potentially critical patients. Nevertheless, a protocolized approach to initiating referral for organ donation from the ED requires minimal effort, increases the likelihood of successful organ donation, and should be within the emergency physician's mission and scope of practice.

Section III: Review of the literature

The gap between the number of individuals awaiting organ transplantation and the number of organs donated has been growing steadily over the past decade. In the United States alone, currently over 10 000 individuals are awaiting organs for transplantation, while fewer than 30 000 organs are transplanted each year.[2,3] As a result of this disparity, the medical and organ procurement communities have endeavored to increase the number of organs available for transplantation.

Emergency medicine has recently been recognized to play an important role in the organ donation process.[4] While referral for organ donation was traditionally viewed as the domain of inpatient critical care providers, recent evidence highlights the importance of emergency providers in the organ donation process. Specifically, potential donors referred to OPOs from the ED are far more likely to undergo successful donation than those referred from inpatient settings.[4]

Meanwhile, clinical advances in transplantation and resuscitation medicine, coupled with efforts to expand the organ donor pool, have raised the possibility of procuring organs from individuals suffering circulatory, rather than neurologic, death. The majority of these donations occur in controlled, inpatient settings after the discontinuation of life-sustaining therapies such as mechanical ventilation. However, uncontrolled donation after circulatory death is also possible, and has taken place throughout the United States as well as in Barcelona, Madrid, Paris, and Tokyo.[5-9] Studies of the feasibility of uncontrolled donation after cardiac death in the prehospital and ED settings are underway.[1,10,11]

This expanding role of emergency medicine in the care of potential organ donors presents unique ethical challenges. This chapter will introduce emergency providers to the ethical challenges of organ donation including issues of determination of death, public perception and trust, patient autonomy and consent, and goals of care.

Determination of death

The majority of donated organs are retrieved from live donors or through donation after neurologic determination of death (DNDD). Determination of brain death typically requires time and the involvement of neurology or neurosurgery specialists, and as a result rarely occurs in the ED setting. Nevertheless, the act of referring a patient for potential organ donation can begin before a formal determination of brain death is made. Indeed, the majority of OPOs require notification **before** the formal determination of brain death is made. An example of one OPO's referral criteria is shown in Box 24.1.

Box 24.1 Sample OPO donor referral guidelines[12]

When to contact the OPO for potential donor referral:

- GCS ≤ 4 in a mechanically ventilated, heart-beating patient
- Discussion of withdrawal of mechanical or pharmacological life support
- Brain death testing is being considered
- Family meeting planned to discuss end-of-life measures
- Family initiates discussion of potential organ donation.

An alternative route to donation, donation after circulatory determination of death (DCDD, formerly referred to as non-heart-beating donation) is becoming more common, but is still far less frequent than DNDD or living donation.[9] In its more common "controlled" form, DCDD takes place when a patient has a devastating condition (but is not brain dead), the family or surrogate has requested the withdrawal of life-sustaining therapies, and it is anticipated that the patient will expire after the discontinuation of these therapies. In controlled DCDD, life-sustaining therapies are then withdrawn, the patient's heart stops beating, they are pronounced dead, and after a brief time interval, a separate team of physicians quickly initiates efforts to preserve and retrieve organs.

With advancements in resuscitation and transplant medicine, "uncontrolled" donation after cardiac death has also entered the realm of possibility. This raises the possibility of a patient suffering a cardiac arrest in the prehospital setting or ED, being pronounced dead after failed resuscitation efforts, and then quickly shifting gears to organ preservation and retrieval. Organized programs to obtain organs after uncontrolled cardiac death are underway in New York City, Pittsburgh, Barcelona, Madrid, Paris, and Tokyo.[1,5–8,10,11]

Emergency physicians are frequently called on to pronounce death. The prospect of declaring death in a patient who will then immediately have organs retrieved for transplantation alters the ethical landscape, however. The declaration of death in such cases should be made by a physician who is caring for the patient, and who is not affiliated with the organ recovery team. This separation of providers is needed to avoid the potential for or perception of conflicting loyalties between the care of the patient and the interests of potential organ recipients. A separation of time between the declaration of death and the organ retrieval process is also required to avoid the perception of conflicts of interest, and to eliminate the likelihood of unexpected return of spontaneous circulation. However, this temporal separation must be kept brief in order to minimize the warm ischemic time of the organs. The Institute of Medicine and the Society of Critical Care Medicine have recommended a minimum time of 2 minutes of asystole be observed before the declaration of death in these circumstances, to ensure that auto-resuscitation will not occur.[9]

Public perception and trust

Breaking the news to a family that their loved one has died is one of the most difficult tasks we face as physicians. Simultaneously approaching family members to inquire about harvesting their loved one's organs for donation can feel like an impossibly cruel gesture. In fact, the rates of obtaining family consent are abysmal when discussions of potential brain death and organ donation are included in the same conversation. Separating, or "decoupling," the notification of brain death from the request for organ donation has been found to be three to eight times more likely to result in family consent to donation compared with coupled requests.[13,14] This dramatic difference in rates of consent may be the result of protecting physicians from the perception of a conflict of interest when concurrently advocating both for a patient's best interests and for the interests of potential organ recipients. Both practical and ethical considerations suggest that the initial discussion of death and the discussion of potential organ donation should be separated both temporally and in terms of the person approaching the family. For this reason, discussions of death are usually led by the physician caring for the patient, while a representative from the OPO later approaches the family about the possibility of organ donation.

It may seem respectful to delay the referral to an OPO until after a patient has left the ED, out of deference to the immediacy of a family's significant grief and their potential vulnerability. However, some have suggested that the process of donating a loved one's organs may in fact be a positive way for some family members to cope with their loss and may help facilitate their bereavement.[15,16] A study of family members of patients who died in the ED finds that the vast majority of relatives would not mind being approached about organ donation in the ED.[16] Moreover, it may be overestimating grief responses to assume that family members of gravely ill or newly deceased patients in the ED are so overwhelmed by emotion or paralyzed by grief, that they would be rendered unwilling or unable to make decisions about organ donation. In fact, rates of consent to organ donation are equal if not better when potential donors are referred from the ED rather than inpatient settings.[4] Therefore, while emergency providers should not broach the issue of organ donation with families of potential donors directly, they should take an active role in referring potential donors to the OPO in appropriate cases.

Patient autonomy and issues of consent

Conflict can arise when an individual's organ donor registry status and the wishes expressed by the individual's family differ. It is helpful to consider the legal, ethical, and practical perspectives in such conflicts. Nearly all US states have adopted the Uniform Anatomical Gift Act, which mandates that the donor registry status printed on most state driver's licenses is considered a legal document, and provides a legal basis that supports using registry status over family wishes when in conflict. Similarly, the ethical principle of respect for autonomy suggests that we should honor the individual's own previously expressed wish regarding organ donation rather than valuing their family members' opinion over their own. However, practical considerations often result in deferring to the family's desires regarding donation. Taking an individual's organs for donation over the wishes of their family, even when the individual would have wanted to become an organ donor, can result in extreme misgivings among the family and has the potential to negatively impact the societal impression of the organ donation process. As a result, most (but not all) OPOs employ the "double veto rule" wherein if either the potential donor's previously expressed wishes or the family's wishes oppose organ donation, then organ retrieval is not pursued.[17]

The double veto rule is ethically controversial. Some authors argue that it is an affront to individual autonomy, while others argue that families' wishes carry more ethical weight than that of their deceased relative. Some believe overriding the wishes of the family to respect an individual's wish to be an organ donor jeopardizes the entire enterprise of organ donation and will result in a societal backlash, yet others cite evidence that, by a 5:1 margin, most individuals believe family objection to organ donation should not override the wishes written on a donor card.[17-20] May et al. write that "asking the family for consent when an organ donor card has been signed actually places an undue, and unnecessary, burden on the family," and conclude that "honoring the documented wishes of a deceased patient to donate, even when the family does not consent, is not only morally permissible, but morally required."[17] In a compromise position that seeks to respect potential donors' autonomy while also addressing the practical issue of family concerns, several OPOs now **inform** families of their deceased relatives' consent to organ donation, address their questions, and describe the benefit of this generous act in positive terms, instead of **asking** for permission to carry out the donor's wishes.

Goals of care

At the ethical foundation of organ donation is the dead donor rule, which states that the organ retrieval process should not cause or hasten death.[21] Once a family has decided to consent to donate the organs of their brain dead relative, several interventions may be used to preserve those organs including a ventilator to ensure oxygenation, vasopressors to maintain hemodynamic stability, bronchoscopy to maximize pulmonary function, and heparin to prevent vascular thrombosis and ischemia.[22] If brain death is diagnosed and organ procurement is in line with the patient's and family's wishes, then it is acceptable to administer the preceding organ-sustaining treatments. Because brain death is almost never determined in the ED, however, emergency physicians cannot ethically administer interventions with the sole purpose of preserving the patient's organs for donation. This is especially true if those interventions would hasten the patient's death or cause the patient harm. As a result, the interventions administered in the ED ought to be those intended to benefit the patient.

As donation after circulatory determination of death becomes more commonplace, however, there may be an increasing need to begin treatments aimed at temporary organ preservation (TOP) in the ED or even in the prehospital setting. In fact, due to the sudden and unpredictable nature of this process, several US states have now passed legislation allowing for initiation of these treatments without explicit consent, while efforts are made to determine the deceased patient's previous wishes and to contact their family.[23] TOP measures may include cardiac compressions, mechanical ventilation, heparin administration, or even extracorporeal membranous oxygenation. The prevailing ethical view is that these practices are ethically acceptable, as they in fact maximize respect for autonomy by preserving the opportunity to donate while efforts are made to identify patient and family wishes.[9,23-25] Without TOP the opportunity to donate would be lost, and individuals who are later found to have wanted to become organ donors will not have had their last wish upheld. The cost of measures aimed solely at TOP are borne by the OPO, and should never be the responsibility of the potential donor or donor's family.[8,26] While treatments intended solely for the preservation of organs are ethically acceptable, they should be initiated by a member of the organ transplant team and not by the emergency provider, whose focus should remain centered on care intended for the benefit of individual patients and their families.

Conclusion

The shortage of available organs for transplant has led to a push to increase the potential organ donor pool. As a result, increasing attention is being paid to the role of emergency medicine in the organ donation process. Emergency medicine plays a key role, as patients referred for potential donation from the ED are more likely to become successful donors, and because efforts to pursue uncontrolled donation after circulatory determination of death are expanding. Public discourse and formal research are needed to assess and inform societal perspectives and attitudes on organ donation from the ED. As efforts to obtain organs from patients dying in the prehospital and ED settings have made clear, organ donation is an ethically, legally, and emotionally charged issue.[1,10,11]

Section IV: Recommendations

• The shortage of organs available for transplantation and the resultant push to increase the size of the potential organ donor pool do not diminish the importance of respecting patient autonomy and of adhering to the principles of non-maleficence, beneficence, and the dead donor rule.
• Organ donation is ethically permissible after death is pronounced by either neurologic or circulatory criteria, but the pronouncement of death should be made by a physician who is caring for the patient and who is not affiliated with the organ recovery team.
• The discussion of organ donation should be initiated by representatives of the OPO and not by the emergency provider caring for the patient.

• Efforts aimed solely at organ preservation are ethically acceptable, but should not be initiated until after death is pronounced and should be performed by members of the organ transplant team rather than by the emergency provider.
• Emergency providers should consult their regional OPO early in the hospital course of any patient they suspect may be an eventual candidate for organ donation, owing to the increased likelihood of successful donation when potential donors are referred from the ED.

References

1. Stein R. (2010) Project to get transplant organs from ER patients raises ethics questions. *Washington Post.* 15, 1.
2. Health Resources and Services Administration. (n.d.) *Organ Procurement and Transplantation Network Data.* Rockville, MD: US Department of Health and Human Services. Available at: http://optn.transplant.hrsa.gov/. Accessed June 15, 2011.
3. United States Health Resources and Services Administration. (2007) *Annual Report of the U.S. Organ Procurement and Transplantation Network and the Scientific Registry of Transplant Recipients: Transplant Data 1997–2006.* Rockville, MD: US Department of Health and Human Services.
4. Michael GE, O'Connor RE. (2009) The importance of emergency medicine in organ donation: successful donation is more likely when potential donors are referred from the emergency department. *Acad Emerg Med.* 16(9), 850–8.
5. Fieux F, Losser MR, Bourgeois E, et al. (2009) Kidney retrieval after sudden out of hospital refractory cardiac arrest: a cohort of uncontrolled non heart beating donors. *Crit Care.* 13(4), R141.
6. Sánchez-Fructuoso AI, Marques M, Prats D, et al. (2006) Victims of cardiac arrest occurring outside the hospital: a source of transplantable kidneys. *Ann Intern Med.* 145(3), 157–64.
7. Mateos-Rodríguez A, Pardillos-Ferrer L, Navalpotro-Pascual JM. (2010). Kidney transplant function using organs from non-heart-beating donors maintained by mechanical chest compressions. *Resuscitation.* 81(7), 904–7.
8. Morozumi J, Matsuno N, Sakurai E, et al. (2010) Application of an automated cardiopulmonary resuscitation device for kidney transplantation from uncontrolled donation after cardiac death donors in the emergency department. *Clin Transplant.* 24(5), 620–5.

9. Institute of Medicine. (2006) Committee on increasing rates of organ donation. In: Childress JF, Liverman CT. (eds) *Organ Donation: Opportunities For Action.* Washington, DC: National Academies Press. Available at: www.nap.edu/openbook.php?record_id=11643. Accessed December 24, 2011.

10. Buckley C. (2008) City to explore a way to add organ donors. *The New York Times.* Available at: www.nytimes.com/2008/06/01/nyregion/01organ.html. Accessed August 23, 2010.

11. Kaufman BJ, Wall SP, Gilbert AJ, et al. (2009) Success of organ donation after out-of-hospital cardiac death and the barriers to its acceptance. *Crit Care.* 13(5), 189.

12. LifeNet Health Organ Procurement Organization. (2011) *LifeNet Health Quarterly Newsletter,* April 2011. Available at: http://lifenethealthopo.org/OPO/uploads/files/4th%20quarter%202010%20The%20Referral%2004122011.pdf. Accessed June 20, 2011.

13. Klieger J, Nelson K, Davis R, et al. (1994) Analysis of factors influencing organ donation consent rates. *J Transpl Coord.* 4(3), 132–4.

14. Franz HG, DeJong W, Wolfe SM, et al. (1997) Explaining brain death: a critical feature of the donation process. *J Transpl Coord.* 7(1), 14–21.

15. Stein A, Hope T, Baum JD. (1995) Organ transplantation: approaching the donor's family. *BMJ.* 310(6988), 1149–50.

16. Wellesley A, Glucksman E, Crouch R. (1997) Organ donation in the accident and emergency department: a study of relatives' views. *J Accid Emerg Med.* 14(1), 24–5.

17. May T, Aulisio MP, DeVita MA. (2000) Patients, families, and organ donation: who should decide? *Milbank Q.* 78(2), 323–36, 152.

18. Corlett S. (1985) Public attitudes toward human organ donation. *Transplant Proc.* 17(6 Suppl 3), 103–10.

19. Kluge EH. (1997) Decisions about organ donation should rest with potential donors, not next of kin. *CMAJ.* 157(2), 160–1.

20. Peters DA. (1986) Protecting autonomy in organ procurement procedures: some overlooked issues. *Milbank Q.* 64(2), 241–70.

21. Robertson JA. (1999) The dead donor rule. *Hastings Cent Rep.* 29(6), 6–14.

22. Wood KE, Becker BN, McCartney JG, et al. (2004) Care of the potential organ donor. *N Engl J Med.* 351(26), 2730–9.

23. Bonnie RJ, Wright S, Dineen KK. (2008) Legal authority to preserve organs in cases of uncontrolled cardiac death: preserving family choice. *J Law Med Ethics.* 36(4), 741–51, 610.

24. Childress JF. (2008) Organ donation after circulatory determination of death: lessons and unresolved controversies. *J Law Med Ethics.* 36(4), 766–71, 610.

25. Motta ED. (2005) The ethics of heparin administration to the potential non-heart-beating organ donor. *J Prof Nurs.* 21(2), 97–102.

26. Association of Organ Procurement Organizations. *Funding.* Vienna: Association of Organ Procurement Organizations. Available at: www.aopo.org/funding-a30. Accessed August 13, 2011.

25 Mandatory and permissive reporting laws: conflicts in patient confidentiality, autonomy, and the duty to report

Joel Martin Geiderman

Co-Chairman, Department of Emergency Medicine, Professor of Emergency Medicine, Cedars-Sinai Medical Center, Los Angeles, CA, USA

Section I: Case presentation

While working in the emergency department (ED), a pharmacy calls you to verify a prescription written by a colleague that the pharmacist thinks may have been altered. You ask for a copy of the prescription. When the prescription is sent to you, you find that it is a valid prescription, but the number of Vicodin (hydrocodone/paracetamol) pills appears to have been changed from 15 to 60. You check the chart, and verify that the physician ordered 15 pills. On further review of the patient's chart, you find that he is a firefighter. You call him to discuss this matter, but find that he is on leave of absence attending paramedic school.

A patient presents with a severe dog bite sustained from her own mastiff. Your county requires reporting of dog bites for epidemiological purposes. The patient asks you not to report the bite because she is currently being sued for a disfiguring bite sustained by a child in her neighborhood, and she fears her dog will be taken away and her homeowner's insurance revoked if you report this injury. She states that her dog is her only companion.

A 45-year-old undocumented immigrant is brought in after his wife hit him over the eye with a glass, causing a laceration to his eyebrow. After you involve the social worker, the patient begs you not to call the police to report this event, fearing deportation of his wife, and perhaps himself.

Section II: Discussion

Dr. Peter Rosen: Would it matter if the occupation of the man in our case was a firefighter or a physician? We have some fairly compelling evidence that a prescription has been forged, and it seems to me that the emergency physician has little option but to report the patient to the police. It is illegal, and, in fact, it is a felony to fake prescriptions or to alter them in any way.

Dr. Joel Geiderman: I have received calls about patients who have forged prescriptions, and I've been notified by pharmacies about fake prescriptions; although we all know this action constitutes a felony, I'm not sure we report every infraction that crosses our desks. I would argue, however, that the person's occupation does matter—what if the patient is an airline pilot? Surely, there should be a greater duty to report a crime as the risk of significant public harm increases.

PR: Although I don't personally care what the agency does with the information I report to them, I do not

---

Ethical Problems in Emergency Medicine: A Discussion-Based Review, First Edition. John Jesus, Shamai A. Grossman, Arthur R. Derse, James G. Adams, Richard Wolfe, and Peter Rosen.

care to place myself or my institution in the path of a criminal investigation, because I failed to live up to a legal mandate to report a crime. On one occasion, I had a physician who was actually on call at the time, brought into the ED for a heroin overdose. I found a way to inform his institution that there was a problem that should be addressed: that one of their staff members was attempting to practice medicine while on mood-altering agents, and was acting in a way that was dangerous to himself and to his patients. What would you do if a patient presenting with his first seizure were an airline pilot?

Dr. James Adams: First, I want to emphasize that we're not primarily agents of social control; rather, we're primarily agents for the patient. Sometimes our patients are distasteful and nasty, but we're still agents for the patient. Regarding the airline pilot, I'm not sure I have a mechanism set up in my ED to facilitate such reporting, and I don't know whom I would contact. If I met this patient today, I would call the hospital legal team and ask for guidance in dealing with an altered, drug-using patient in a high-risk occupation. The patient in our case is trying to manipulate us in order to gain access to drugs. In some ways, this is a matter of fact situation. That said, I believe we shouldn't approach his care with a pure punitive stance. Perhaps the best we can do for the patient is to facilitate his admission into a drug addiction treatment center. The first appropriate action is to ask the pharmacy not to fill the prescription, and then flag his name, so that pharmacists may scrutinize the patient's future narcotic prescriptions more closely.

PR: Isn't there a legal responsibility of the physician to report the patient to the authorities?

Dr. Arthur Derse: Some states do require reporting, and some do not. The physician should be protected from litigation if he chooses to report the patient's activity. Nevertheless, I agree with the notion that we have a greater responsibility to report patients who place other people in danger. The responsibility to report patients who endanger other people also extends to our own colleagues. The *Washington Post* recently featured an article that focused on the rate of doctors reporting other doctors whom they feel might be a danger to their patients; the article found that doctors do not report other doctors very often.[1]

In our attempt to mitigate this risk however, we ought to be careful to avoid judging our patients' behaviors, and to protect their confidentiality to the greatest degree possible.

When I have found a patient's behavior to constitute a danger to others, such that I am willing to breach my duty of confidentiality, I have not always found the report to be helpful. For example, I reported a patient who had a new-onset seizure while driving, and received a letter back saying: "Thank you very much for reporting this, the patient's license has already been revoked." The patient was already driving without a license, and my report did nothing to mitigate the danger posed to the public.

Dr. John Jesus: Though I agree that we should attempt to prevent patients from endangering others, I feel some discomfort with our focus on seizures and drug use, as there are many other conditions that might impair patients with even greater frequency, for which there are no mandated reporting laws. For example, the fatigue associated with shift work and overnight call place a physician at high risk of falling asleep while on the road, endangering self and the public. One could make an argument that physicians in this state expose the public to a greater risk than a patient with a seizure disorder stable on antiepileptic medications. If a coercive reporting policy exists that forces physicians to report patients who endanger the public, then it ought to be based on consistent findings of impairment rather than on particular, arbitrarily chosen disease processes.

Dr. Shamai Grossman: There are times when we are forced to breech patient confidentiality, because our obligations as members of a moral and lawful society outweigh our obligation to any individual patient. Sometimes we are fortunate to have the law on our side, and sometimes we don't have legal backing—but we still have a moral obligation to report patients who endanger the health and lives of the public. Even though the patient may lose his job as a result of the physician report, he may also end up crashing an airplane full of people if we don't report him, which is a far more egregious ethical lapse.

JA: While our discussion concerning the threshold to report is important, the mechanism of reporting is equally important. When we speak about reporting a dangerous patient, we're not talking about calling any random person. Physicians should think hard about the agencies to whom they report their patients, and set up policies and mechanism for doing so thoughtfully and appropriately.

PR: In response to Dr. Jesus's point about the lack of consistency with which we are, by law, forced to report patients, the argument is, unfortunately, irrelevant. It doesn't matter if the law is a good law or a bad law, a just law or a complete law—it's a law under which we live and must abide. Fortunately, in most states physicians are able to use some judgment about whether the patient reaches their threshold of threatening public safety.

I can't change the number of drug addicts who exist, and I can't change the number of people becoming drug addicts; therefore, I don't go out of my way to try and change this element of society. I also feel that there is danger in a physician who actively flaunts a law because he feels that the law is somehow inappropriate. I understand the motives behind a physician who attempts to protect a basketball player by not reporting his gunshot wound, but I can't see why he would risk his career for this patient. However, when we come across illegal information, especially if it represents a felony, we have a duty to report it. On the other hand, I don't go looking to make problems for patients, nor do I go looking to make problems for myself either. I don't owe so much to a patient that I have to break the law to meet whatever the patient's needs.

When I treated a pilot who feared losing his license after he had a seizure for the first time, I called his wife in and sat them both down. I said, "This is hard news for you, but you're going to have to face this now, or after you've crashed a plane that kills 350 people. I think that there are clearly other options for you rather than to continue flying while you are at risk for further seizure activity." I didn't report it to the airline, but I didn't have to because he reported himself. It turned out that putting him together with his wife, and giving him time to sit down and reflect, proved more useful than trying to personally take control of the situation. Let us move on to the second and the third cases, as they add other complexities and issues.

JG: Regarding the case of the dog bite—there are many locales where the reporting of animal bites is legally required.

PR: Only in the very rare instance am I willing to break the law in order to protect a patient. How does everyone else feel?

JG: We shouldn't tell people to break the law, but the real question is what is our ethical obligation? Now in this case, this dog had a history of aggressive behavior in the past, and therefore one could argue that the dog's aggressive tendencies put people around it at risk. If this had been a nip on the finger by a small dog, I might have been willing to comply with the patient's wishes.

PR: Laws are rules of conduct established by an authority that has the power to enforce them. If you choose to break the law, you are putting yourself at risk for punishment by the authority that established the law. Ethics are rules of behavior that are established by societal populations, or small groups such as a professional organization or a hospital group, which don't necessarily have the power to enforce the behavior or punish you, except to expel you from the group. There are limits to and tension between my ethical and legal obligations I am willing to tolerate. If there exists a law that requires me to report every Jew so that he can be killed, then clearly I will refuse to divulge such information, even if it requires me to break the law.

Only once have I disregarded the law in favor of patient care: I had a patient who had a gunshot wound to the leg [see also Chapter 6]. He was brought to me in the custody of police with a court order to remove the bullet from his leg, in order to retrieve evidence important to a criminal case against the patient. First, an X-ray study demonstrated that the bullet had shattered and would not provide any useful evidence. Secondly, the operation would not provide any benefit to the patient as it was not causing him any problem that would alter his health or life. Therefore, I refused to remove the bullet. The police officer said, "But the judge will be very angry!", and I said, "Well, let the judge operate on him then." I felt the judge did not have the right or the need to practice medicine in a way that I felt was unethical. The judge can't make me operate unnecessarily, and I was willing to go to prison rather than perform that operation. This was an extraordinary case. In general, I may not agree with the law, but for the most part, I'm not going to jeopardize my professional standing.

JJ: I will concede to you that we ought not to disobey laws unless we are willing to suffer the consequences to our reputation, personal standing, or our freedom. My comment about the inconsistencies in the laws that require me to report a pilot who has had a seizure without also reporting a non-compliant diabetic, serves more to criticize law-makers than as a recommendation for subversion. We see people every day who suffer from conditions that impair their judgment or their senses, and yet we are required to report nothing for the vast majority of those conditions to the US Department of Motor Vehicles or elsewhere. How is that fair, for example, to patients who are singled out after their first seizure?

PR: There is no ethical principle that doesn't collapse in some special circumstance, and I think that part of practical ethics is to decide what's most important to each case and whether or not you can live with your decisions. I do not believe that there are Kantian categorical moral imperatives that can be applied universally. In our third case, we have an example of a patient who has a medical problem, and a fear that if the injury is reported to immigration, he and his family will be put at risk of deportation. Once again, this decision may end up being a personal choice. That said, most of the clinicians in California hospitals ignore the proposition passed in California requiring such reporting, and nothing untoward ever seems to occur. Healthcare is simply extended to anyone who presents to the ED whether or not the patients are considered "illegal."

JG: Actually, the whole category of mandatory reporting for domestic abuse is rather controversial. The American College of Emergency Physicians has a policy that says we oppose mandatory reporting of domestic violence. In fact, such reporting can cause many other problems for a patient who doesn't consent to have the abuse reported, and some people believe that we should honor the patient's decision. Another concern is that victims of domestic violence may not seek appropriate medical care if they know that the clinicians will report the incident without their consent. Given that, there are reasonable arguments for and against reporting domestic violence—this remains an issue with which emergency physicians continue to struggle.

JJ: I support emergency physicians who are hesitant to report domestic abuse when the patient refuses to give consent for the report. When victims of domestic violence present to the ED, their decision-making authority has often been violated, and their sense of helplessness may be at its most poignant. In this state, we should support the recovery of those comfort zones rather than adding insult to injury that may result in disrupting the trust between patient and physician. Physicians ought to be looking out for their patients' interests and protecting their patients' privacy and confidentiality. Victims of domestic violence need our compassion, a safe bed, and resources that will facilitate their ability to remove themselves from a situation. An automatic or mandatory reporting of domestic violence may serve to cause more harm than benefit.

PR: We need to at least be cognizant of the reality that just because we are inclined to help a patient doesn't mean that the patient will react well to our efforts. I was involved in a lawsuit in which a victim of domestic violence was advised by a physician to be admitted to a safe bed, in order to separate her from an abusive partner. She refused and left the institution with the partner, who doused her in gasoline and set fire to her 2 hours later. She survived her horrendous burns and sued the emergency physician for not admitting her.

SG: It sounds like you're saying that there are some patients who will benefit from acting in what we feel are their best interests, and there are other patients for whom this approach will not be true. A physician must develop a certain sense of ethics that are his own, and hope that they are consistent with how society wants you to care for patients. When this approach is not consistent with societal mores, each physician must make decisions according to a personal set of ethical principles.

PR: That explanation suggests that I would place my own beliefs above the authorities around me, and in some instances that may well be true. I believe at times that is the duty of every physician. I do my best to help my patient; I do my best to obey the law; and when they are in conflict, I make a decision about which I will honor, and that decision will be based on the individual circumstances of each individual case.

AD: The underlying purpose of these mandatory reporting laws, in theory, is to decrease the risk to life and health of others. In the first case we wouldn't necessarily report drug use for its own sake, but rather because drug use may represent a danger to other people. One reason dog bites are reported is for epidemiologic purposes. Should there be a case of rabies, we might be able to prevent an outbreak with a robust method of tracking communicable diseases. This system was set up for the purpose and logic of preventing disease spread and in the spirit of promoting public health. For these reasons, I can appreciate the logic behind mandatory reporting laws.

JJ: Though we have brought up the example of reporting laws in California, the law is entirely silent in most US states. In fact, only six of 50 states as of 2007 mandate reporting of domestic violence, and only five as of 2007 require reporting of impaired driving.[2] While the law may require reporting in many categories of impairment and abuse, the aspects of our discussion which focus on doing the best for our patients when there is no legal guidance is perhaps of greatest concern to most emergency physicians today.

PR: It is near universally true that any law will have consequences that were not intended. As a result, even though those enacting laws may have good intentions, these laws are rarely enacted in a way that makes them useful. It's easy to become cynical about the utility of law, and feel that you are in an appropriate position to decide whether or not to follow it. When faced with a difficult patient or a difficult situation where there is a law that can help you decide how to address the situation, then use it. The fact that all 50 states don't have mandatory reporting doesn't help the doctors who work in the six states that do, and I think that you have to be cognizant of your local regulations and laws, and do your best not to break local rules while also practicing ethical medicine.

JG: Although we have discussed issues surrounding mandatory reporting, there are equally important issues regarding the practice of permissive reporting, which introduces the possibility of bias and prejudice. A physician may suspect abuse in one culture more than another, and he may therefore be more likely to report instances associated with a particular group of people. Permissive reporting laws introduce a slippery slope down which lie issues far worse than are found with mandatory reporting laws.

JA: The point we all can agree upon is that our primary purpose is to take care of patients, and none of us appreciate a lot of interference with that aim. We have to protect the integrity of our profession, which really is to care for people and primarily be agents for the patient. Sometimes there are laws that direct us to break the duty to protect our patients' confidentiality. Even though we have good ethics in place and good laws to direct some of our professional decisions, there will be situations in which they come into conflict. The resultant decisions will be hard to make, and physicians will need to utilize their best judgment to guide their actions and treatment.

Section III: Review of the literature

Ethical versus legal

The discussion above focused heavily on the legal rather than the ethical considerations at hand. A simple reading of the law will inform us of what is and is not legally required according to various mandatory reporting laws, some of which are controversial, and vary from state to state. The questions however, are: What are the ethical considerations when it comes to reporting? In what situations are we bound by a higher duty to respect patient autonomy and confidentiality rather than to accede to some other consideration? Arriving at the proper conclusion involves ethical reasoning and a closer examination of the underlying issues.

The very fact that some (but not all) mandatory reporting laws in the United States vary from state to state gives rise to the notion that the reasoning behind some of them is suspect and may need to be questioned. Presumably, medical judgments may vary from situation to situation—but not from state to state; the notion of personal integrity mandates that we apply the same ethical concepts to all patients equally. Why would a physician be expected to act differently from an ethical perspective if he or she resided in California rather than in Texas or Massachusetts?

How is it that what may be considered immoral and illegal is different? A simple example is the situation in which a person who cannot swim falls in the water with little risk to the witness in trying to assist the victim. In the United States (unlike in other parts of the world), on the one hand, there is generally no legal obligation to help the victim. On the other hand, there is a strong moral obligation to try to rescue the victim. To further illustrate the difference, a law that required the sole parent of small children to unduly place his or her own life at risk by jumping off a bridge into a cold river in an attempt to save an unrelated immersion victim could be questioned and understandably disobeyed on moral grounds.

What are mandatory reporting laws and why are they necessary?

Mandatory reporting laws are deemed necessary for both societal and individual purposes. The rationale for enacting such laws includes:
• Gathering information for either epidemiological or statistical purposes
• Protecting members of the public from harm from a communicable disease
• Protecting members of the public from harm from a violent/criminal act (reporting of gunshot wounds) or an accident (seizure reporting)
• Protecting an individual patient from further harm caused by a perpetrator
• Assisting law enforcement in solving crimes or preventing future acts.[3]

The reason mandatory reporting laws are discussed in the ethics literature is because they set aside both patient autonomy and the physician's duty to protect confidentiality. Reporting is required by the government without a necessary legal requirement to obtain the patient's permission to disclose personal health information. Many ethical codes on confidentiality carve out an exception for situations where there is a higher duty or in order "to obey the law."

Less controversial mandatory reporting laws

Suspected or confirmed child abuse
All 50 US states have laws on the books requiring the reporting of suspected or confirmed child abuse.[2] Forty-six states have criminal penalties for failure to comply with these laws. In 2009, there were 3.5 million referrals in the United States for suspected child abuse to child protective services or an equivalent agency according to the Child Abuse and Neglect Data System (NCANDS).[4] In a quarter of these cases there was found do be at least one victim of abuse.

Eighty-one percent of the perpetrators were parents and 6% were other relatives. The incidence of child abuse (or neglect) that year was estimated at 894 000 and 1770 children died as a result of abuse.

Children are considered particularly vulnerable, and in many cases are not free to express their own free will or are deemed capable of protecting, defending themselves, or changing their own circumstances. In these instances, it is quite reasonable for the physician to set aside "autonomy," which does not exist in such cases, and act paternalistically, i.e., *in loco parentis* (in the place of a [responsible] parent).

Nevertheless, reporting of suspected child abuse is not without its controversies and critics, especially in individual cases.[5-8] Parents who are reported often complain or threaten lawsuits. Generally, however, there are immunity laws that protect physicians so long as they report in good faith. Ethically, physicians are also bound to tell the truth. Therefore when suspected child abuse is reported, parents should be informed regardless of the aforementioned immunity from litigation. Aside from being the right thing to do ethically, most guardians will be appreciative if physicians take the time to express their concerns and actions in an honest way and explain their duty to report. This may also serve to diminish hard feelings toward the physician afterwards, should the investigation clear the parents of suspicion. In any event, even at the risk of angering a parent, the duty to protect a potentially vulnerable child trumps all other considerations.

Communicable diseases
The control and prevention of infectious disease has traditionally been a primary mandate for governmental health authorities. Routine reporting of various diseases in the United States began when the State Board of Health of Massachusetts initiated a plan for the weekly voluntary reporting of prevalent diseases by physicians by postcard in 1874.[9] In 1883, Michigan became the first US jurisdiction to mandate the reporting of specific infectious diseases. By 1901, all US states required notification of certain communicable diseases to local health authorities.

Under American law, the authority to require notification of diseases resides with the states. Variation among states exists among conditions and diseases to be reported, time frames for reporting, agencies receiving reports, persons required to report, and

---

Box 25.1 Reportable infectious diseases in California

Title 17, California Code of Regulations, Sections 2505 and 2641.5—2643.20 (Revised 12/08/2009)

To be reported to the local health officer by telephone within 1 hour:

- Anthrax
- Avian influenza
- Botulism
- Brucellosis
- *Burkholderia mallei* and *B. pseudomallei*
- Plague, animal or human
- Smallpox (variola)
- Tularemia
- Viral hemorrhagic fever agents (e.g., Crimean-Congo, Ebola, Lassa and Marburg viruses)

To be reported to the local health officer in writing within 1 working day:

- Acid-fast bacilli
- Anaplasmosis/ehrlichiosis
- *Bordetella pertussis*
- *Borrelia burgdorferi*
- Chlamydia trachomatis infections, including lymphogranuloma venereum (LGV)
- Coccidioidomycosis
- Cryptosporidiosis
- *Cyclospora cayetenensis*
- Diphtheria
- Encephalitis, arboviral
- *Escherichia coli* STEC, including O157:H7 infection
- Gonorrhea
- *Haemophilus influenzae* (from sterile site in patient <15 years old)
- Hepatitis A, acute infection, by IgM antibody test or positive viral antigen test
- Hepatitis B, acute infection, by IgM anti-HBc antibody test
- Hepatitis B surface antigen positivity
- Hepatitis C
- *Legionella pneumophila*
- *Listeria monocytogenes*
- Malaria
- Measles (Rubeola), acute infection, by IgM antibody test or positive viral antigen test
- *Mycobacterium tuberculosis*
- *Neisseria meningitidis*
- Poliovirus
- Rabies, animal or human
- Rubella, acute infection by IgM antibody test or culture
- *Salmonella* species, including S. *typhi*
- Shiga toxin (in feces)
- *Shigella* sp.
- Syphilis
- *Vibrio* sp. infections
- West Nile virus infection

---

conditions under which reports are required. In many states, healthcare providers are encouraged to report diseases directly to local health departments charged with rendering epidemiologic services rather than to the state health department. As an example, Box 25.1 lists conditions currently required to be reported to local health authorities in California; in some cases this is within an hour of diagnosis and in other circumstances during the first business day.[10]

The federal Quarantine Act of 1878 authorized the US Public Health Service to collect morbidity data for use in quarantine measures against yellow fever, smallpox, and cholera.[9] The Quarantine Act of 1893 authorized the US Public Health Service to collect morbidity information each week from state and local

public health authorities throughout the United States.[9]

The poliomyelitis epidemic in 1916 and the influenza pandemic of 1918 heightened interest in reporting requirements, resulting in the participation of all US states in national morbidity reporting by 1925. Since 1961, the Centers for Disease Control (CDC) in Atlanta has had the responsibility of operating the National Notifiable Diseases Surveillance System, for the purpose of tabulating and disseminating summary morbidity data. Today, all US states participate in a national morbidity reporting system and regularly report data for 49 infectious diseases and related conditions to the CDC.[11] Box 25.2 lists conditions currently notifiable under federal law.

Box 25.2 Nationally notifiable infectious conditions in the United States (2010)

- Anthrax
- Arboviral neuroinvasive and non-neuroinvasive diseases:
  - California serogroup virus disease
  - Eastern equine encephalitis virus disease
  - Powassan virus disease
  - St. Louis encephalitis virus disease
  - West Nile virus disease
  - Western equine encephalitis virus disease
- Botulism:
  - Botulism, foodborne
  - Botulism, infant
  - Botulism, other (wound and unspecified)
- Brucellosis
- Chancroid
- *Chlamydia trachomatis* infection
- Cholera
- Cryptosporidiosis
- Cyclosporiasis
- Dengue:
  - Dengue fever
  - Dengue hemorrhagic fever
  - Dengue shock syndrome
- Diphtheria
- Ehrlichiosis/anaplasmosis:
  - *Ehrlichia chaffeensis*
  - *Ehrlichia ewingii*
  - *Anaplasma phagocytophilum*
  - Undetermined
- Giardiasis
- Gonorrhea
- *Haemophilus influenzae*, invasive disease
- Hansen disease (leprosy)
- Hantavirus pulmonary syndrome
- Hemolytic uremic syndrome, post-diarrheal
- Hepatitis:
  - Hepatitis A, acute
  - Hepatitis B, acute
  - Hepatitis B, chronic
  - Hepatitis B virus, perinatal infection
  - Hepatitis C, acute
  - Hepatitis C, chronic
- HIV infection[a]:
  - HIV infection, adult/adolescent (age ≥13 years)
  - HIV infection, child (age ≥18 months and <13 years)
  - HIV infection, pediatric (age <18 months)
- Influenza-associated pediatric mortality
- Legionellosis
- Listeriosis
- Lyme disease
- Malaria
- Measles
- Meningococcal disease
- Mumps
- Novel influenza A virus infections
- Pertussis
- Plague
- Poliomyelitis, paralytic
- Poliovirus infection, non-paralytic
- Psittacosis
- Q fever:
  - Acute
  - Chronic
- Rabies
  - Rabies, animal
  - Rabies, human
- Rubella
- Rubella, congenital syndrome
- Salmonellosis
- Severe acute respiratory syndrome-associated coronavirus (SARS-CoV) disease
- Shiga toxin-producing *Escherichia coli* (STEC)
- Shigellosis
- Smallpox
- Spotted fever rickettsiosis
- Streptococcal toxic-shock syndrome
- *Streptococcus pneumoniae*, invasive disease
- Syphilis:
  - Primary
  - Secondary
  - Latent
  - Early latent
  - Late latent
  - Latent, unknown duration
  - Neurosyphilis
  - Late, non-neurological
  - Stillbirth
  - Congenital

- Tetanus
- Toxic-shock syndrome (other than streptococcal)
- Trichinellosis (trichinosis)
- Tuberculosis
- Tularemia
- Typhoid fever
- Vancomycin—intermediate *Staphylococcus aureus* (VISA)
- Vancomycin—resistant *Staphylococcus aureus* (VRSA)

- Varicella (morbidity)
- Varicella (deaths only)
- Vibriosis
- Viral hemorrhagic fevers:
  - Arenavirus
  - Crimean-Congo hemorrhagic fever virus
  - Ebola virus
  - Lassa virus
  - Marburg virus
- Yellow fever

[a]AIDS has been reclassified as HIV stage III.

Source: United States Department of Health and Human Services Centers for Disease Control and Prevention, February 10, 2011. Accessed May 15, 2011. http://www.cdc.gov/osels/ph_surveillance/nndss/phs/infdis2010.htm.

While the reporting of most infectious diseases is not controversial or problematic, this has not always been the case with regard to the human immunodeficiency virus (HIV) epidemic that began in 1982. In the early days of the epidemic, the stigma of being homosexual, the most common factor associated with contracting the disease, caused people to shy away from wanting to report the illness. Reporting was avoided because of the very real fear of discrimination, both economically and socially, even when the disease was contracted in a non-sexual fashion. In more enlightened times this situation has changed. Legislatures have also changed, and, in recent years, physicians have been required to report HIV to try to alleviate its spread. There are also funding implications for accurate reporting as society allocates limited dollars for diseases that are most prominent in the population, both for research and supportive services. For these reasons, the reporting of HIV, once shunned, is now commonly required by law and well accepted. Also helpful is legislation that serves to deter discrimination.

Reportable injuries and causes of death

In many states, reportable conditions include traffic accidents, residential fires, penetrating trauma, falls, occupational injuries, poisoning, sexual assault, suicides, and drowning (Box 25.3). Most of this reporting is aimed at either preventing future injuries, enforcing statutes designed to protect the public, or solving crimes. In most cases, there are few ethical objections

Box 25.3 Reportable crimes and causes of injury and death in some or all US states

- Alleged or proven sexual assault
- Suspected or proven child abuse
- Traffic accidents
- Impaired driving
- Residential fires
- Burns
- Penetrating trauma
- Falls
- Occupational injuries
- Suspected involvement in terrorism
- In-hospital events such as impersonation of a physician or pharmacist; patient or infant abduction; or alleged adult abuse by the institution
- Poisoning
- Natural death
- Homicide
- Suicide
- Accidental death
- Drowning

to such reporting, though some exist.[12] In general, the dead have a more limited right to confidentiality. In fact, the cause of death is routinely reported on death certificates (a public record) without the consent or permission of the deceased or their next of kin.

Duty to warn

Tort law has established that if a patient discloses to a physician that they intend to inflict harm on a third party, the physician has a "duty to warn" the patients who can be identified as being in imminent danger of physical harm. In the index 1974 case, *Tarasoff* v. *Regents of the University of California*, the Tarasoff family sued after their daughter, Tatiana Tarasoff, was murdered by a man who, while under psychological care in the university counseling center, had expressed his intention of killing Tatiana.[13] Few people question the ethics of breaching confidentiality in order to protect a third party from foreseeable harm, as long as the suspicion is reasonable. Should a clinician do so, they are generally protected from legal retribution.

More controversial mandatory reporting laws

Elder abuse and neglect

Forty-three US states have elder abuse and neglect mandatory reporting laws, and the majority of them have accompanying legislation that legally shields those who report it.[2] Similar to child abuse laws, elder abuse laws carry criminal penalties for failure to comply but they are rarely enforced. The true incidence of elder abuse is difficult to ascertain with a wide range of estimates, from 700 000–2.5 million annually in the United States.[14-16] State statistics vary widely as there is no uniform reporting system and national data are not collected. Adding to the uncertainty, definitions of elder abuse vary in the literature. Another reason estimates vary is because elder abuse is a category under which one can file negligence suits against facilities and individuals who care for the elderly.[17] In this case, arguments arise as to whether certain acts of omission or commission constitute elder abuse, with financial consequences for both sides further confusing the definitions of abuse. Whatever the true current incidence, as the population gets older and resources remain scarce, both the numbers of people at risk and the incidence of elder abuse are expected to rise.

Proponents of mandatory elder abuse reporting argue that elderly people constitute a vulnerable population that is either unable (due to incapacity) or unwilling (because of the fear of retribution or shame) to report abuse or neglect on their own.[18,19] Aside from protecting the index case for their own protec-tion, there is an argument for mandating reporting for societal benefit if the reporting leads to exposing facilities or individuals who are in fact abusing or neglecting others under their care.

Opponents of routine mandatory reporting are concerned that reporting of competent patients who could otherwise act on their own behalf violates their autonomy and confidentiality. Consequently, these patients may place less trust in their physicians. Under such circumstances, patients may avoid the ED for their care.[12,14] Other barriers to mandatory reporting include lack of time and knowledge; vague definitions; fear of offending patients, families or private physicians; uncertainty; and the reluctance to be drawn into civil lawsuits.[2,15]

Elder abuse is among a number of conditions whose mandatory reporting is opposed under a policy statement on domestic violence of the American College of Emergency Physicians (ACEP). Instead, ACEP "encourages reporting . . . to local social services, victim's services, the criminal justice system, or any other appropriate resource agency (in order) to provide confidential counseling and assistance, in accordance with the patient's wishes."[20]

Domestic violence

Domestic violence, also termed as intimate partner violence, spousal abuse, and battering, refers to the victimization of a person with whom the abuser has had an intimate or romantic relationship.[21] According to the American Medical Association, domestic violence may take the form of physical, sexual, or psychological abuse and often escalates over time. While much of the published literature assumes that women are the usual victims of domestic abuse, there is ample evidence to assume that men are frequently the victims as well.[22]

The legal duty to report some cases of domestic violence is implicit in laws that require the reporting of crimes committed with guns, knives, and other deadly weapons. Such laws exist in 45 US states.[23-25] Laws that require the reporting of suspected sexual assault may also encompass some cases of domestic violence. A small minority of states have laws that specifically mandate the reporting to law enforcement of all suspected cases of domestic violence, regardless of mechanism. California has been at the vanguard of such laws, fueling heated controversy.

Proponents of these laws cite the duty to protect vulnerable victims who may be reluctant to report on their own behalf out of shame or fear of reprisal. Further, they argue that the ED offers an opportune, and even unique, setting to address this problem for several reasons.[25] Underserved patients are seen disproportionately in the ED as compared with other settings and this may offer an opportunity to screen for domestic violence; in addition, the long times patients experience waiting to be seen affords an opportunity for screening without causing unnecessary delays. Theoretically, some patients may also feel more comfortable disclosing abuse in the secure setting offered by the ED, particularly to strangers with whom they have no relationship.[26]

Opponents of laws requiring the reporting of all domestic violence to law enforcement authorities point to the fact that there is little evidence that such reporting uniformly contributes to the safety of victims or facilitates access to appropriate resources.[23,24,27-31] In fact, it is argued that mandatory reporting may paradoxically put abused patients at increased risk by deterring them from telling their providers about the abuse or from seeking care at all.[22,31] In such cases, care and referrals to appropriate resources and counseling will not occur. Furthermore, if there is no effective response to reporting, the presence of a mandatory reporting law may produce a false sense of security on the part of the patient.[32]

Routine reporting to law enforcement may produce other unwanted consequences including physical danger, loss of a job (for the alleged abuser), deportation, family separation, or other circumstances that may be less acceptable than solutions that could be worked out without police involvement.[32] The issue of deportation could especially impact the willingness of undocumented immigrants to seek care in the ED, where much of their care is routinely provided.

Setting aside the issue of mandatory reporting, physicians and other providers have an affirmative moral duty to be familiar with domestic violence, reasonably screen for it, detect it, treat it, and provide appropriate referrals to shelters and other resources. Caregivers must set aside biases and misconceptions about domestic violence and not let these interfere with the diagnosis and management of abuse. Physicians must have adequate training in these issues. Medical societies should put their resources into helping to reduce the scourge of abuse and assuring the proper care and protection for its victims. Finally, individual doctors who are situated to do so should look for opportunities within their communities to help address all these issues.

Like elder abuse, domestic violence is also among the conditions whose mandatory reporting is opposed by ACEP.[19] The American Medical Association takes a more nuanced position on mandatory reporting of domestic violence.[33] It recommends:
• That physicians comply with the law in jurisdictions where reporting is mandatory
• Physicians within these jurisdictions should advocate to change the law if evidence suggest that mandatory reporting laws are not in the best interest of the patients (author's note: this shifts the burden of proof to physicians who must show evidence that these laws cause harm, rather than leaving it with law-makers to show they have benefit)
• In jurisdictions without mandatory reporting laws, reporting requires the informed consent of the patient. In this author's opinion, the fact that in the absence of mandatory reporting laws the policy recommends obtaining consent makes clear that from an ethical rather than legal point of view, the patient's informed consent is preferred.

Seizures and other lapses of consciousness
Mandatory reporting of seizures is required in six US states.[34] In some states, the laws are drawn more broadly, e.g., California, where the law requires the reporting to the department of motor vehicles of all conditions characterized by a lapse of consciousness, including seizures.[35,36] A survey of physicians in California finds that of 14 possible conditions that can cause a lapse of consciousness, only seizures are consistently reported; the others are rarely or never reported.[37] This may be partly because it is unclear when an event is an isolated event and when it becomes a condition. For instance, if a patient has an episode of syncope that is felt to be most likely vasovagal, this may be interpreted as a single episode rather than a condition. Similarly, what should one do about a patient with diabetes who experiences hypoglycemia and has their drug regimen changed? Existing guidelines are vague. Oregon has a broadly written law that requires the reporting to the department of motor vehicles of "functional and cognitive impairments" that are "severe and uncontrollable,"[2]

widely interpreted to include drug and alcohol abuse if they result in a motor vehicle crash, subject to interpretation by the physician.

Patients whose condition is reported against their will are subject to suspension of their driver's license and require medical follow-up, supervision, monitoring, and a release to be able to return to driving. Overriding the patient's desire to keep their episode or illness confidential frequently results in dissatisfaction or anger toward the physician who files the report. This may be minimized in some cases by taking the time to address the issue with the patient, empathizing with them, and stressing that they are being reported, in part, in order to prevent future harm to them or someone else, and to comply with the law. In fact, physicians are morally obligated to be truthful and tell patients who are conscious and possess capacity that their condition will be reported.

Opponents of mandatory reporting argue that this compromises patient confidentiality and trust with little potential gain. They point out that the risk of a patient with seizures having an accident is barely greater than for those without seizures, and that the loss of driving privileges can have severe consequences on someone's life, such as loss of independence, compromised ability to work and provide for one's self and family, social isolation, limited participation in community, decreased quality of life, and diminished self-worth.[34] Another concern is that patients with seizures will withhold crucial information about themselves from doctors at routine visits and potentially not receive optimal care for their condition.[38]

The ACEP policy on reporting of potentially impaired drivers states that reporting should be individualized to the patient's clinical condition and the risk posed to the patient and public by continued driving.[39] ACEP opposes mandatory reporting of entire classes of patients or diagnoses (e.g., epilepsy) unless compelling evidence exists for a public health benefit for such reporting. The AMA policy is similar.[40]

Permissive reporting laws

Permissive reporting laws allow but do not compel physicians to report certain conditions, e.g., the use of alcohol or drugs during a serious motor vehicle accident. California's mandatory reporting law for lapse of consciousness law also has a permissive clause:

103900. (a) Every physician and surgeon shall report immediately to the local health officer in writing, the name, date of birth, and address of every patient at least 14 years of age or older whom the physician and surgeon has diagnosed as having a case of a disorder characterized by lapses of consciousness. However, if a physician and surgeon reasonably and in good faith believes that the reporting of a patient will serve the public interest, he or she may report a patient's condition even if it may not be required under the department's definition of disorders characterized by lapses of consciousness pursuant to subdivision.[35]

Such laws raise ethical concerns. When individuals can pick and choose whom to report, they may be more likely to choose members of one socioeconomic or cultural group over another. Human nature is likely to lead one to be more suspicious of someone who appears, acts, or speaks differently than they do. Even mandatory laws are subject to these concerns, since there may be a bias with regard to whom one is suspicious of, and suspicions only must be reported.

At the heart of all of these situations is the moral responsibility of physicians to weigh and balance the duties to protect confidentiality; to respect patient autonomy; to protect society and third parties; and to follow the law. As seen, arriving at the right balance is often difficult. It is also important that physicians receive proper education and training in these areas, and are familiar with the principles of ethical reasoning. Medical societies, hospital medical staff, and those outside the profession can also play useful roles in guiding physicians as to the proper course.

Mandatory reporting laws and civil disobedience: conscience over law

Just as confidentiality is not inviolate, neither is it always a clear or absolute duty to report a "mandatory" condition. A physician's professional duty is primarily to the patient. A moral hazard is created when a physician becomes an agent of the state.

During the Nazi era in Germany, 1933–1945, physicians were integral to implementing key Nazi policies, all of which were "legal" under the regime of the Third Reich. These included the Nuremberg race laws (e.g., physicians headed up racial offices and conducted examinations required under the Marital

Health Law); the Sterilization Act, under which 360 000 sterilizations were performed on patients suspected of carrying "genetic defects" (in addition to performing the procedures, physicians were expected to report potential candidates for sterilization), and the "Operation T-4" euthanasia program, which initially required physicians and midwives to register any child born with congenital deformities, and who were then euthanized at one of 28 institutions, including some of the most venerable hospitals in Germany (the program was eventually expanded to include children with acquired diseases, and later to undesirable adults).[41] All of the aforementioned laws had a "mandatory reporting" component. In addition, physicians had a role in the "final solution," resulting in the mass genocide of Jews, and others, and conducted unethical experiments on forced subjects in the concentration camps. Indeed, it is safe to say that the full scope of the atrocities that transpired during the Holocaust could not have been carried out had physicians not been co-opted as agents of the state, and had they resisted the laws of the day.[41]

In California in recent years, voters passed proposition 187, a statewide ballot initiative allegedly designed to deter illegal immigration into the United States from its southern border.[42] In part, the measure required medical personnel to report anyone "reasonably suspected" of being an illegal alien to state and federal agencies. Left to individual discretion, "reasonable suspicion" might be based on a patient's appearance, surname, skin color, or spoken language. Fortunately, this law was challenged in the courts and was never implemented. Had it been implemented, in the opinion of the author, physicians would have been morally obligated to commit civil disobedience and not follow it, since following it would have produced clear harm to patients and likely would have deterred them from seeking care in the first place.

Section IV: Recommendations

• Confidentiality is not absolute and may be breached under certain circumstances involving mandatory reporting laws.
• Physicians should be familiar with mandatory reporting requirements within the jurisdictions in which they practice. Reporting conditions in order to improve the public health by infection control, injury prevention, etc. is an affirmative obligation since it is designed to confer good and prevent harm.
• Child abuse laws should be followed in order to protect vulnerable patients who are not situated to act autonomously to protect themselves.
• Adult patients with decision-making capacity should give informed consent before suspected domestic violence or elder abuse is reported, unless the physician is legally compelled to report.
• Physicians working in states with mandatory reporting laws for domestic violence and elder abuse (regardless of consent) should try to balance their duty to follow the law with the special ethical concerns and needs of each patient, and should seek to have these statutes revised to allow for consent.
• Physicians should report certain lapses of consciousness as required by law in order to avoid civil lawsuits and licensure issues. However, physicians in these states should seek to change laws that require the reporting of entire classes of patients or diagnoses.
• Permissive reporting should be viewed skeptically. Discrimination in reporting is a potential pitfall.
• Physicians have a duty to disobey laws they believe are ethically wrong, and to follow their conscience.

References

1. Stein R. (2010) Do doctors rat on each other? *Washington Post.* July 14. Available at: http://voices. washingtonpost.com/checkup/2010/07/do_doctors_rat_on_each_other.html. Accessed August 29, 2011.
2. Gupta M, Madsen T. (2006) Mandatory reporting laws and the emergency physician. *Ann Emerg Med.* 49(3), 369–76.
3. Geiderman JM, Moskop JC, Derse AR. (2006) Privacy and confidentiality in emergency medicine: obligations and challenges. *Emerg Med Clin North Am.* 24, 633–56.
4. Child Welfare and Information Gateway. *National and State Child Abuse and Neglect Statistics.* Rockville, MD: US Department of Health and Human Services. Available at: www.childwelfare.gov/systemwide/statistics/can/stat_natl_state.cfm. Accessed June 30, 2011.
5. Melton GB. (2005) Mandated reporting: a policy without reason. *Child Abuse Negl.* 29, 9–18.
6. Faller KC. (1985) Unanticipated problems in the United States child protection system. *Child Abuse Negl.* 9, 63–9.

7. Fortune MM. (2010) Confidentiality and mandatory reporting: a clergy dilemma? *Faith Trust Inst.* 19, 1–6.

8. Buckley H. (2011) Mandatory reporting may not be right for a child. *The Post. IE* July 24. Available at: www.iasw.ie/index.php/misc-folder/444-mandatory-reporting-may-not-be-right-for-child-abuse-dr-helen-buckely-july-2011. Accessed August 30, 2011.

9. Chorba TL, Berkelman RL, Safford SK, et al. (1990) Mandatory reporting of infectious diseases by clinicians. *MMWR Recomm Rep.* 39(RR-9), 1–17.

10. California Department of Public Health. (2011) *Reportable Infectious Diseases. Reporting by Laboratories.* Available at: www.cdph.ca.gov/HealthInfo/Documents/TITLE_17_SECTION_2505.pdf. Accessed August 30, 2011.

11. Centers for Disease Control and Prevention. (2010) *Nationally Notifiable Infectious Conditions.* Rockville, MD: US Department of Health and Human Services. Available at: www.cdc.gov/osels/ph_surveillance/nndss/phs/infdis2010.htm. Accessed August 30, 2011.

12. Robinson DJ, ONeil D. (2007) Access to health care records after death: balancing confidentiality with appropriate disclosure. *JAMA.* 297(6), 634–6.

13. Tarasoff *v.* Regents of the University of California, 17 Cal. 3d 425, 551 P.2d 334, 131 Cal. Rptr. 14 (Cal. 1976).

14. Kleinschmidt KC. (1997) Elder abuse: a review. *Ann Emerg Med.* 30(4), 463–72.

15. Jones JS, Veenstra TR, Seamon JP, et al. (1997) Elder mistreatment: national survey of emergency physicians. *Ann Emerg Med.* 30(4), 473–9.

16. National Center on Elder Abuse. (2005) *Elder Abuse Prevalence and Incidence. Fact sheet.* Washington, DC: National Center on Elder Abuse.

17. The Law Offices of Young & Wallin. (2006) *Elder Law Information From Elder Abuse Lawyers in California.* Available at: www.elderabusepractice.com/elderlaw.html. Accessed May 22, 2011.

18. Moskowitz S. (1998) Saving granny from the wolf: elder abuse and neglect: the legal framework. *Connecticut Law Rev.* 31, 77–204.

19. Jgers GJ, Daly JM, Brinig MF, et al. (2003) Domestic elder abuse and the law. *Am J Public Health.* 93, 2131–6.

20. American College of Emergency Physician. (2007) *Policy Statement on Domestic Family Violence.* Washington, DC: American College of Emergency Physician. Available at: www.acep.org/content.aspx?id=29184. Accessed May 22, 2011.

21. Council on Scientific Affairs, American Medical Association. (1992) Violence against women relevance for medical practitioners. *JAMA.* 267(23), 3184–9.

22. George MJ. (1997) Riding the donkeys backwards: men as the unacceptable victims of marital violence. *J Men's Stud.* 32, 137–59.

23. Hyman A, Schillinger D, Lo B. (1995) Laws mandating reporting of domestic violence. *JAMA.* 273(22), 1781–7.

24. Hyman A. (1996) Domestic violence: legal issues for healthcare practitioners and instoitutions. *JAMWA.* 51(3), 101–5.

25. Houry D, Sachs CJ, Feldhaus KM, et al. (2002) Violence-inflicted injuries: reporting laws in the fifty states. *Ann Emerg Med.* 39(1), 56–60.

26. Koziol-McLain J, Campbell J. (2001) Universal screening and mandatory reporting: an update on two important issues for victims/survivors of intimate partner violence. *J Emerg Nurs.* 27(6), 602–6.

27. Rodriguez MA, Craig AM, Mooney DR. (1998) Patient attitudes about mandatory reporting of domestic violence implications for health care professionals. *West J Med.* 169, 337–41.

28. Iavicoli L. (2005) Mandatory reporting of domestic violence: the law, friend or foe? *Mount-Sinai J Med.* 72(4), 228–31.

29. Hayden SR, Barton ED, Hayden M. (1997) Domestic violence in the Emergency department: how do women prefer to disclose and discuss the issues? *J Emerg Med.* 15(4), 447–51.

30. Rodriguez MA, McLoughlin E, Nah G, et al. Mandatory reporting of domestic violence injuries to the police what do emergency department patients think? *JAMA.* 2001;286(5), 580–3.

31. Geiderman JM. (2000) Mandatory reporting laws do not deter patients from seeking medical care [letter]. *Ann Emerg Med.* 35, 11–16.

32. Bauer H, Mooney D, Larkin H, et al. (1999) Culture and medicine California's mandatory reporting of domestic violence injuries: does the law go too far or not far enough? *West J Med.* 171, 118–24.

33. American Medical Association. (2007) *Amendment to opinion E-2.02, physicians' obligations in preventing, identifying, and treating violence and abuse.* CEJA Report 6-I-07, pp. 1–7.

34. Lee W, Wolfe T, Shreeve S. (2002) Reporting epileptic drivers to licensing authorities is unnecessary and counterproductive. *Ann Emerg Med.* 39, 656–9.

35. California Department of Motor Vehicles. (2011) *Health and Safety Code Section 103900. Reporting Disorders Characterized by Lapses of Consciousness.* Sacramento, CA: California Department of Motor Vehicles. Available at: http://dmv.ca.gov/pubs/vctop/appndxa/hlthsaf/hs103900.htm. Accessed July 8, 2011.

36. California Department of Motor Vehicles. (2011) *Health and Safety Code Section Article 2.4, Sections*

110.01 and 110.02 of title 13. *Driver Safety Information Lapses of Consciousness Disorder*. Sacramento, CA: California Department of Motor Vehicles. Available at: http://dmv.ca.gov/dl/driversafety/lapes.htm. Accessed July 8, 2011.

37. Vierra DA, Turnipseed SD, Panacek EA. (2005) Reporting of lapses of consciousness by emergency physicians. *Ann Emerg Med*. 46(3), 33.

38. Salinsky MC, Wegener K, Sinnema F. (1992) Epilepsy, driving laws, and patient disclosure to physicians. *Epilepsia*. 33(3), 469–72.

39. American College of Emergency Physicians. (2011) *Physician Reporting of Potentially Impaired Drivers. Policy Statement*. Washington, DC: American College of Emergency Physicians. Available at: www.acep.org/Content.aspx?id=78585. Accessed May 22, 2011.

40. American Medical Association. (2000) *Impaired Drivers and Their Physicians. Code of Medical Ethics Opinion 2.24*. Chicago, IL: American Medical Association. Available at: www.ama-assn.org/ama/pub/physician-resources/medical-ethics/code-medical-ethics/opinion224.page. Accessed July 16, 2010.

41. Geiderman JM. (2002) Physician complicity in the Holocaust: historical review and reflections on emergency medicine in the 21st century—Part I. *Acad Emerg Med*. 9, 223–31.

42. Geiderman JM. (2002) Physician complicity in the Holocaust: historical review and reflections on emergency medicine in the 21st century—Part II. *Acad Emerg Med*. 9, 232–40.

26 Ethics of care during a pandemic

John C. Moskop

Wallace and Mona Wu Chair in Biomedical Ethics, and Professor of Internal Medicine, Wake Forest School of Medicine, Winston-Salem, NC, USA

Section I: Case presentation

The medical director of the emergency department (ED) at a leading academic medical center is also chair of a pandemic influenza taskforce created to develop medical center policies and procedures for responding to a severe influenza pandemic. Today the taskforce is struggling with a difficult issue. The group is aware that, should a severe pandemic reach its city, the number of patients with life-threatening illness presenting to the ED would far exceed the hospital's capacity. They have discussed several options for responding to this situation of extreme scarcity, but cannot reach consensus on which one to incorporate into their plan. Options they have discussed are:

1. When ED and hospital beds are fully occupied, they would close the ED, and inform arriving patients that there is no room for them and that they should seek care elsewhere or return home.

2. Avoid turning patients away from the hospital, even though they will have to be cared for in conference rooms, hallways, the hospital cafeteria, and on the floors of already occupied patient rooms, and the care provided to each patient will be limited by the availability of staff and resources.

3. Direct "overflow" patients to an alternative care facility. (This option would require the institution to

identify and prepare this facility in advance, including stockpiling of material resources and recruitment of personnel to staff the facility.)

4. Do nothing, e.g., Ignore the possibility that more patients may seek care than the hospital can accommodate and offer no advice about what to do with these patients.

Which option should the taskforce choose?

Section II: Discussion

Dr. Peter Rosen: The most recent experience we all had with the flu epidemic is fairly typical of what happens when we try to make plans for an event about which we have poor information. I really don't see this as an ethical dilemma as much as I see it as a communications dilemma. Epidemiologists have been predicting a reoccurrence of the 1918 pandemic every 12 years. We've had two major scares. The first was during President Gerald Ford's administration, when national immunization was commenced because of a single case of swine flu in a soldier who, it turns out, died of the flu because he had been forced to march 5 miles with a 103° fever. The second involved the recent H1N1 flu strain, which despite the hype, actually produced very little in the way of major illness. What we did see was a tremendous overload

Ethical Problems in Emergency Medicine: A Discussion-Based Review, First Edition. John Jesus, Shamai A. Grossman, Arthur R. Derse, James G. Adams, Richard Wolfe, and Peter Rosen.
© 2012 John Wiley & Sons, Ltd. Published 2012 by John Wiley & Sons, Ltd.

of ED occupancy, and a major problem with dispositions driven largely by the high density of college and university students.

Dr. James Adams: We always want to consider the worst-case scenarios, but often resources are not actually overstretched. In fact, if we look at past disasters, both infectious disasters and natural disasters, it's very rare that the resources of the medical community in the United States are really authentically outstretched. Nevertheless, let's assume that we are dealing with that very rare situation where our resources are outstretched by the demand. We then face the ethical dilemma of deciding who really must stay in the hospital and what information we should use to make these decisions. A shift in our thinking may help us understand that our resources are not that limited.

PR: I've been involved in a number of civilian disasters, but not on the magnitude of a natural disaster or a terror attack where hospital resources throughout a city are destroyed. We had an instance in San Diego, during which a nursing home next to the hospital caught fire. We didn't know the extent of the fire, but a tremendous amount of smoke billowed into the hospital. We faced the decision of whether or not we would be forced to close the hospital and evacuate all patients. I was quite surprised at how easy it was to find facilities to which we could move patients, and empty the ED. We made an announcement about the possibility of dangerous toxic smoke inhalation. "If any of you need immediate care we will make sure that you receive it, but if not, could you possibly see fit to come back later?" Ninety percent of the patients in the ED went home, and didn't even ask for alternative help.

Dr. John Moskop: In the pandemic flu plans I have reviewed, public health and hospital authorities typically make several key assumptions. The first assumption is that the virulence of a pandemic influenza strain can vary greatly, and that a severe pandemic would produce large numbers of patients who require hospitalization. The second assumption is that there will not be much outside assistance available, because surrounding hospitals and communities will also be overwhelmed with the surge of pandemic flu patients. The third is that hospitals can and should implement several measures to increase their surge capacity. For example, hospitals should

discharge patients who no longer require hospital care. They should screen and divert patients with minor illness who don't need hospitalization. They should cancel elective admissions and other procedures that aren't immediately needed. They can convert some units within the hospital in order to meet expected needs of severely ill flu patients. The fourth assumption is that despite all those measures, hospital capacity may ultimately be insufficient to meet patient demand. A fifth assumption is that hospitals may expect their employees to fulfill their job responsibilities during a pandemic. The final assumption is that at least some advance preparation for a pandemic situation is desirable, because it will enable a more organized and consistent response to the situation, and will be more likely to achieve the priority goals of the hospital and of the society than an ad hoc, unplanned response.

PR: If you study historical epidemics, employee participation in disaster relief, because of the natural dangers involved, has been variable. During the great plague epidemics in the twelfth century, as well as with the AIDS epidemic, there was significant unwillingness of medical personnel to care for these patients. I don't think there is a way of knowing how medical staff will respond to an epidemic.

Dr. Arthur Derse: There are uncertainties in the response of medical staff in any given disaster situation. We had some experience with this in the SARS [severe acute respiratory syndrome] epidemic in Toronto, during which a number of employees chose not to return to work. Some of those people were later fired from their positions for that decision. We might expect similar occurrences, and should also expect that if a pandemic occurs, a certain percentage of healthcare workers will be sick and unable to work.

Dr. John Jesus: There are some morally relevant reasons why physicians and other healthcare professionals might not show up to work. In addition to a conflicting duty of providing care for sick children and the elderly, there is also the issue of whether or not physicians have a right to protect themselves from the risk of harm to themselves. How much personal risk can we expect medical personnel to accept? I think that will end up being a personal value judgment. Though those clinicians may be fired for breach of duty, I don't know if I can judge their decisions as ethically inappropriate. There is also a lot of uncertainty about who may or may not show up for work. I think that an institution can go a long way towards trying to limit the amount of attrition by focusing on planning and communication. The goal of this would be to reduce the likelihood of medical personnel making decisions based on either irrational fear or incorrect information.

PR: You have raised the point of ethical duty. When you take on the job of a physician or nurse you do so for a variety of reasons. At least one of those reasons is that you want the rewards of being a health professional and that carries a price tag. The price is that you are exposed to dangers and stresses that you otherwise would not be. I personally think that it's unethical to assume those responsibilities only when it is convenient, lucrative, and without risk. If that is your attitude towards being a physician, then you should find a different profession. It is your duty as a physician to accept the reality that you care for patients at some personal risk. I converted my tuberculosis skin test after a patient spat in my face in an ED, for example.

AD: The generation ahead of yours was fully aware that they could contract TB [tuberculosis] by taking care of patients. Today, however, the prevalence of infectious diseases is drastically lower than it had been, and what has become "out of sight" is now also "out of mind." We have to make sure that physicians are aware of the professional responsibility that goes along with their professional status. Despite their inexperience with personal risk, it is my understanding that in a number of epidemics, most health professionals did come to work to care for patients. If schools are closed, however, children will remain at home, and someone will have to take care of them. Many of the nurses and physicians in our institutions will then be torn between having to care for their children at home and going to work. We expect professionals to put themselves on the line, but if they have other familial responsibilities, they may not honor a duty to report to work. Finally, while there is an acceptance of a more utilitarian approach to disaster response within medical ethics, the same legal obligations exist regardless of the situation. There is no waiver of liability during a disaster; negligence and duty to an individual do not change.

PR: I'm specifically interested in the difference in response to polio and to HIV [human immunodeficiency virus] epidemics. I lived as a medical student through the last years of non-immunized America, and as a student helped to care for some of the last patients with polio. I didn't witness any hesitation from professionals caring for patients with polio despite its communicability. The exact opposite was true for HIV. The stigma attached to a disease that was, at the time, transmitted via male homosexual intercourse, resulted in a very different cultural response.

In regards to disaster planning, the focus has been on "single impact" disasters—an earthquake, for example. We have been unprepared for those that occur from infectious disease. A good disaster plan could provide solutions for the kind of finite resource dilemma that we would face when dealing with a pandemic. There are a few challenges, however, that we will face when trying to develop an effective plan. First, we have a major lack of accurate data. We really don't have the data necessary to estimate the resources required or the amount of hospital bed space needed to accommodate the influx of inpatients. The second problem is that we assume we can plan for everything. We attempt to model disease spread and numbers affected to handle unusual resource allocations for a pandemic, but there will be continued spread of disease over time, uneven distribution of patients across a given area, public hysteria, and other factors we aren't able to imagine that will impede our ability to prepare for the event ahead of time.

JM: Planning for pandemic healthcare would require weighing the likely consequences of different decisions, and would be similar to the kind of decisions public health directors make in implementing social distancing measures like closing schools, churches, theaters, and other public gathering places in a particular city. Each decision has a price, and the issue then becomes when is it worth paying that price in order to control the spread of this disease or to mitigate the consequences of the disease. I agree with the importance of open communication within a hospital about the plans for different stages in response to a pandemic. Should such planning be shared with the community for public input? Is this kind of transparency desirable or necessary for this kind of planning?

PR: Each institution has to look at what population it serves while making pandemic response plans. For example, in Boston it might be useful to work with the dozens of universities and schools around each hospital. Every institution serves a unique population, and it shouldn't make unilateral plans for that population without involving the surrounding institutions. One issue that arose during our recent flu epidemic was the willingness of parts of the institution to inflict extra work on other parts of the institution unilaterally. For instance, the infectious disease department refused to admit any pandemic flu patients to inpatient hospital beds and demanded that they remain in the ED. Actions like these demonstrate a complete lack of understanding of what boarding dozens of patients in the ED means to the function of that department, its patients, and the patients in the waiting room not yet seen.

Communication should extend to include all hospitals in a given metropolitan area. Even if hospitals communicate, I fear that we are so busy competing with one another that we will have very few collaborative plans. There have been instances, however, when I have seen collaborative efforts between multiple hospitals work. For example, when I worked in San Diego, we had a cruise ship arrive with 300 passengers with food poisoning. In order to handle the patient load, we set up a network of buses that transported a certain number of patients to multiple hospitals, in order to better distribute patients.

I've learned over the years that public health is political health. We live in a society where the response to any disaster is to assign blame. In order to avoid becoming victim of this societal slant, regardless of how irrational it may seem, you need to show that you've thought about the problem, and you have come up with a rational plan.

AD: Another factor to consider in planning for a flu pandemic is the need for ventilator support. There are only so many ventilators in each hospital. Even if one is able to coordinate heroic efforts from healthcare responders and a network of hospitals, the pandemic response will be limited by the resources at your disposal.

PR: My experience with attempting to set up advance protocols for how finite resources will be distributed is that it raises much anger and animosity. Regarding the question of limited number of ventilators, we tried to make rules that would be fair using age and likelihood of survival, but we were never able to reach an agreement. In the end, we agreed to use the ventilators on whom we thought it was appropriate, and when we ran out we would give relatives the option of standing there and hand bagging their relatives.

JJ: Along these lines, one should note that during a national disaster, the first responders to a disaster will be the public themselves. It is worth trying to include them in a conversation about ways they can help or prevent their families from becoming ill. Involving the public early is a worthwhile endeavor, but this should be done by departments of public health rather than individual institutions.

PR: Though this approach may appear desirable on paper, it may be plagued with misinformation. Last winter's flu epidemic, for example, involved information disseminated by public health departments that changed daily. The information was more likely to scare the public, and ensure that they present immediately to the ED than it was to give them useful information regarding how to respond.

JA: The words used to describe and inform the public are critical to controlling fear. The media, however, depend on this fear to maintain the public's attention. This approach often works against our public health goals. The healthcare community can be very resilient, but we need everyone involved to be on the same page. Public health departments and the media need to be responsible with what words they use to inform the public and the manner in which they do so.

PR: We are reliant on television, newspapers, and radio to disseminate information broadly and quickly. Unfortunately, we can count on the media to present the worst possible picture. During our recent flu epidemic, the media predicted millions of deaths but as it turned out, this just wasn't true. Providing accurate information about the situation will be essential for responding properly as the needs for care change.

JA: This case addresses the worst-case scenario in which we have done all we can do to increase capacity and to respond to patient surge, and yet are still unable to meet the needs of the patients before us. Clearly, there will be no easy solution to that situation. There will be loss and dissatisfaction, and there won't be consensus. We can think about the pros and cons of the different options, and the position of not taking a position because it's just too sensitive. I think there are different values at stake.

PR: Should we try to plan for the worst possible scenario? I would answer "No." The reason is that because it's so rare to encounter the worst possible case, we don't know what the response to it should be. We have to wait and see. Look at the national response to 9/11. For a couple of months we had a unity in America that we hadn't experienced since Pearl Harbor. That was unpredictable and unsustainable. Now, if you tried to get people to reach the same kind of consensus about a response to a terrorist attack it would be virtually impossible. We should set up a response that involves changing normal behavior to enable us to utilize our resources. Some care is better than no care. When we reach the point where we have exhausted what we can do, we determine the next steps. This will mean making different decisions than we would on the first day of the epidemic. Trying to get an agreement for that in advance just polarizes people and creates anger instead of generating useful plans.

JA: There are opportunity costs for resources that are used in preparation. They may have a big pay off and they may not. It's very difficult to predict.

PR: One of the preparation events which has bothered me for years is the disaster drill. My personnel who are trying to take care of actual patients with real diseases are asked to stop and take care of fake patients with fake diseases, because they have to get ready for an event that probably isn't going to happen. At the same time, I don't want to be unprepared to respond to a disaster. I just don't know how to do it in a way that makes it effective.

JJ: The ED does, in fact, experience periods of time when its resources are very limited and restricted on a regular basis. Just this past winter, when dealing with the influx of parents with sick children, it was important to have a plan before seeing them. It's much easier for an individual caregiver to refuse to treat a child with oseltamivir if the clinician has a rational basis for the refusal. Having accurate information and departmental agreement is also important to stem the natural clinician impulse to treat every patient with all resources available. This is clearly impossible during a true pandemic, but may also be

true of a flu season with a shortage of vaccine as occurred during our last flu season.

Dr. Shamai Grossman: Ultimately no matter what the disease or epidemic with which we are confronted, we are obligated to do as much as possible for each individual; ultimately we could never ignore the idea that we may be overwhelmed, nor could we tell patients to "go home, we will not care for you". We are ethically obligated, either through advance planning or overextension of our resources, to save as many lives as we can.

Section III: Review of the literature

Beginning in 2005, reports appeared in the medical literature and popular media about a new and highly pathogenic strain of avian influenza A (H5N1).[1,2] In addition to killing millions of poultry in southeast Asia, this new viral strain could cause serious illness and death in humans, and early evidence suggested that the virus had been transmitted from one human to another in a few cases. These reports raised fears that this H5N1 avian flu viral strain might soon fulfill the three necessary conditions for pandemic spread, namely: (1) a novel viral strain to which humans lack resistance, (2) a strain that causes disease in humans, and (3) a strain that is transmitted efficiently from humans to other humans.[3] H5N1 avian flu has a 60% case fatality rate in humans despite medical treatment, and this fact, together with a patient profile similar to that of the 1918–19 flu pandemic, suggested that this virus could produce a severe flu pandemic; perhaps as severe as the 1918–19 pandemic, with its worldwide death toll of 40–50 million people, including some 550 000 in the United States.[4] Public health officials responded rapidly in 2005 and 2006—the World Health Organization (WHO) made major revisions to its International Health Regulations and Global Influenza Preparedness Plan.[5,6] The US Department of Health and Human Services published a national pandemic influenza plan, and every state prepared its own statewide pandemic flu plan.[7,8] These early pandemic plans addressed a variety of issues, including disease surveillance and reporting, travel restrictions, pandemic stages and planning assumptions, command, control, and communication systems, and operational plans. Most did not, however, explicitly address the difficult ethical issues likely to arise in a severe flu pandemic.[9]

Drawing on their experience during the SARS outbreak in Toronto in 2003, scholars at the University of Toronto Joint Centre for Bioethics published a report in November 2005, describing key ethical values and issues in pandemic planning.[10] This report identifies four major issues: (1) healthcare workers' duty to provide care during a pandemic, (2) restrictions on personal liberty in the interest of public health, (3) allocation of scarce medical resources during a pandemic, and (4) international governance and cooperation in pandemic response. This widely circulated report helped US public health officials and scholars recognize that a severe influenza pandemic could pose virtually unprecedented moral challenges for healthcare workers, and they devoted considerable effort over the next few years to analysis of central moral issues in pandemic planning and response, especially the first three issues listed above.

Professional duties to provide pandemic care

Physicians and other healthcare professionals have well-established professional and legal duties to provide care for their patients. Caring for patients with serious communicable diseases can pose significant health risks to their caregivers, however. In the early years of the AIDS epidemic and in the 2003 SARS outbreak, some healthcare professionals chose not to accept the risk of caring for infected individuals.[11–13] The threat of a severe flu pandemic raises once again the question whether healthcare professionals have a special or greater duty to provide care in a situation of great need than at other times, despite high risks to themselves.

Many commentators conclude that physicians and other healthcare professionals do have a special duty to provide care during a flu pandemic.[14–16] These commentators appeal to several reasons in defense of this duty. They point out that flu patients will have great needs for care, and that professionals have special expertise to address those needs. Some commentators argue that healthcare professionals have an implied contract with society to provide care, in return for the social privileges they receive. In addition, some professionals have entered into specific contractual agreements to provide care in emergency situations. Finally, health professionals may have a duty to their colleagues to bear a fair share of the increased workplace risks encountered in a pandemic.

Other commentators question the scope of the professional duty to provide care, and conclude that this duty may be limited in significant ways during a pandemic.[17–19] These writers often argue that professionals have a right to protect themselves from grave danger, and point out that self-protection may enable them to care for future patients. They also assert that professionals may have a duty to care for family members during a pandemic that overrides their duty to work.

To support claims for a duty of healthcare professionals to provide pandemic care, several reports propose that healthcare institutions and government assume reciprocal duties to professionals.[16,20] These reports ascribe duties to healthcare institutions to provide their workers with appropriate personal protective equipment, preventive care, training, compensation, and support services in pandemic situations. They ascribe to government a duty to protect the good faith efforts of professionals to provide health services in extreme circumstances by altering legal standards of care or providing qualified immunity from liability.[21,22] In response to the latter proposal, however, Annas argues that altering legal standards of care during an emergency is not necessary to induce healthcare workers to respond, nor is it justifiable on moral grounds.[23]

Restrictions on personal liberty

For more than a century, US law has given public health officials the authority to restrict personal liberty in order to protect the public's health.[24] To prevent transmission of serious communicable diseases, travel restrictions can be imposed, infected patients can be isolated and required to undergo treatment, and patient contacts can be quarantined. Widespread vaccination is likely the most effective measure to prevent flu transmission, but current vaccine development and production processes take 6 months or longer to complete, and so will not be immediately available in a pandemic caused by a novel viral strain.[25] In the earliest days of a flu pandemic, travel restrictions, isolation of patients, and quarantine of exposed persons may slow disease transmission, but cannot prevent the spread of flu because infected persons can transmit disease before symptoms appear and the incubation period is very short, averaging 2 days.[26] Once illness is widespread, public health measures targeting individuals or small groups will not effectively prevent disease transmission. In these situations, pandemic plans recommend implementation of community-wide "social distancing measures" to limit disease transmission by reducing person-to-person contact.[27,28]

Proposed social distancing measures include closing of schools and day care centers, cancellation of public events such as church services, concerts, theater performances, and sporting events, and implementation of work-at-home arrangements. Evidence from the 1918–19 pandemic suggests that these social distancing measures can be effective in slowing the progression and reducing the severity of a flu pandemic. Studies comparing the responses of multiple US cities to the flu pandemic show that cities that implemented school closures and public gathering bans sooner and maintained these measures longer had delayed peak mortality and reduced overall mortality rates.[29–31]

Government and public health officials cannot take decisions to impose social distancing measures lightly, however, since these measures also have significant moral and social costs. Such measures curtail basic personal freedoms, especially freedom of association and rights to work. They may also have severe economic consequences, as businesses are forced to close by public order or due to high rates of absenteeism. Imposition of these measures will certainly heighten public fear, and may lead to isolation and neglect of vulnerable citizens. If healthcare workers and employees in other socially essential positions, such as law enforcement, food production and distribution, telecommunication, and public utilities, choose not to work in order to protect themselves from infection, basic social services will be severely disrupted.[32]

Allocation of scarce medical resources

Probably the most widely discussed ethical issue in pandemic planning in recent years has been the allocation of scarce medical resources. Pandemic healthcare will likely employ a variety of resources, including vaccines, antiviral drugs, outpatient medical services, inpatient care, and intensive care. Depending on several factors, including the severity of the pandemic, the resulting demand for care, and the available supply of resources, any of the above resources may

be in short supply. When demand outstrips supply, some patients will receive the care they need, and others will not. Several terms, including "allocation," "rationing," and "triage," are commonly used to refer to decisions about which patients will receive scarce medical resources.[33]

US legislators, and the American public, have long been extremely reluctant to acknowledge and confront the potential scarcity of healthcare resources. A notable example of this reluctance was the sustained attention devoted to tenuous political charges that a proposed provision of the US federal healthcare reform legislation would create "death panels" empowered to refuse patient desires for life-sustaining treatment.[34] Hospital pandemic planners such as those described in the case introducing this chapter may be tempted to avoid this controversial subject by simply ignoring the possibility of having to ration scarce resources in a severe pandemic. This strategy has its own risks, however, since hospitals have specific legal obligations, and licensing and accreditation requirements, to develop comprehensive emergency response plans. In March 2011, Tenet Healthcare reached an out-of-court settlement with plaintiffs who argued that Tenet's failure to prepare for a foreseeable emergency at its Memorial Medical Center in New Orleans caused harm to them after Hurricane Katrina.[35]

Although the problem of resource scarcity in an emergency may be obvious, the appropriate response may remain controversial. The moral difficulty of rationing or triage decisions derives in part from the existence of multiple competing values, guiding principles, and plausible candidates for treatment priority.[36] Table 26.1 lists six different allocation principles and the groups that would be likely to receive treatment priority under each principle. Plausible arguments can be marshaled for each of these candidate principles and priority groups, but none enjoys clear or consensus superiority over the others, and so there is no single or simple solution to rationing problems.

Vaccine allocation

The first pandemic resource allocation issue to receive explicit consideration was the allocation of vaccines and antiviral medications. An appendix to the 2005 federal pandemic response plan contains recommendations from two federal advisory committees, the

Table 26.1 Candidate allocation principles and corresponding priority groups

Allocation principle	Corresponding priority group
Preserve basic societal functions	Workers in "critical industries"
Save the most lives	Patients at greatest risk of death
Maximize the number of years of life saved	Patients with the longest life expectancy
Prevent the most suffering	Patients with the most severe symptoms
Promote the opportunity to live through the major stages of life	Children and young adults
Give all in need an equal chance for care	Patients selected by a lottery or other random method

Advisory Committee on Immunization Practices (ACIP) and the National Vaccine Advisory Committee (NVAC), regarding the distribution of pandemic flu vaccines. These committees recommended that healthcare workers and groups at highest risk for severe disease receive priority for vaccination.[37] Writing in *Science* in 2006, Emanuel and Wertheimer challenged the NVAC/ACIP recommendations for vaccine distribution. These authors would give priority for vaccination to healthy adolescents and young adults over patients at highest risk for severe disease, arguing that while adolescents and young adults have already made a significant investment in their lives, they also have a significant portion of their lives still to live.[38]

A major revision of federal pandemic flu vaccine allocation guidelines appeared in 2008.[39] The revised guidelines add two new groups, deployed military personnel and infants and toddlers 6–35 months old, to the highest priority category, and relegate adults with high-risk conditions to a much lower (tier 4) priority for vaccination.

Antiviral allocation
Treatment with the neuraminidase inhibitor drugs oseltamivir (Tamiflu) and zanamivir (Relenza) has been shown to shorten the duration of influenza and to reduce influenza mortality rates when administered

within 48 hours of symptom onset.[40,41] These drugs are also effective in preventing illness in persons exposed to influenza patients. Use of these antiviral drugs to treat and prevent infection is therefore an important element of a pandemic flu response. In addition to the flu vaccine allocation recommendations described above, the 2005 federal pandemic flu plan also included NVAC recommendations for distribution of antiviral drugs.[37] These recommendations, published when the national supply of antivirals was quite limited, proposed that antiviral drugs be used primarily for treatment of infected persons, and not for prophylaxis. Antiviral drug production expanded rapidly in the next few years; by 2008, the US federal government had purchased and added to the Centers for Disease Control and Prevention (CDC) strategic national stockpile a total of 50 million regimens of antiviral drugs for use in a flu pandemic, and individual states, businesses, and healthcare institutions had established their own stockpiles.[42]

In 2008, the federal government issued revised guidelines for the use of antiviral drugs in an influenza pandemic.[43] The revised federal guidelines recommend expansion of antiviral drug use to include prophylaxis as well as treatment. Three priority prophylactic uses are identified: (1) initial containment of pandemic flu outbreaks overseas and at the US border, (2) administration to healthcare workers at high risk of occupational influenza exposure, and (3) postexposure prophylaxis for other healthcare workers, immunocompromised persons, and persons living in residential settings such as nursing homes, prisons, and homeless shelters.

Allocation of hospital and intensive care services

In its 2007 document entitled *Community Strategy for Pandemic Influenza Mitigation*, the CDC introduced a "pandemic severity index" to guide pandemic planning and response efforts.[44] This index uses the case fatality ratio (the ratio of fatal to total influenza cases) to divide pandemics into five categories: a category 1 pandemic, with a case fatality ratio of <0.1%, would be similar in severity to seasonal influenza, and a category 5 pandemic, with a case fatality ratio of >2.0%, would be as severe as the 1918 flu pandemic. Care for patients in categories 1 and 2 pandemics, where the vast majority of illness is mild and does not require hospitalization, can be provided in the US healthcare system as currently configured. Categories 3, 4, and 5 pandemics, however, would produce large numbers of patients with severe illness requiring hospitalization and intensive care that would likely exceed existing hospital capacity.

Recognizing that H5N1 avian flu causes severe disease in humans, and could produce a severe pandemic, commentators writing after 2005 urged health systems and hospitals to develop strategies to respond to a possibly massive pandemic surge of seriously ill patients.[45–48] The case discussed in this chapter poses a question about how hospital officials should prepare for such a potential surge of pandemic patients. Beginning with Ontario in 2005, multiple governmental planning groups have included detailed hospital guidelines for mass critical care and for triage in their pandemic plans.[49–53] These guidelines typically offer recommendations in two general areas. First, they recommend strategies hospitals can implement to increase surge capacity. These strategies include deferral of elective procedures, discharge of inpatients who can be safely cared for in another setting, purchase and stockpiling of portable ventilators and ventilator supplies, reconfiguration of hospital units with oxygen capacity into temporary critical care units, and cross-training and redeployment of staff from deferred services to influenza care. In an influenza pandemic, these strategies would be implemented first in order to expand capacity to meet patient needs for care.

Second, federal and most state pandemic plans call for the creation of alternative care facilities to augment pandemic surge capacity.[54] The value of this strategy, however, depends entirely on the makeup and capabilities of the alternative care facility. Lam et al. note that government pandemic plans assign a variety of tasks to alternative care sites, from simple lodging facilities to provision of "a full range of hospital services."[54] If the facility provides only alternative lodging for its patients, like an emergency storm shelter, it will be relatively easy and inexpensive to establish, but the benefits it can provide to seriously ill patients will also be very limited, and most patients will likely be better off returning to their homes (recall the dangers faced by those directed to the Superdome in New Orleans following Hurricane Katrina). If the facility provides a full range of hospital services, it will obviously be able to provide the kind of care needed by seriously ill patients, but the

advance costs of planning, equipping, stocking, and staffing what would amount to a new acute care hospital would be enormous, and those resources might never be needed. More appropriate tasks for alternative care facilities might be initial triage of suspected flu patients, or step-down care for stable non-influenza patients, but these tasks would make only a modest contribution to increasing hospital surge capacity, at best.

Despite implementation of these measures to expand capacity, the volume of seriously ill patients at the height of a category 4 or 5 pandemic will almost certainly exceed available hospital resources, both locally and nationally.[55] To address this situation, existing guidelines offer additional recommendations in a second area, namely, triage. These guidelines focus primarily on triage decisions for the limited number of mechanical ventilators and intensive care unit beds. Drawing on an initial brief triage protocol developed by a working group for the Ontario Department of Health and Long Term Care,[46] all of the pandemic intensive care triage plans cited above recommend the same basic approach, as follows: A triage officer or team assesses whether the patient meets established inclusion criteria (to determine that critical care is needed). If so, the triage officer assesses whether the patient meets established exclusion criteria (to determine whether the patient can benefit from critical care). If the patient does not meet an exclusion criterion, the patient is evaluated using the Sequential Organ Failure Assessment (SOFA) scoring system[56] and assigned to a triage category based on his or her SOFA score; patients with lower SOFA scores are considered most likely to survive with critical care interventions, and therefore receive highest priority for care. Patients receiving critical care are reassessed at regular intervals, and may be withdrawn from critical care if their condition deteriorates or fails to improve.

Writing in 2009, White et al. offer a different strategy for pandemic triage of intensive care services.[57] These authors argue that, because the SOFA score is an indicator of short-term survival, triage systems based on SOFA scores implement the allocation principle "save the most lives." In contrast, they propose a multiprinciple triage scoring system in which priority would be awarded on the basis of (younger) patient age and long-term life expectancy in addition to short-term survivability.

A twenty-first century pandemic

The first influenza pandemic of the twenty-first century emerged very suddenly, and from an unexpected source. A novel swine-origin H1N1 influenza virus was identified as the source of a flu outbreak in Mexico in April 2009.[58] After rapid worldwide spread of the novel H1N1 viral strain over the next several months, WHO announced the existence of a pandemic in June.[59] During the first spring surge of the new pandemic, hospital intensive care units in several affected cities reported "significant stress" on their operations, and some expressed fear that the new virus could be a virulent one.[60] In the United States, the CDC released a fourth of its strategic national stockpile supply of antiviral drugs to the states in April 2009.[41] In the northern hemisphere, pandemic influenza cases peaked in October and November 2009, just before large quantities of pandemic flu vaccine were released.[61] Despite the early fears, however, the 2009 H1N1 flu pandemic proved to be a mild one, with a case fatality ratio of about 0.05%.[62] In August 2010, WHO announced that the 2009–10 H1N1 influenza pandemic was over.[63]

Section IV: Recommendations

- Recognize that the occurrence of a severe influenza pandemic would pose unprecedented moral challenges for governments, institutions, and healthcare professionals.
- Review your institution's pandemic response plans and identify responsibilities you may have in those plans.
- If existing institutional pandemic response plans are deficient, propose ways to improve them.

References

1. The Writing Committee of the World Health Organization (WHO) Consultation on Human Influenza A/H5. (2005) Avian influenza A (H5N1) infection in humans. *N Engl J Med.* 353, 1374–85.
2. Specter M. Nature's bioterrorist. (2005) *The New Yorker* 81(2), 50ff. Available at: www.newyorker.com/archive/2005/02/28/050228fa_fact_specter. Accessed July 6, 2011.
3. Asamoa-Baah A. (2004) *Technical Consultation on Influenza Pandemic Preparedness: Opening Address.* Geneva: World Health Organization. Available at: http://www.who.int/csr/disease/avian_influenza/adgspeech/en/. Accessed July 6, 2011.
4. McNeil DG Jr. (2006) Avian flu tends to kill youths as in 1918 wave, study finds. *NY Times* (July 2). Available at: www.nytimes.com/2006/07/02/world/02flu.html?scp=1&sq=Avian%20flu%20tends%20to%20kill%20youths%20as%20in%201918%20wave&st=cse. Accessed July 6, 2011.
5. World Health Organization. (2008) *International Health Regulations (2005).* 2nd ed. Geneva: World Health Organization. Available at: http://whqlibdoc.who.int/publications/2008/9789241580410_eng.pdf. Accessed July 6, 2011.
6. World Health Organization. (2005) *WHO Global Influenza Preparedness Plan.* Geneva: World Health Organization. Available at: www.who.int/csr/resources/publications/influenza/en/WHO_CDS_CSR_GIP_2005_5.pdf. Accessed July 6, 2011.
7. Department of Health and Human Services. (2005) *HHS Pandemic flu Plan.* Rockville, MD: US Department of Health and Human Services. Available at: www.hhs.gov/pandemicflu/plan/pdf/HHSPandemicInfluenzaPlan.pdf. Accessed July 6, 2011.
8. Council of State and Territorial Epidemiologists. (2006) *CTSE State Pandemic Influenza Plans.* Atlanta GA: Council of State and Territorial Epidemiologists.
9. Thomas JC, Dasgupta N, Martinot A. (2007) Ethics in a pandemic: a survey of the state pandemic influenza plans. *Am J Public Health.* 97, S26–S31.
10. University of Toronto Joint Centre for Bioethics Pandemic Influenza Working Group. (2005) *Stand on Guard for Thee: Ethical Considerations in Preparedness Planning for Pandemic Influenza.* Report. Toronto: University of Toronto Joint Centre for Bioethics. Available at: www.jointcentreforbioethics.ca/publications/documents/stand_on_guard.pdf. Accessed July 6, 2011.
11. Arras JD. (1988) The fragile web of responsibility: AIDS and the duty to treat. *Hastings Cent Rep.* 18(2 Suppl), 10–20.
12. Emanuel EJ. (1988) Do physicians have an obligation to treat patients with AIDS? *N Engl J Med.* 318, 1686–90.
13. Ruderman C, Tracy CS, Bensimon CM, et al. (2006) On pandemics and the duty to care: whose duty? who cares? *BMC Med Ethics.* 7, 5. Available at: www.biomedcentral.com/1472-6939/7/5. Accessed July 7, 2011.
14. American Medical Association. (2004) Opinion 9.067—Physician obligation in disaster preparedness and response. In: *AMA Code of Medical Ethics.*

Chicago, IL: American Medical Association. Available at: www.ama-assn.org/ama/pub/physician-resources/medical-ethics/code-medical-ethics/opinion9067.page? Accessed July 7, 2011.

15. Iserson KV, Heine CE, Larkin GL, et al. (2008) Fight or flight: the ethics of emergency physician disaster response. *Ann Emerg Med*. 51, 345–53.

16. North Carolina Task Force on Ethics and Pandemic Influenza Planning. (2007) *Stockpiling Solutions: North Carolina's Ethical Guidelines for an Influenza Pandemic*. Durham, NC: North Carolina Institute of Medicine. Available at: www.nciom.org/wp-content/uploads/2007/04/flureport.pdf. Accessed July 7, 2011.

17. Reid L. (2005) Diminishing returns? Risk and the duty to care in the SARS epidemic. *Bioethics*. 19, 348–61.

18. Sokol DK. (2006) Virulent epidemics and scope of healthcare workers' duty of care. *Emerg Infect Dis*. 12, 1238–41.

19. Malm H, May T, Francis LP, et al. (2008) Ethics, pandemics, and the duty to treat. *Am J Bioethics*. 8, 4–19.

20. Meslin EM, Alyea JM, Helft PR. (2008) Healthcare workforce management and pandemic influenza preparedness. In: *Pandemic Influenza Preparedness: Ethical Issues and Recommendations to the Indiana State Department of Health*. Indianapolis, IN: Indiana University Center for Bioethics, pp. 67–81. Available at: https://scholarworks.iupui.edu/bitstream/handle/1805/1912/pandemic_TADs-ABs_2008.pdf?sequence=1. Accessed July 7, 2011.

21. Gostin LO, Hanfling D. (2009) National preparedness for a catastrophic emergency: crisis standards of care. *JAMA*. 302, 2365–6.

22. Institute of Medicine. (2009) *Guidance for Establishing Crisis Standards of Care for Use in Disaster Situations: A Letter Report*. Washington, DC: National Academies Press.

23. Annas GJ. (2010) Standard of care—in sickness and in health and in emergencies. *N Engl J Med*. 362, 2126–31.

24. Parmet WE, Goodman RA, Farber A. (2005) Individual rights versus the public's health—100 years after *Jacobson v. Massachusetts*. *N Engl J Med*. 352, 652–4.

25. Harris KM, Maurer J, Kellermann AL. (2010) Influenza vaccine—safe, effective, and mistrusted. *N Engl J Med*. 363, 2183–5.

26. Toner E. (2006) Do public health and infection control measures prevent the spread of flu? *Biosecur Bioterror*. 4, 84–86.

27. World Health Organization Writing Group. (2006) Nonpharmaceutical interventions for pandemic influenza, national and community measures. *Emerg Infect Dis*. 12, 88–94.

28. Centers for Disease Control and Prevention. (2007) *Community Strategy for Pandemic Influenza Mitigation*. Atlanta, GA: Centers for Disease Control and Prevention. Available at: www.pandemicflu.gov/professional/community/commitigation.html. Accessed July 8, 2011.

29. Hatchett RJ, Mecher CE, Lipsitch M. (2007) Public health interventions and epidemic intensity during the 1918 influenza pandemic. *Proc Natl Acad Sci*. 104, 7582–7.

30. Bootsma MCJ, Ferguson NM. (2007) The effect of public health measures on the 1918 influenza pandemic in U.S. cities. *Proc Natl Acad Sci*. 104, 7588–93.

31. Markel H, Lipman HB, Navarro JA, et al. (2008) Nonpharmaceutical interventions implemented by US cities during the 1918–1919 influenza pandemic. *JAMA*. 298, 644–54.

32. Middaugh JP. (2008) Pandemic influenza preparedness and community resiliency. *JAMA*. 299, 566–8.

33. Iserson KV, Moskop JC. (2007) Triage in medicine, part I: Concept, history, and types. *Ann Emerg Med*. 49, 275–81.

34. Corn BW. (2009) Ending end-of-life phobia—a prescription for enlightened health care reform. *N Engl J Med*. 361(27), e63.

35. Hodge JG Jr, Fuse Brown E. (2011) Assessing liability for health care entities that insufficiently prepare for catastrophic emergencies. *JAMA*. 306, 308–9.

36. Moskop JC, Iserson KV. (2007) Triage in medicine, part II: Underlying values and principles. *Ann Emerg Med*. 49, 282–7.

37. Department of Health and Human Services. (2005) Appendix D: NVAC/ACIP recommendations for prioritization of pandemic influenza vaccine and NVAC recommendations on pandemic antiviral drug use. *HHS Pandemic flu Plan*. Rockville, MD: Department of Health and Human Services. Available at: www.hhs.gov/pandemicflu/plan/pdf/AppD.pdf. Accessed July 11, 2011.

38. Emanuel EJ, Wertheimer A. (2006) Who should get influenza vaccine when not all can? *Science*. 312, 854–5.

39. Department of Health and Human Services, Department of Homeland Security. (2008) *Guidance on Allocating and Targeting Pandemic Influenza Vaccine*. Rockville, MD: US Department of Health and Human Services. Available at: www.flu.gov/individualfamily/vaccination/allocationguidance.pdf. Accessed July 11, 2011.

40. Genentech USA. (2011) *Tamiflu Package Insert*. San Francisco, CA: Genentech USA, Inc. Available at: www.gene.com/gene/products/information/tamiflu/pdf/pi.pdf. Accessed July 12, 2011.

41. GlaxoSmithKline. (2010) *Relenza Package Insert.* Research Triangle Park, NC: GlaxoSmithKline. Available at: http://us.gsk.com/products/assets/us_relenza.pdf. Accessed July 12, 2011.

42. Patel A, Gorman SE. (2009) Stockpiling antiviral drugs for the next influenza pandemic. *Clin Pharmacol Therap.* 86, 241–3.

43. Department of Health and Human Services. (2008) *Guidance on Antiviral Drug Use during an Influenza Pandemic.* Rockville, MD: US Department of Health and Human Services. Available at: www.pandemicflu.gov/vaccine/antiviral_use.pdf. Accessed July 12, 2011.

44. Centers for Disease Control and Prevention. (2007) Pre-pandemic planning: the Pandemic Severity Index. *Community Strategy for Pandemic Influenza Mitigation.* Atlanta, GA: US Centers for Disease Control and Prevention. Available at: www.flu.gov/professional/community/commitigation.html#IV. Accessed July 13, 2011.

45. Hick JL, O'Laughlin DT. (2006) Concept of operations for triage of mechanical ventilation in an epidemic. *Acad Emerg Med.* 13, 223–9.

46. Christian MD, Hawryluck L, Wax RS, et al. (2006) Development of a triage protocol for critical care during an influenza pandemic. *CMAJ.* 175, 1377–81.

47. Levin PJ, Gebbie EN, Qureshi K. (2007) Can the health-care system meet the challenge of pandemic flu? Planning, ethical, and workforce considerations. *Public Health Rep.* 122, 573–8.

48. Devereaux A, Christian MD, Dichter JR, et al. Summary of suggestions from the Task Force for Mass Critical Care Summit, January 26–27, 2007. *Chest.* 133, 1S–7S.

49. Ontario Ministry of Health and Long-Term Care. (2008) Chapter 17. Acute care services. In: *Ontario Health Plan for an Influenza Pandemic.* Toronto, ON: Ministry of Health and Long-Term Care. Available at: www.health.gov.on.ca/english/providers/program/emu/pan_flu/ohpip2/ch_17.pdf. Accessed July 13, 2011.

50. Utah Department of Health. (2009) *Utah Pandemic Influenza Hospital and ICU Triage Guidelines.* West Salt Lake City, UT: Utah Department of Health. Available at: http://pandemicflu.utah.gov/plan/med_triage081109.pdf. Accessed July 13, 2011.

51. New York State Workgroup on Ventilator Allocation in an Influenza Pandemic. (2007) *Allocation of Ventilators in an Influenza Pandemic: Planning Document.* New York, NY: New York State Department of Health. Available at: www.health.state.ny.us/diseases/communicable/influenza/pandemic/ventilators/docs/ventilator_guidance.pdf. Accessed July 13, 2011.

52. Vawter DE, Garrett JE, Gervais KG, et al. (2010) *For the Good of Us All: Ethically Rationing Health Resources in Minnesota in a Severe Influenza Pandemic.* Minnesota Pandemic Ethics Project Report. St. Paul, MN: Minnesota Center for Health Care Ethics. Available at: www.health.state.mn.us/divs/idepc/ethics/ethics.pdf. Accessed Jul7 13, 2011.

53. Pandemic Influenza Ethics Initiative Work Group, VHA National Center for Ethics in Health Care. (2010) *Meeting the Challenge of Pandemic Influenza: Ethical Guidance for Leaders and Health Care Professionals in the Veterans Health Administration.* Available at: www.ethics.va.gov/docs/pandemicflu/Meeting_the_Challenge_of_Pan_Flu-Ethical_Guidance_VHA_20100701.pdf. Accessed July 13, 2011.

54. Lam C, Waldhorn R, Toner E, et al. (2006) The prospect of using alternative medical care facilities in an influenza pandemic. *Biosecur Bioterror.* 4, 384–90.

55. Toner E, Waldhorn R. (2006) What hospitals should do to prepare for an influenza pandemic. *Biosecur Bioterror.* 4, 397–402.

56. Ferreira FL, Bota DP, Bross A, et al. (2001) Serial evaluation of the SOFA score to predict outcome in critically ill patients. *JAMA.* 286, 1754–8.

57. White DB, Katz MH, Luce JM, et al. Who should receive life support during a public health emergency? Using ethical principles to improve allocation decisions. *Ann Intern Med.* 150, 132–8.

58. Perez-Padilla R, de la Rosa-Zamboni D, Ponce de Leon S, et al. (2009) Pneumonia and respiratory failure from swine-origin influenza A (H1N1) in Mexico. *N Engl J Med.* 361, 680–9.

59. Chan M. (2009) *World Now at the Start of 2009 Influenza Pandemic* (WHO Director-General statement, June 11, 2009). Geneva: World Health Organization. Available at: www.who.int/mediacentre/news/statements/2009/h1n1_pandemic_phase6_20090611/en/index.html. Accessed July 20, 2011.

60. Funk DJ, Siddiqui F, Wiebe K, et al. (2010) Practical lessons from the first outbreaks: Clinical presentation, obstacles, and management strategies for severe pandemic (pH1N1) 2009 influenza pnuemonitis. *Crit Care Med.* 38(4 Suppl), e30–e7.

61. Centers for Disease Control and Prevention. (2010) Update: influenza activity in the United States, 2009–2010 season. *MMWR.* 59, 901–8.

62. Nishiura H. (2009) The virulence of pandemic influenza A (H1N1): an epidemiological perspective on the case-fatality rate. *Expert Rev Respir Med.* 4, 329–38.

63. World Health Organization. (2010) *H1N1 in Post-Pandemic Period* (Director-General statement, August 10, 2010). Geneva: World Health Organization. Available at: www.who.int/mediacentre/news/statements/2010/h1n1_vpc_20100810/en/index.html. Accessed July 20, 2011.

Education and research

27 Practicing medical procedures on the newly or nearly dead

Ajay V. Jetley,[1] Catherine A. Marco[2]

[1]Resident Physician, Department of Emergency Medicine, University of Toledo College of Medicine, Toledo, OH, USA

[2]Professor, Department of Emergency Medicine, University of Toledo Medical Center, Toledo, OH, USA

Section I: Case presentation

An 89-year-old Caucasian woman is transferred to the emergency department (ED) from an elderly care facility after she develops chest pain unresponsive to her usual sublingual nitroglycerin. En route to the ED, the patient becomes non-responsive, and cardiac monitoring reveals ventricular fibrillation. Cardiopulmonary resuscitation (CPR) is delayed by approximately 9 minutes as the patient is still in transport, and she develops asystole and respiratory arrest. On arrival to the ED, it is discovered that the patient has a do-not-resuscitate and comfort care (DNR-CC) order, as she has multiple comorbidities. The family, who is also en route, confirms that their mother wanted to "go peacefully," and state that they want the DNR-CC order to be honored, and that they will arrive in approximately 45 minutes. On hearing this, the attending emergency physician calls the medical students rotating through the ED that month, to practice placement of central lines, intubations, arterial lines, intravenous lines, lumbar punctures, and chest thoracostomy tubes.

Section II: Discussion

Dr. Peter Rosen: Practicing procedures on newly dead cadavers has only recently been an ethical conundrum. As I look back on my emergency medicine career, it didn't appear to be a problem until the mid 1980s. Nevertheless, we never thought about doing procedures like lumbar punctures or procedures that would not have been a customary part of the patient's resuscitation. The issues surrounding this practice commenced with the nursing staff who were not comfortable with procedures performed on these patients. When the issue first surfaced, while I was at Denver General Hospital, we resolved it by not pronouncing the patient dead until we had done all the resuscitative procedures that we felt were indicated. What do you do at your institution? Is there an opportunity to practice intubations or other resuscitative procedures on the dead or nearly dead, or has this teaching resource been permanently lost?

Dr. James Adams: The educational opportunity has been permanently lost in the majority of cases. There has been much discussion in the recent past about obtaining permission from the family, but I don't know anyone who does it. What people have continued to do, however, is to perform procedures during the resuscitation. It seems to me that the ethical issues involved are not resolved when the procedures performed have a very low likelihood of being successful. Although we want to maintain the trust of the patient, we've also lost something in the process. We no longer perform procedures after the patient has died.

Ethical Problems in Emergency Medicine: A Discussion-Based Review, First Edition. John Jesus, Shamai A. Grossman, Arthur R. Derse, James G. Adams, Richard Wolfe, and Peter Rosen.
© 2012 John Wiley & Sons, Ltd. Published 2012 by John Wiley & Sons, Ltd.

PR: Dr. Jesus, have you noticed procedures being practiced on cardiac arrest patients in your training?

Dr. John Jesus: Within my institution, procedures are not done after the person is pronounced dead. There are procedures, however, that are performed peri-resuscitation. That said, just today I polled 6–10 of my colleagues to see how many of them had witnessed or taken part in postmortem procedures without the consent of family, and many of them had. Many of them suggested that it was a common practice in their training program. This practice is still occurring across the United States, though with an increasing level of controversy.

PR: We've made too big a deal out of this issue. As a result, we have lost a valuable educational resource. There comes a time when we have to remember that it's not an ideal world, and if you ask people what they're most comfortable with, they will not understand the need for education. I've had many patients' relatives ask me, "Why can't you learn your procedures on a computer?"

Dr. Catherine Marco: In our institution, we don't practice procedures on the newly dead, although I remember this practice occurring when I was a medical student. There was a series of bad press surrounding this practice, and a few years ago, the practice evaporated. Even the most vocal proponent of practicing postmortem procedures stopped allowing the residents to perform them. Nevertheless, people find ways around it by not pronouncing the patient "dead" until someone has had an opportunity to do all the procedures that are feasible.

PR: I find the suggestion that we ask families for their permission, to be at best naïve, and at worst somewhat dishonest. I believe almost no family will give permission. To say we're going to practice procedures when my attention is focused on teaching rather than on the resuscitation, and even though the procedures have a very low probability of success is dishonest. The procedure that I still practice, and believe we all should practice, is intubation. You never see enough anatomy, and I think everybody ought to have a chance to hone that skill, because (a) it does not cost anything, (b) it produces no defect to the cadaver, and (c) it's a practice from which everybody profits. I've always been reluctant to perform surgical procedures

that have no chance of success. I feel particularly uncomfortable performing a procedure for which the patient and their family will be charged but has no chance to benefit the patient. Despite popular belief that residents don't have to practice on humans, nobody wants a physician who is inexperienced. Now we are faced with the difficulties of acquiring expert experience and providing adequate educational experiences for our residents, while also attempting to meet unreasonable public demand for experienced practitioners at all times.

JJ: There are several studies published in which investigators interviewed family members, and found them amenable to postpartum procedures. In one study conducted in a neonatal intensive care unit, the majority of the parents asked, soon after infant death, consented to procedures like intubation and line placement.[1] In another study, a strong majority of people (75%) answered that they would be "upset" if procedures were done without their consent.[2] Taken together, it seems that we may be avoiding the question because we're not comfortable approaching families, not because families would refuse to give their consent.

PR: I'm not familiar with this literature, but I don't believe it. I think that in real death circumstances, relatives I have interacted with don't want anyone experimenting with their loved one. I found that nursing staff members were much more comfortable with practicing intubation when they were asked to take part in the practice, and I don't see this as something that really needs consent. I also have a problem with a lot of the literature pertaining to having families as spectators during major resuscitations in which major invasive procedures are being performed. We're not a sporting event, and we don't need the adulation of a crowd. Survey research trying to figure out how people feel about this is fraught with all the perils and all the cautions of surveys, and I don't think they provide any useful evidence.

JA: The limited data supporting these practices are extremely biased toward people who are interested in the subject matter, and the interviewers participating in these studies are very skilled and are highly motivated to obtain the answers for which they are looking. In addition, the research participants have a very different experience when they are answering a hypothetical survey than the real-life experience of overwhelming grief of losing a loved member of their family. Do they really know to what they are consenting? Can they even hear anything after their loved one has just died? I do agree that part of the barrier lies with the inertia of attending physicians and residents, who find the act of approaching grieving families with a request to practice procedures on their newly dead family members distasteful and emotionally difficult. If this practice was clearly the right thing to do, it would be easier. The practice has had the benefit of time to work out the issues, and yet instead of continuing the practice, we are slowly eliminating it as a training opportunity.

Should it be eliminated? We're intubating a lot fewer times each shift than I did when I was in residency, yet it seems that there are more and more difficult intubations with a growing obese population. Although we've gotten a lot better at intubating, and are able to utilize different airway adjuncts, most of the physicians I know haven't had the opportunity to use these airway adjuncts. Consequently, we have very limited skills and limited experience even though we have abundant tools. Simulation is a great resource, but it has limited applicability when dealing with the performance anxiety of a real-world situation. The experience that would closest mimic real-world situations involves participation in real resuscitations. If my relative comes in extremis, I really want a skilled operator to do that intubation. What remains an open question, however, is how do we train people with the skills they need for these emergent circumstances?

CM: I have mixed feeling about practicing medical procedures on the newly or nearly dead. Ken Iserson was a strong proponent of this type of education, because it is the one situation in which there is literally no risk to the patient, while simultaneously providing a great deal of educational benefit to our residents and indirectly to their future patients. I believe most family members, however, would be upset if they knew this was going on with their recently deceased loved one's body. It is also important to recognize that in lieu of this opportunity, it has become commonplace to avoid pronouncing a patient dead until several invasive procedures have been performed. If the procedure performed offers absolutely no chance of benefit to the patient, then

this tactic is also intellectually dishonest. In an attempt to consider these points simultaneously, I favor performing procedures when there is **some** possibility of benefiting the patient. Despite the importance of resident education, I believe that once we extend beyond the set of interventions that may potentially benefit the patient, we must ask the family for consent.

JA: I struggle with the need to guarantee our graduates have the airway skills they need. I have the benefit of a 4-year residency, which provides more opportunities to ensure that residents learn to use different adjuncts and techniques. The question, however, is whether all residencies provide the same opportunities? Another critical issue to consider, is what fewer learning opportunities will mean for the care of patients in extremis. In those situations when patients' lives are at stake, will the newest intern be allowed to take the first crack at the intubation? If I knew that inexperienced residents were performing procedures on my family members that they could practice nowhere else with the same sort of situational stress, I would be at least as upset as I would be if I knew residents were practicing on a newly deceased family member. I'm not sure which is worse.

PR: When it comes to a difficult airway, the first attempt should go to the most experienced hands in the room, not the least. If that resuscitation fails, however, then there exists an opportunity for a number of people to become familiar with a difficult airway. In this scenario, the patient is not pronounced dead until everybody in the room has the opportunity to intubate the patient. That said, we must to be careful on whom we choose to practice certain procedural techniques. If the patient has clearly stated a preference through DNR orders, then we should respect those wishes and refrain from resuscitation efforts, never mind practicing resuscitation techniques. I have no trouble waiting to pronounce the patient dead if that makes people comfortable. I am not comfortable, however, with approaching a grieving relative to say, "Your mother just died; she's a difficult airway and I would like my people to practice their airway skills on her newly dead body." I can't conceive of the circumstances in which it would be reasonable to expect relatives to grant such permission.

There are times when I do not agree with the modern notion that physicians have to be completely communicative about every phase and detail of medical practice. There are times when we have to use some judgment about what and how much we share with patients, so that we can provide them and society with appropriate medical care. There are many facets of medical education that families would find appalling if they knew the details of how that education is obtained. As a resident in surgery, we performed many operations that families assumed were performed by the attending physician. Had they known residents were performing the operation, they never would have given their consent for the procedure. The same is true in the field of emergency medicine.

Dr. Shamai Grossman: Would you feel the same way if you were taking care of a patient whose religious beliefs precluded practicing medical procedures on the newly dead unless there was some immediate life-saving benefit to another patient in the ED?

PR: If I understand the question, you are asking about practicing because there is an immediate need for education. That doesn't change the ethical issues, merely heightens the conflict between education and patient preference. There is still no way to be completely honest with patients and relatives and achieve our educational goals.

SG: Frankly, I believe that we have no right to use patients without their implicit consent to do procedures on them that have no possible benefit to them. If the patient is already dead, this is always the case; if the patient is not yet dead, then I believe the procedure is appropriate ethically, only if it has some possibility of sustaining the patient's life. If this ultimately results in inferior medical education, this may be one of the unfortunate cases where ethics trumps education.

JJ: In my training, one of the alternatives to practicing on nearly or newly dead patients that I found most helpful was a mandatory anesthesia rotation during which we were supervised in controlled settings and practiced with every tool imaginable under expert oversight. In 3 weeks I was able to perform 60 intubations, giving me a considerable amount of experience with the anatomy and the tools of airway management. This sort of experience is an important bridge between practicing on manikins and animals and performing intubations on crashing patients in the ED.

JA: Do you think though that patients and families know that there is gong to be an inexperienced operator doing the intubation, rather than the attending anesthesiologist? I don't think they do.

JJ: Part of every consent procedure includes the idea that trainees will be present and involved. To what extent they probably don't know. For that reason, it is not full informed consent.

SG: The very idea that patients are seeking care at a teaching institution should allow for some expectation among patients that their care will be provided by training physicians.

PR: We've had anesthesia rotations at every residency in which I have been attached. When I was program director in San Diego, we also had a mandatory requirement that residents gain a minimum of an additional 12 intubations every year by going to same-day surgery. I am still not convinced this was enough. Experience with difficult airways, however, will not be acquired through the anesthesia rotation. The place to practice rare intubation skills, like digital intubation, is in the resuscitation rooms of the ED. It's not that I make a practice of lying to patients; I simply don't make a practice of sharing every thought I have with the patient. I also don't make a practice of explaining in detail what education takes place with every patient, because I don't feel that information will benefit them or the teaching program we represent. There comes a time when society members ought to trust and rely on the fact that residents and attending physicians alike are working in their best interests, whether it's for immediate benefit or whether it's for their long-term interests. If that were not the case, we would never be able to educate anyone.

In point of fact, patients' benefit greatly from having less experienced trainees involved in their care. An example of this from personal experience comes from an experience I had as a patient in the coronary care unit; it wasn't the experienced cardiologist who made rounds on me once an hour throughout the night of my admission, it was the intern. When I was a patient in a private community hospital for an episode of pneumonia, I didn't see my attending physician until 24 hours after I was admitted. I think that there is real value to being a patient in a training facility, a value that is also associated with some responsibilities to the educational program.

JJ: Though we can no longer technically harm a patient who has died, we can potentially "wrong," or treat unjustly the bodies, and the relatives' memories of the life that used to occupy them. While this concept has no impact on the deceased, it does have a significant impact on the surviving relatives and the public image of the physician, department, and institution in which the perceived injustice occurred. Similar to the affront on trust and legitimacy of the efforts of an institution with a perceived conflict of interest, a physician can engender a great deal of animosity and distrust from having the perception of treating the bodies of the newly dead unjustly. This may lead to public protest and subsequent administrative punitive action against the physician or department. Public outcry over perceived injustice of the PolyHeme trial in the mid 1990s, for example, ultimately led to the severe regulatory restriction of Exception from Informed Consent Research (EFIC) and its funding. Given the slow decline and elimination of the practice of learning procedures on the newly dead, I would argue that invoking the slippery slope argument in this instance may be appropriate.

PR: By and large, people want to trust professionals, and it is incumbent upon the professional to behave in a way that is trustworthy. But can I guarantee that a physician will be trustworthy?—I cannot. If what you mean by invoking the slippery slope argument is that inappropriate actions are likely to happen, then I agree with you. There are times when you will encounter people, like the attending physician in this case, who argues that we ought to be doing lumbar puncture, and maybe another physician responds by saying that we ought to perform a laparotomy and teach the residents how to perform a splenectomy. These are examples of exceeding the trust placed in you to act in the best interests of our patients. I have read too much ethical literature trying to produce perfection and attempting to overcome the lack of trust that is generated by the unethical actions of a misguided few, rather than the actions of the great majority of physicians who behave and treat their patients appropriately. The consequence is similar to what we have seen happen with the practice of learning on the newly dead—a loss of a great opportunity to learn useful skills.

JA: The reason people still attempt to justify practicing medical procedures on the newly or nearly dead

is that attending clinicians are trying to fulfill their responsibility to train their residents. The integrity of the teaching institution really depends on having highly skilled practitioners and trainees who are expected to advance their skills rapidly. On the other hand, the family has the option of preventing us from performing any procedure, and I argue that is as it should be. First and foremost we must have the respect and trust of our patients and that of society; but secondly, we experience conflict due the loss of potential learning opportunities without the ability to measure whether that loss is meaningful or not.

PR: We have developed a dependency on data that are not derivable. You can't prove that training makes a difference, but why should you have to? It's intuitively obvious that it does. When we remove elements of training from our residency programs we can't prove that we have harmed the programs. That said, there's no question that if you don't have the expertise to care for a difficult airway, you will not do as good a job the first time you are faced with one for which you are responsible. I don't think we need a double-blinded prospective study to prove an obvious point.

I am very concerned about having the respect of patients I care for, and I am very concerned about having the respect of society. We must strike a fine balance between permitting restrictions to the adequacy of our training, in order to respect individual and societal interests, and taking steps to ensure that our residents are adequately trained to become competent physicians. Each of us will have a different level of comfort about how we handle perimortem and postmortem procedures—upon which is all that we are likely to agree. I may allow more procedures to be practiced than another physician, but that doesn't make me right and the other physician wrong or vice versa. Have you actually asked a patient's relative permission for practicing on a cadaver?

CM: No, I haven't. I also don't know anyone who routinely requests consent from families to perform postmortem procedures. In addition, I agree with prior comments about alternative educational methods of obtaining procedural experience. I am the residency director at our program, and we don't have any trouble obtaining what I consider adequate numbers of intubations or central venous lines. The few procedures that we have trouble acquiring adequate experience involve pericardiocentesis or floating a pacing wire, which we make a point of addressing in a pig lab.

PR: I am convinced that the best way to learn how to intubate is to intubate a patient who truly needs and would benefit from the intervention. What I would like to see are residents in EDs that are busy enough with critically ill patients to acquire proficiency with all procedures. No matter how many critically ill patients to which our residents are exposed, however, we have fewer and fewer indications for rare procedures such as a thoracotomy, pericardiocentesis, and internal pacing. Those are, however, the procedures that I am not inclined to practice on a recently dead cadaver, as the procedure itself mutilates the body without any benefit to the patient. On the other hand, I don't have any problem with practicing techniques such as oral intubation, nasal intubation, or digital intubation that clearly doesn't harm the cadaver.

JJ: Taking advantage of all the alternatives to practicing postmortem procedures is important. Animal laboratories, anesthesia rotations, and procedure simulation with manikins all approximate the skills necessary for procedures in the ED. I would also acknowledge that absolutely nothing will give you the experience of working and trying to do difficult procedures on patients who need them and need them quickly. I would recommend that residents seek out procedures and learn all they can from each of them as if they would need to perform the next one on their own in a single coverage community ED at 4 am. Proactively seek out critically ill patients, and be the first to volunteer to try those procedures with which you are least comfortable.

JA: We've had probably a decade or more of discussion, and my observation of the discussion today is that we are in a similar place as we were when we started. The struggle is important as it reminds us of the responsibilities and duties we have to our practice, our patients and their families, and to our residents, who represent the future of our discipline.

PR: Ultimately this is one of the harder ethical dilemmas, because I don't think there is a way to come to consensus, and I think in most of the difficult cases so far, that has not been the case. Regardless of the challenges that face medical education, we have an obligation to train the next generation of physicians. If we fall short, the result will be a single generation of very experienced physicians who are not universally available, leaving open the question of what should be done for the next generation of patients.

Section III: Review of the literature

Education for procedural competency, such as central line placement and endotracheal intubation, cannot be taught solely from a book or a lecture. Procedural competency necessitates first-hand education, experience, and expertise. There are many avenues for learners to gain this experience, including manikin simulators, preserved cadavers, and animal models.[3–5] In the past, it has been accepted practice for educators to allow learners to practice these techniques on newly and nearly dead patients.[6] Additionally, studies show that this education is often practiced without obtaining consent from the survivors.[7] The argument about whether this practice is acceptable centers around two major themes: is it ethical to perform these procedures on the newly deceased, and is it ethical to perform these procedures without obtaining informed consent from the next of kin? In this chapter, we will examine these themes from both sides, focusing on the arguments presented by the proponents of each side and present the authors' opinion of the best course of action for the practicing emergency physician.

Ethical arguments supporting teaching procedures on the newly dead

The basis for performing procedures on the newly deceased is simple to understand. Invasive and semi-invasive procedures, such as endotracheal intubation, central line placement, and chest thoracostomies are all life-saving procedures in the critically ill patient. It is therefore important that the emergency physician can perform these procedures. It has been shown that an effective medium available to teach these procedures is on the newly dead. While alternatives to a fresh corpse do exist, some believe that these alternatives are inferior teaching tools in comparison.[8,9] One can learn intubation skills working in an anesthesiology department, but these departments may have limited resources to train learners, and one may not be able to practice other life-saving techniques.

Simulation models and animal models are also helpful, but do not provide a true human simulation. In fact, it has been shown that emergency medicine services (EMS) personnel trained solely on manikins have lower success rates of emergency intubation when compared with those trained on animals and live patients.[10] Finally, preserved cadavers are rendered stiff and rigid to the point where the learning experience may be significantly degraded.[11]

Besides providing the most realistic experience, there are additional benefits to the practice of these procedures on the newly deceased. Each procedure may have significant complications that are more likely to occur when these techniques are performed by an inexperienced clinician. It would therefore be unethical to perform them on living patients for educational purposes alone; they must have some direct benefit to the patient.[12] Since it is impossible to physically harm a corpse, many consider practicing these procedures on the newly dead the ideal opportunity.[13-15] One of the primary tenets of medicine is "first do no harm." If this is the case, then a physician should use the best available methods to develop and maintain skills, as an incompetent physician performing a procedure with significant and dangerous complications would directly breach this rule. Some might argue that the benefit that society enjoys (having competent physicians) outweighs any of the negative ramifications associated with practicing on the newly dead.

Furthermore, one must consider the feelings of anxiety experienced by both the learner and the patient in educational settings. If a patient has already expired, the anxiety experienced by the learner is reduced as the patient will have no adverse effects if the procedure were to fail or produce a complication. In these ways, practicing procedures on the newly dead ensures that society will have an ample supply of competent physicians, with optimal learning experience, coupled with minimal risk and discomfort to any of the parties involved.

Ethical arguments against teaching procedures on the newly dead

There are several arguments that may be presented against teaching procedures on the newly dead. The first and foremost argument against practicing on the newly dead, especially without obtaining consent, is that it may damage the already waning public trust in physicians.[16,17] The concern is that this may be seen as a violation of the rights of the body, and, to a lesser degree, a physical violation as well. While some may argue that one loses all rights in death, to perform these actions in a veiled manner may be seen as an admission of wrong-doing, and therefore undermines future patient–physician relationships. Synonymous to this is the public misperception of seeing these actions as disrespectful toward the body. While respect for the corpse is taught in medical schools and is extensively described in bioethical literature, it is easy to understand why a family member may experience emotional distress at images of "lining up" medical students and residents to insert catheters and tubes into the body of their loved one.[18-20]

From the medical training perspective, however, many argue that practicing on the corpse is a sign of respect. Iserson describes "postmortem practice as the ultimate respect for the corpse," as this practice allows the patient to provide a genuine service to society and honors the memory of the newly deceased.[21] Despite respect for the corpse being taught ubiquitously within the medical field, the fact remains that the public rejects this practice without knowledge and consent. In 2001, there was an incident regarding organ procurement without public knowledge that led to a full investigation of a hospital's organ procurement protocols as well as examining the professional practice of hospital staff.[22] Medicolegal concerns also influence this potential practice. Some US state laws govern the handling of corpses, and such practices may potentially result in an actionable offense.[23]

Another argument against practice without consent is that many studies show that the majority of family members will consent if approached, especially when the question is framed in a sensitive manner and it is explained to them that the outcome is to help save a life in the future.[24] In two studies specifically addressing endotracheal intubation on deceased infants and wire-guided retrograde tracheal intubation, 73% and 59% of families granted consent, respectively.[1,25] Other studies have explored procedures such as cricothyrotomy, central line insertions, chest tube insertions, and endotracheal intubations, with similar results but lower rates of consent with more invasive procedures.[26-29] Moreover, surveys of patients find that a majority would allow their own body to be used for practice but they would be less likely to allow a family member's corpse to used for training purposes.[2,7]

Legal considerations

At the time of the writing of this chapter, there are limited data available regarding the practicing of procedures on the newly deceased. While it has been generally accepted that the family holds no real property rights to the corpse, some courts do recognize a less-inclusive "quasi-property right."[30] This "right" essentially safeguards the family's ability to put into effect the final wishes of the deceased, and to allow for funeral and burial arrangements. However, in the United States, the Supreme Courts of Georgia, Florida, and Michigan have all ruled that the family has no constitutional rights to the body, and that the rights of the deceased ended with their death.[31–33] Other US states have passed laws allowing for medical personnel to remove the corneas and adrenal glands of the deceased without the consent of the family. While there have been several court cases in which the plaintiff asserted their loved ones' corneas were removed without consent or notice, the courts have upheld these statutes, based on their compliance with public law that a corpse cannot have its rights violated, that the family does not have any rights to the body, and that the procedure did not disfigure the corpse to an extent that would cause "unbearable emotional distress."[21]

In *Lacy* v. *Cooper Hospital/University Medical Center*, a pericardiocentesis was performed on the body of a child who had been pronounced dead. The family claimed emotional distress. In this case, the court found that "the mental distress found by the family was not severe enough to meet the requirements for intentional or negligent infliction of emotional distress," and the hospital was not held liable for the procedures.[34] While it is not known how future court cases may evolve, in the absence of hospital policy and specific legal guidelines, hospitals and physicians who continue to train on the newly dead corpse without consent may be at risk for future litigation. Patient or family consent prior to practicing procedures is the most prudent medicolegal defense of this practice.

Existing policies and guidelines

The American Medical Association (AMA) has issued an opinion entitled "Performing procedures in the newly deceased for training purposes", which states that[35]:

Physicians should work to develop institutional policies that address the practice of performing procedures on the newly deceased for purposes of training. Any such policy should ensure that the interests of all the parties involved are respected under established and clear ethical guidelines. Such policies should consider rights of patients and their families, benefits to trainees and society, as well as potential harm to the ethical sensitivities of trainees, and risks to staff, the institution, and the profession associated with performing procedures on the newly deceased without consent.

Regarding consent for procedures, the AMA opinion states[35]:

Physicians should inquire whether the deceased individual had expressed preferences regarding handling of the body or procedures performed after death. In the absence of previously expressed preferences, physicians should obtain permission from the family before performing such procedures. When reasonable efforts to discover previously expressed preferences of the deceased or to find someone with authority to grant permission for the procedure have failed, physicians must not perform procedures for training purposes on the newly deceased patient.

The American College of Emergency Physicians (ACEP) has published an information paper "Teaching procedures using the newly dead",[36] which recommends specific principles, including:
• Medically appropriate procedures should be performed on all patients, including dying patients; these should be documented in the medical record and appropriately billed.
• All procedures performed by learners should be appropriately supervised by qualified emergency physicians.
• Caregivers should respect the dignity of each patient until the time of death and should show respect for the body of the patient after death.
• Teaching procedural skills must not interfere with family visitation, autopsy, or forensic evidence collection.

In the ACEP paper, the controversy regarding obtaining consent is discussed but no definitive policy is suggested regarding consent from families to perform procedures following pronouncement of death.

The issue has also been addressed in the American Heart Association (AHA) 2005 guidelines for cardiopulmonary resuscitation, which state that "The consent of family members is both ideal and respectful of the newly dead but not always possible or practical at the time of cardiac arrest."[37]

Other countries have also addressed this issue. The British and Norwegian medical association guidelines strictly prohibit the use of the newly dead. The British guidelines make an exception for endotracheal intubation in the case of patients with extreme craniofacial injuries because it is an exceptional learning experience that cannot be readily replicated by any simulation.[38] Canada and Israel both have legislation that allows physicians to practice procedures on the newly deceased if the patient or the family give permission prior to the time of the patient's death.[39]

Conclusions

Procedural competency can be taught to learners through a variety of settings, including procedures on patients, manikin simulation, and cadaver and animal models. Procedural training on the newly or nearly dead can be performed ethically, following patient or family consent. Faculty supervision is imperative for all models of training in procedural competency.

Section IV: Recommendations

- Assess institutional resources for procedural education, including simulation, cadaver, and animal models.
- Obtain consent from family prior to practicing procedures on the newly or nearly dead.
- Demonstrate respect of the body and family.
- Provide appropriate faculty supervision of procedural education.

References

1. Benefield DG, Flaskman RJ, Lin TH, et al. (1991) Teaching intubation skills using newly deceased infants. *JAMA.* 265, 2360–3.

2. Manifold CA, Storrow A, Rodgers K. (1999) Patient and family attitudes regarding the practice of procedures on the newly deceased. *Acad Emerg Med.* 6, 110–15.

3. Gilbert MK, Hutchinson CR, Cusimano MD, et al. (2000) Regehr G.A computer-based trauma simulator for teaching trauma management skills. *Am J Surg.* 179, 223–8.

4. Wik K, Thowsen K, Steen PA. (2001) An automated voice advisory manikin system for training in basic life support without an instructor. A novel approach to CPR training. *Resuscitation.* 40, 167–72.

5. Kaufmann C, Liu A. (2001) Trauma training: virtual reality applications. *Stud Health Technol Inform.* 81, 236–41.

6. Kaldijan LC, Wu BJ, Jekel JF, et al. (1999). Insertion of femoral-vein catheters for practice by medical house officers during cardiopulmonary resuscitation. *N Engl J Med.* 341, 2088–91.

7. Denny CJ, Kollel D. (1999) Practicing procedures on the recently dead. *J Emerg Med.* 17, 949–52.

8. Orlowski JP, Kanoti GA. (1988) The ethics of using newly dead patients for teaching and practicing intubation techniques. *N Engl J Med.* 319, 439–41.

9. Nelson MS. (1990) Models for teaching emergency medicine skills. *Ann Emerg Med.* 19, 333–5.

10. Stewart, RD, Paris PM, Pelton GH, et al. (1984) Garretson D. Effect of varied training techniques on field endotracheal intubation success rates. *Ann Emerg Med.* 13, 1032–6.

11. Tachakra S, Ho S, Lynch M, et al. (1998) Should doctors practice resuscitation skills on newly deceased patients? A survey of public opinion. *J R Soc Med.* 91, 576–8.

12. Berger JT, Rosnder F, Cassell, EJ. (2002) Ethics of practicing medical procedures on newly dead and nearly dead patients. *J Gen Int Med.* 17, 774–8.

13. Burns JR, Reardon FE, Truog RD. (1994) Using newly deceased patients to teach resuscitation procedures. *N Engl J Med.* 331, 1652–5.

14. Iserson KV. (1991) Requiring consent to practice and teach using the recently dead. *J Emerg Med.* 9, 509–10.

15. Morag RM, DeSouza S, Steen PA, et al. (2005) Performing procedures on the newly deceased for teaching purposes. *Arch Intern Med.* 165, 92–6.

16. Schmidt T, Abbott J, Geiderman J, et al. (2004) Ethics seminar: The ethical debate on practicing procedures on the newly dead. *Acad Emerg Med.* 11, 962–6.

17. American College of Emergency Physician. (n.d.) *Code of Ethics for Emergency Physicians.* Available at: www.acep.org/practres.aspx?id=29144. Accessed July 1, 2010.

18. Annas G. (1989) *The Rights of Patients*. Carbondale, IL: Southern Illinois University Press, pp. 234–6.

19. American Medical Association, Council on Ethical and Judicial Affairs. (1997) *Code of Medical Ethics*. Chicago, IL: American Medical Association, pp. 30–1.

20. American Medical Association, Council on Ethical and Judicial Affairs. (2002) Performing procedures on the newly deceased. *Acad Med*. 77, 1212–16.

21. Iserson KV. (1994) Life versus death: exposing a misapplication of ethical reasoning. *J Clin Ethics*. 5, 261–3.

22. Woodman R. (2001) Storage of human organs prompts three inquiries. *BMJ*. 320, 77.

23. Kerns AF. (1997) Better to lay it out on the table than do it behind the curtain: hospitals need to obtain consent before using newly deceased patients to teach rescuscitation procedures. *K Cont Health Law Pol*. 13, 581–612.

24. Orloski JP. (1994) Politically correct ethical thinking and intubation practice on cadavers. *J Clin Ethics*. 5, 256–60.

25. McNamara RM, Monti S, Kelly JJ. (1995) Requesting consent for an invasive procedure in newly deceased adults. *JAMA*. 273, 310–12.

26. Oman KS, Armstrong JD, Stoner M. (2002) Perspectives on practicing on the newly dead. *Acad Emerg Med*. 9, 786–90.

27. Brattebo G, Wisberg T, Solheim K, et al. (1993) Public opinion on different approaches to teaching intubation techniques. *BJM*. 307, 1256–7.

28. Alden AW, Ward KLM, Moore GP. (1999) Should post-mortem procedures be practiced on recently deceased patients? A survey of relatives' attitudes. *Acad Emerg Med*. 6, 749–52.

29. Olsen J, Spigler S, Windisch T. (1995) Feasibility of obtaining family consent for teaching cricothyrotomy on the newly dead in the emergency department. *Ann Emerg Med*. 25, 660–5.

30. Hayes, GJ. (1994) Issues of Consent; the use of the recently deceased for intubation training. *J Clin Ethics*. 5, 211–16.

31. State of Florida v. Powerll, 497 So.2d 1188–1198 (1986).

32. Georgia Lions Eye Bank, Inc v. Lavant, 335 S.E.2d 127–129 (1985).

33. Tillman v. Detroit Receiving Hospital, 360 N.W.2d 275–279 (Mich. Ct. App. 1984).

34. Lacy v. Cooper Hospital/University Medical Center, 745 F. Supp. 1029 (D.N.J. 1990).

35. American Medical Association. (n.d.) *Opinion 8.181—Performing Procedures in the Newly Deceased for Training Purposes*. Available at: www.ama-assn.org/ama/pub/physician-resources/medical-ethics/code-medical-ethics/opinion8181.shtml. Accessed June 15, 2010.

36. American College of Emergency Physicians Ethics Committee. (n.d.) *Teaching procedures using the newly dead*. Available at: http://www.acep.org/content.aspx?id=30104&terms=practicing%20procedures. Accessed June 15, 2010.

37. Emergency Cardiac Care Committee and Subcommittee, American Heart Association. (2005) 2005 American Heart Association guidelines for cardiopulmonary resuscitation and emergency cardiovascular care, Part 2: Ethical issues. *Circulation*. 112, IV6–IV11.

38. Tonks A. (1992) Intubation practice on cadavers should stop. *BMJ*. 305, 322.

39. Sperling D. (2004) Breaking through the silence: Illegality of performing resuscitation procedures on the newly-dead. *Ann Health Law*. 13, 393–426.

28 Ethics of research without informed consent

Dave W. Lu,[1] Jonathan Burstein,[2] John Jesus[3]

[1]Acting Instructor, Department of Medicine, Division of Emergency Medicine, University of Washington School of Medicine, Seattle, WA, USA

[2]OEMS Medical Director, Commonwealth of Massachusetts, Assistant Professor, Harvard Medical School, Department of Emergency Medicine, Boston, MA, USA

[3]Chief Resident, Department of Emergency Medicine, Beth Israel Deaconess Medical Center, Boston, MA, and Clinical Instructor, Department of Emergency Medicine, Christiana Care Health System, Newark, DE, USA

Section I: Case presentation

A 20-year-old man is rushed by paramedics to a local emergency department (ED) after he is found unconscious at the scene of a motor vehicle collision. In the ED, while awaiting operating room availability, it is discovered that the patient has multiple sources of massive hemorrhage. Despite aggressive efforts with crystalloid and blood product administration, it becomes evident the patient is failing standard resuscitation therapy. At this point, it is brought to the attention of the emergency physician that the hospital is part of an ongoing randomized controlled trial investigating the efficacy of a novel pro-hemostatic agent in patients with uncontrollable hemorrhage. The study has been approved by the hospital's institutional review board (IRB). The comatose patient is clearly unable to give informed consent to be a part of this trial, and there is no immediate family member available. The emergency physician after consultation with the trauma surgeon decides to enroll the patient into this trial, and he is randomized to receive the experimental drug.

Section II: Discussion

Dr. Peter Rosen: The requirement for an IRB is something fairly recent in American research, and it follows a public relations exposure of inappropriate research. A few highly publicized cases include one involving orphan children being deliberately exposed to hepatitis B and another where mental hospital patients were deliberately exposed to syphilis.[1-4] Most journals will not accept an article without IRB approval or without an IRB waiver. It is very difficult to achieve rapid IRB turnaround, and convincing the IRB to permit research without prospective informed consent is even more difficult. Are there any legal exceptions to standard rules that allow us to perform research in emergency situations?

Dr. Arthur Derse: The code of federal regulations 45 CFR 46 was created mainly to prevent people from having research done upon them without their direct knowledge or consent.[5] The cases that you mentioned were part of the impetus to ensure that research subjects had protection that required the recognition of the difference between a research subject and a patient. When these regulations were enacted, there were no exceptions made for emergency research. The lack of a plan for emergency research came to a head in the 1990s, when a number of acute care researchers sought to study cardiac arrest and resuscitation. Through their efforts to educate legislators about the fact that there was no exception or waiver for informed consent for patients who were unable to consent for treatment during an emergency, a waiver was granted that allows emergency research without consent, though it is rigorously circumscribed.

Ethical Problems in Emergency Medicine: A Discussion-Based Review, First Edition. John Jesus, Shamai A. Grossman, Arthur R. Derse, James G. Adams, Richard Wolfe, and Peter Rosen.
© 2012 John Wiley & Sons, Ltd. Published 2012 by John Wiley & Sons, Ltd.

The application of a research protocol ensures only the promise of treatment, without a guarantee. The fact that clinical investigators do not know which treatment arm confers more benefit than the other, or any benefit at all for that matter, is termed a state of clinical equipoise. Equipoise is necessary for any ethical research protocol that involves more than minimal risk.

Another important consideration in performing emergency research concerns the difference in responsibilities between the physician and the investigator. Normally a physician has the fiduciary responsibility to act in the patient's best interest, and to provide the standard of care. When an investigator is conducting a research protocol, the relationship with the research participant is such that ensuring proper medical treatment is no longer the primary goal. When the physician and the investigator are the same individual, the situation can become ethically challenging.

Dr. John Jesus: The dual role of physician-investigator is ethically problematic. In the best of circumstances, patients frequently do not understand the concept of equipoise or randomization, and they generally make a therapeutic misconception when choosing to participate in a research study. The situational stress of a medical emergency, in combination with the confusion patients may experience when approached by an individual describing himself as both physician and researcher, would only exacerbate the difficulty of obtaining truly informed and voluntary consent.

PR: How can we expect people in the middle of a medical emergency to make rational choices about their participation in a protocol? Though such research might use a specific research team with pre-established protocols, the research would be more likely to succeed with protocols that do not require individual patient consent.

AD: In some research involving critical illness and resuscitation, however, the intervention under study is no longer a known treatment, but rather an experimental treatment that may or may not confer benefit to the patient. Yet patients in these situations may see this as their best hope for actual treatment in a setting where they have no other choices.

JJ: This speaks to another issue, which is the assumption that people in a disaster or emergency are somehow vulnerable and unable to make an autono-

mous decision. This assumption appears in the literature frequently, yet there is little data indicating that victims of disaster actually are unable to make autonomous choices. As a result, an attempt should be made to acquire voluntary informed consent from every patient approached. The issue of vulnerability should be assessed on a case-by-case basis. It may, in fact, be true that some critically ill patients would be unable to make autonomous decisions for themselves, but it is also possible that they could, despite the situational stress in which they might find themselves.

Jonathan Burstein: The sociological literature has actually assessed the question of whether disaster victims are capable of making autonomous decisions, and finds that people in disasters actually tend to make better decisions.[6,7]

AD: To quote Samuel Johnson, "Nothing concentrates the mind better than the prospect of a hanging."

JJ: Historically, vulnerability has been used as a way to prevent research in women, children and pregnant patients, but since then we have come to realize that research in these populations is important to the development of medical treatments for these populations. Moreover, labeling a population "vulnerable" does not represent an *a priori* exclusion from research.[8] Rather, vulnerability here means that additional measures to ensure the protection of subjects from exploitation are required.

PR: The patients injured enough to be incapacitated are much fewer in number, and are so obviously in distress that it is unlikely they will be asked to make a decision. In addition the nature of their injuries may often require swift intervention. How should we prioritize patients to the research protocol while simultaneously prioritizing their clinical status? Moreover, are there suggestions on how we can capture and retain public trust before, during, and after the research?

JB: My answer to the latter question, after significant experience in disaster response and a long period of consideration, is that the answer lies in early education. We must educate our children about the basics of what happens when things go wrong, and what one can do to help. The more short-term strategy lies with building trust ahead of time. Attempting to engender public trust during an emergency does not work well.

AD: The media is a double-edged sword and can be incensed that a possible life-saving treatment, as during the HIV [human immunodeficiency virus] epidemic, is being withheld from individuals. At the same time, the fact that research is being conducted without the consent of individuals enrolled in the study can lead to public outrage, regardless of the circumstances and lengths the researchers may have gone to protect subjects. In this case, the public message could focus on equipoise, attempting to educate the media and the public that we do not know if the drug actually works, and the reason for the clinical trial is to assess if the drug actually confers benefit.

JJ: AIDS patients faced a similar argument when they requested access to experimental therapies, and their counterargument was that they had nothing to lose—they were going to die anyway. I imagine that if people in this scenario knew about the experimental therapy, and knew their death was almost certain, a reasonable person in a similar situation might use the same argument.

PR: That is also a dangerous argument. Cancer patients have been preyed upon by a lot of quackery under the guise that they are dying, and a new experimental therapy is their only hope of survival. Laetrile, the apricot cyanide medication, is an example that comes to mind. I think that we need to be cautious about arguing from emotions—just because an individual wishes to try an experimental agent before dying of an incurable disease does not mean that an untested agent should be administered, which has at least as much chance of hurting the individual as it does of helping.

Section III: Review of the literature

Traditionally, studies involving human subjects require the voluntary participation and prospective informed consent of enrolled individuals. In clinical trials involving critically ill patients, however, researchers face considerable challenges in obtaining informed consent from subjects whose decision-making abilities are compromised by their emergent medical condition.

In 1996, new regulations developed by the US Food and Drug Administration (FDA) and the Department of Health and Human Services (DHHS) were instituted to permit certain emergency and resuscitation research involving human subjects to take place without obtaining prospective informed consent.[5,9] Collectively known as the Final Rule, these regulations were the result of a multidisciplinary effort led by the specialty of emergency and allowed resuscitation research to proceed with a "waiver of informed consent" or an "exception for emergency treatment" in specific circumstances and under stringent safeguards.[10] In the decade and half since passage of the Final Rule, however, there have been significant controversy and debate among researchers and members of IRBs over the proper application of the regulations in actual clinical trials.

This chapter will provide a brief review of the history and standards of the Final Rule, followed by a discussion of the ethical considerations of conducting human subjects research without obtaining prospective informed consent. Remaining ethical challenges to the provisions of the Final Rule are then examined, and recommendations for the Final Rule's future implementation are proposed.

History of the Final Rule

The FDA first addressed clinical research involving the exception for emergency treatment in 1981 by requiring investigators to fulfill a number of specific conditions: (1) the subject must be in a life-threatening situation; (2) informed consent cannot be obtained from the subject; (3) time is not sufficient to obtain consent from a surrogate; and (4) no alternative therapy is available to provide an equal or greater likelihood of saving the subject's life.[9] These guidelines were similar, although different in significant ways, to a separate set of regulations concurrently issued by the DHHS, which required: (1) the research entails minimal risk; (2) the waiver of informed consent does not adversely affect patients' rights and welfare; (3) the research could not be done without a waiver; and (4) subjects will be informed after their participation.[5] Although both sets of guidelines aimed to protect human subjects in research wherein their prospective informed consent may not be possible, investigators quickly found that each set of rules were too restrictive and impractical to reasonably permit them to successfully conduct critical care research.[11,12]

In an attempt to overcome these conflicting and prohibitive rules, investigators in the 1980s frequently invoked the concept of "deferred consent," rather than a waiver or exception, in order to obtain IRB approval for studies that enrolled subjects incapable of immediately providing informed consent.[13] This circumvention, however, was eventually determined to be unacceptable in 1993 by the Office for Protection from Research Risks—since renamed the Office for Human Research Protection (OHRP)—because critics argued that for subjects to later consent to actions that have already been performed was ethically problematic. As a result of this decision, all research involving subjects who were unable to provide prospective informed consent was essentially shut down in the United States.[12,14]

The environment surrounding research without informed consent became even more contentious in 1994, with the release of a US House Subcommittee report entitled "Human guinea pig research in emergency rooms: how some drug and device manufacturers use patients who can't say no."[15] This controversial publication, coupled with the moratorium on all critical care research when consent was not possible, led researchers in resuscitation medicine to establish the Coalition of Acute Resuscitation and Critical Care Researchers. Spearheaded by the Society for Aca-demic Emergency Medicine (SAEM), the coalition aimed to provide recommendations to address the challenges of informed consent in resuscitation research.[15] The coalition's deliberations ultimately resulted in a consensus conference in 1994, and its recommendations provided the impetus for the FDA and DHHS to amend their guidelines and to release the Final Rule in 1996.[10]

Guidelines of the Final Rule

The provisions of the Final Rule permit research on human subjects without their prospective informed consent under a specific and narrow set of conditions (Box 28.1). The fundamental criterion of the Final Rule is that the subject must be unable to provide informed consent as a result of his or her life-threatening medical condition. The researcher, however, should make every reasonable attempt to contact as early as possible the subject's legally authorized representative (LAR) or family in order to obtain consent.

The Final Rule also requires that the treatment under study be in clinical equipoise with current treatment. The condition of equipoise requires that the patient is just as likely to benefit from the treatment under study as the standard treatment, while

---

Box 28.1 Provisions of the Final Rule (21 CFR 50.24)[16]

- The human subjects are in a life-threatening situation, available treatments are unproven or unsatisfactory, and further research is necessary to determine the best therapy.
- Obtaining informed consent is not feasible because:
  - Subjects are not able to give informed consent because of their medical condition
  - The intervention under investigation must be administered before consent from the subjects' legally authorized representatives is feasible
  - There is no reasonable way to identify prospectively the individuals likely to become eligible for participation in the clinical investigation.

- Participation in the research holds out the prospect of direct benefit to the subjects because:
  - Subjects are facing a life-threatening situation that necessitates intervention
  - Animal and preclinical studies show the intervention may directly benefit subjects
  - Risks and benefits associated with the investigation are reasonable in relation to what is known about the medical condition of the potential class of subjects and the risks and benefits of standard therapy.
- The clinical investigation could not practicably be carried out without the waiver.
- The protocol defines the length of the therapeutic window, and the investigator has committed to attempt to contact a legally authorized repre-

sentative for each subject within that window and to ask for consent.

- The IRB has reviewed and approved informed consent procedures and an informed consent document consistent with the Common Rule.
- Additional protections will be provided, including, at least:
  - Consultation with representatives of the communities in which the clinical investigation will be conducted and from which subjects will be drawn
  - Public disclosure of plans for the investigation and its risks and expected benefits
  - Public disclosure following completion of the investigation to apprise the community and researchers of results
  - Establishment of an independent data monitoring committee to exercise oversight of the investigation
  - If a legally authorized representative is not available, the investigator will attempt to contact another family member for permission to enroll the subject.

Reprinted by permissin from Macmillan Publishers Ltd: *Academic Emergency Medicine*. McRae A, Weijer C. (2008) US Federal Regulations for emergency research: a practical guide and commentary. *Acad Emerg Med*. 15, 88–97. Copyright 2008.

not incurring any additional risk.[17] If one treatment has been shown to be superior to another treatment, equipoise does not exist and the study cannot take place without informed consent as outlined by the Final Rule. Additional important elements of the Final Rule include: researchers must conduct consultation with the community from which subjects are likely enrolled; investigators must notify the public of the planned study at least before initiation of the study and after the study's completion; and ongoing review of the study's progress must be performed by an independent data monitoring committee. These provisions of the Final Rule do not ultimately sanction human subject research without informed consent in the United States; they only allow an exception under life-threatening medical and emergent conditions.[15]

Ethical arguments supporting resuscitation research without informed consent

There are several arguments in support of permitting human subjects research without prospective informed consent as outlined in the Final Rule. Chief among them is that continued research in acute and critical care medicine is necessary to improve current therapies, many of which remain inadequate or are poorly supported by evidence.[18] Many critical care and resuscitation studies simply cannot be successfully and reasonably performed without the use of the exception from informed consent. For example, as illustrated in the case at the start of the chapter, the emergent and unpredictable nature of trauma care frequently prohibits researchers from procuring prospective informed consent using traditional means.

Another important argument in favor of research without informed consent is that the absence of consent does not automatically make a study unethical. Informed consent is not an end in and of itself; its presence is not always necessary, nor is it sufficient to demonstrate ethically sound research methods.[17,19] Studies involving children, for example, can be ethically conducted without the express consent of the pediatric patient.[20,21] Similar to critically ill adults who are incapable of giving consent as a result of their medical condition, children are not able to provide informed consent as a result of their limited cognitive, emotional, and psychological capacity. Research on pediatric subjects, however, is still ethically permissible through the route of obtaining parental consent. Parents are allowed to make decisions on behalf of their children because it is assumed that they have their children's best interests in mind. Ethicists argue that just as parents are allowed to expose their children to the sometimes greater than minimal risks of daily life (bungee jumping or riding in roller coasters, for instance), they may similarly subject them to medical research when the risks are commensurate with associated benefits, or when the risks are not more than a minor increase above minimal risk.[17]

One important difference between research in children and that in acutely ill adults incapable of giving consent is that the latter group of subjects often does not have a readily available proxy to provide consent. Moreover, even if a proxy was available to consent for the patient, the emergent nature of the process would make a truly informed decision difficult. To overcome this barrier, ethicists propose that research

without patient or proxy consent is still permissible if the entailed level of risk is appropriate.

To better understand the ethics of research without consent, the issue of risk must first be addressed. One organized approach to ethically analyze the benefits and risks of human subjects research, called **component analysis**, separates the interventions proposed in a study into therapeutic and non-therapeutic procedures (Figure 28.1).[22–24] Therapeutic procedures (the placement of a device or administration of a drug, for example) are performed under the premise that they may benefit the research subject. On the other hand, non-therapeutic procedures (collecting data from

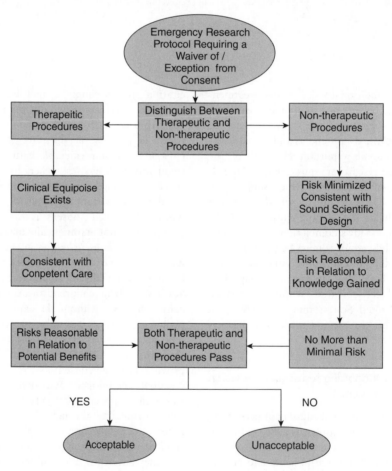

Fig. 28.1 Algorithm for risk analysis, using component analysis.[22] Redrawn by permission from Macmillan Publishers Ltd: *Nature Medicine*. Weijer C, Miller PB. (2004) When are research risks reasonable in relation to anticipated benefits? *Nat Med.* 10, 570–3. Copyright 2004.

medical records or the use of blood samples for analysis, for example), are conducted only to help answer the research question, and do not immediately or directly benefit the subject.

Using component analysis, therapeutic procedures are only ethically permissible if they are in clinical equipoise with the standard of care. Ethicists argue that in a state of equipoise there would be no difference at face value between receiving standard medical care and participating in a research study. Although in critically ill patients the risks of an experimental procedure may be high, if the intervention under study is in clinical equipoise with current therapy, which is expected to have similarly high rates of unsatisfactory outcomes, the risks of the study intervention are ethically acceptable.[19] In fact, some proponents of emergency research suggest that current therapies for certain grave and critical medical conditions are so poor that the use of an experimental therapy with the prospect of significant benefit may actually be in the best interest of the patient, and to forbid that would be unethical.[25]

This accounting of risk is in stark contrast to non-therapeutic procedures, wherein the risk to subjects who will not directly or immediately benefit from their participation must be minimized. When studies of non-therapeutic interventions involve subjects who cannot consent, many ethicists argue that the level of acceptable risk should be limited to minimal risk, defined as that associated with activities of daily life.[23,24] The standard of minimal risk is an even higher level of protection than that found in pediatric research, where the level of acceptable risk is not more than a minor increase above minimal risk. Because critically ill adults frequently will not have parental or proxy consent available, they are even more vulnerable than pediatric research subjects. Therefore, in research of non-therapeutic interventions involving subjects who cannot consent, the level of risk that can be incurred by these subjects should be no more than that encountered in daily life or as part of routine physical examinations. Just as individuals are not asked for informed consent prior to accepting the minimal risks of crossing the street, or driving a car in daily life, studies involving a similar minimal level of risk may not require this consent in resuscitation research when obtaining it is not possible.

Besides informed consent, other equally important ethical principles and values that determine if a study can be ethically conducted include issues of justice, value of the research, scientific validity, and respect for subjects.[19,26] When these other values are promoted by the research effort under consideration, the absence of prospective informed consent does not automatically make the study ethically prohibitive. Just as it would be unjust for physicians and scientists to not perform research on children or dementia patients due to their inability to provide informed consent, the systematic exclusion of critically ill adults from medical research and advances would be unjustly discriminatory and similarly inappropriate.[27] The enrollment of critically ill individuals in research without their prospective informed consent may be considered an essential act of altruism, with their participation ultimately contributing to the good of future vulnerable patients like themselves and to society at large.[26]

Ethical challenges of resuscitation research without informed consent

There are several arguments against the performance of research on human subjects without their prospective informed consent. Some ethicists argue that such research violates the principles of autonomy and respect for persons, and therefore can never be ethically carried out.[28] The first principle outlined by the Nuremberg Code, considered by many to be the most important document in the history of medical research, states: "The voluntary consent of the human subject is absolutely essential."[29] From the infamous Tuskegee Study of Untreated Syphilis that continued up until 1972, to the more recent trials investigating the vertical transmission of HIV infection in Third World countries, many ethicists are reminded that no matter how important the research question, or how altruistic the ultimate research goal, if the methods are not ethically sound, the study cannot proceed.[30,31]

Informed consent is paramount because it protects subjects from the conflicting interests of the researcher. Unlike clinical care wherein both the patient and the physician have common interests devoted to the well-being of the patient, in the setting of medical research, the interests of the investigator may be focused on performing and completing the study rather than on the benefit of the subject.[26] When individuals become research subjects, they are more vulnerable to exploitation by investigators due to divergent interests. No matter what the potential benefits of the experimental intervention may be, critics of research without consent warn that medical care under a researcher–subject relationship is fundamentally and perhaps insurmountably different from care under a physician–patient relationship.[26]

Some ethicists propose that even the condition of clinical equipoise does not exempt researchers from seeking informed consent from patients.[32] Although researchers and members of IRBs may view an experimental therapy as clinically equivalent to treatment considered the standard of care, the subject may not view the situation similarly. The subject, even when offered two choices that are said to be clinically equivalent, ought still be able to choose the one he or she prefers.[32] This may be in keeping with the public's current attitudes on emergency research without prospective informed consent. Available data from limited survey studies in the United States reveal that around half of the public does not agree generally with research without consent in emergency situations.[33] A study of ED patients and visitors demonstrates that almost half of the respondents viewed research subjects as "human guinea pigs."[34]

Investigators aiming to meet the requirements of the Final Rule in order to perform emergency research without consent face many challenges. Chief among them is the requirement for community consultation. Researchers have pointed out the lack of a universally accepted definition of the term "community," the absence of recommendations on how consultation with the community—if successfully identified—should be performed, and what actions should be taken with feedback obtained from community consultations.[35] The requirement for community consultation can also be significantly burdensome in terms of the extra time and financial costs it will add onto studies seeking an exemption from informed consent, all the while without demonstrable evidence of meeting the intended goals of the Final Rule.[36,37] Finally, there is significant concern over whether there is a correct and adequate understanding of how to apply the Final Rule among researchers and members of IRBs.[15] The history of how the Final Rule came to its current form, as well as the details and nuances of its provisions, can be difficult to fully understand, particularly for inexperienced users. This state of affairs has raised fears that researchers may relocate trials requiring an exception from informed consent to less-developed countries in order to evade Final Rule requirements.[38]

Conclusions

Research and innovation in the care of the critically ill are challenging, but must proceed in order to demonstrate the safety and efficacy of potentially life-saving therapies. Obtaining prospective informed consent is the standard by which all human subjects research should proceed. In situations wherein patients are unable to provide this consent as a result of their critical illness, the Final Rule provides a mechanism for these patients to participate in and potentially benefit from experimental therapies while ensuring respect and protection for their role as research subjects. Although there are many recognized challenges to implementation of the Final Rule, the intent of the regulations is not to make research without informed consent as easy as possible for researchers. Rather, the goal is to ensure the highest level of protection to subjects who are perhaps the most vulnerable of all in medical research. The informed consent of a voluntary and autonomous individual to participate in medical research is one of the most powerful forms of protection against research abuse and exploitation. Its absence in trials invoking the Final Rule cannot and should not be considered lightly. Members of the research community must remember that "research is a privilege not to be presumed or exploited, but earned through building and maintaining the public trust."[39]

Section IV: Recommendations

• Critical care and resuscitation research with patients who cannot provide prospective informed consent should be ethically permissible. To prevent investigative work in this area of medicine from taking place would be detrimental to medical science and patients alike.
• Researchers seeking an exemption from informed consent need a thorough understanding of the history and provisions of the Final Rule.
• Members of the resuscitation and critical care research community, including study sponsors and constituents of IRBs, need to continue to refine the

Final Rule to further facilitate scientific endeavors without compromising the ethical protections that all research subjects deserve.

References

1. Krugman S. (1971) Experiments at the Willowbrook State School. *Lancet*. 1, 966–7.
2. Krugman S. (1986) The Willowbrook hepatitis studies revisited: ethical aspects. *Rev Infect Dis*. 8, 157–62.
3. Rothman DJ. (1982) Were Tuskegee & Willowbrook "studies in nature"? *Hastings Cent Rep*. 12, 5–7.
4. Jones JH. (1993) *Bad Blood: The Tuskegee Syphilis Experiment*. New York, NY: Free Press.
5. Code of Federal Regulations. *Title 45 Public Welfare. Part 46 Protection of Human Subjects*. 45 CFR 46. Washington, DC: Department of Health and Human Services.
6. Quarantelli EL. (2008) Panic. In: Darity Jr. WA. (ed.) *International Encyclopedia of the Social Sciences*, 2nd ed. Detroit, MI: Macmillan Reference, pp. 122–4.
7. Quarantelli, EL. (2008) Disaster crisis management: a summary of research findings. In: Boin A. (ed.) *Crisis Management*. Los Angeles, CA: Sage, pp. 45–56.
8. Moreno JD. (1998) Convenient and captive populations. In: Kahn JP, Mastroianni AC, Sugarman J. (eds) *Beyond Consent: Seeking Justice in Research*. New York, NY: Oxford University Press, pp. 111–29.
9. Code of Federal Regulations. *Title 21 Food and Drugs. Part 50 Protection of Human Subjects*. 21 CFR 50. Washington, DC: Department of Health and Human Services.
10. Biros MH, Runge JW, Lewis RJ, et al. (1998) Emergency medicine and the development of the Food and Drug Administration's final rule on informed consent and waiver of informed consent in emergency research circumstances. *Acad Emerg Med*. 5, 359–68.
11. Bateman BT, Meyers PM, Schumacher HC, et al. (2003) Conducting stroke research with an exception from the requirement for informed consent. *Stroke*. 34, 1317–23.
12. Bircher NG. (2003) Resuscitation research and consent: ethical and practical issues. *Crit Care Med*. 31, S379–84.
13. Abramson NS, Safar P. (1990) Deferred consent: use in clinical resuscitation research. Brain Resuscitation Clinical Trial II Study Group. *Ann Emerg Med*. 19, 781–4.
14. Levine RJ. (1995) Research in emergency situations. The role of deferred consent. *JAMA*. 273, 1300–2.
15. Biros MH. (2003) Research without consent: current status. *Ann Emerg Med*. 42, 550–64.
16. McRae A, Weijer C. (2008) US Federal Regulations for emergency research: a practical guide and commentary. *Acad Emerg Med*. 15, 88–97.
17. McRae AD, Weijer C. (2002) Lessons from everyday lives: a moral justification for acute care research. *Crit Care Med*. 30, 1146–51.
18. Biros MH, Lewis RJ, Olson CM, et al. (1995) Informed consent in emergency research: consensus statement from the Coalition Conference of Acute Resuscitation and Critical Care Researchers. *JAMA*. 273, 1283–7.
19. Emanuel EJ, Wendler D, Grady C. (2000) What makes clinical research ethical? *JAMA*. 283, 2701–11.
20. McCormick RA. (1976) Experimentation in children: sharing in sociality. *Hastings Cent Rep*. 6, 41–6.
21. Freedman B. (1978) On the rights of the voiceless. *J Med Philos*. 3, 196–210.
22. Weijer C, Miller PB. (2004) When are research risks reasonable in relation to anticipated benefits? *Nat Med*. 10, 570–3.
23. Weijer C. (2000) The ethical analysis of risk. *J Law Med Ethics*. 28, 344–61.
24. Weijer C. (2004) The ethical analysis of risk in intensive care unit research. *Crit Care*. 8, 85–6.
25. Morrison CA, Horwitz IB, Carrick MM. (2009) Ethical and legal issues in emergency research: barriers to conducting prospective randomized trials in an emergency setting. *J Surg Res*. 157, 115–22.
26. Adams JG, Wegener J. (1999) Acting without asking: an ethical analysis of the Food and Drug Administration waiver of informed consent for emergency research. *Ann Emerg Med*. 33, 218–23.
27. Baren JM, Fish SS. (2005) Resuscitation research involving vulnerable populations: are additional protections needed for emergency exception from informed consent? *Acad Emerg Med*. 12, 1071–7.
28. Ramsey P. (1976) The enforcement of morals: nontherapeutic research on children. *Hastings Cent Rep*. 6, 21–30.
29. Shuster E. (1997) Fifty years later: the significance of the Nuremberg Code. *N Engl J Med*. 337, 1436–40.
30. Angell M. (1997) The ethics of clinical research in the Third World. *N Engl J Med*. 337, 847–9.
31. Kottow M. (2004) The battering of informed consent. *J Med Ethics*. 30, 565–9.
32. Farnell SM. (2002) Medical research: why trouble the patient for informed consent? *Med Pediatr Oncol*. 39, 207–11.
33. Lecouturier J, Rodgers H, Ford GA, et al. (2008) Clinical research without consent in adults in the emergency setting: a review of patient and public views. *BMC Med Ethics*. 9, 9.
34. Wilets I, O'Rourke M, Nassisi D. (2003) How patients and visitors to an urban emergency department view clinical research. *Acad Emerg Med*. 10, 1081–5.

35. Maitland K, Molyneux S, Boga M, et al. (2011) Use of deferred consent for severely ill children in a multicentre phase III trial. *Trials*. 12, 90.

36. Kremers MS, Whisnant DR, Lowder LS, et al. (1999) Initial experience using the Food and Drug administration guidelines for emergency research without consent. *Ann Emerg Med*. 33, 224–9.

37. McClure KB, Delorio NM, Gunnels MD, et al. (2003) Attitudes of emergency department patients and visitors regarding emergency exception from informed consent in resuscitation research, community consultation, and public notification. *Acad Emerg Med*. 10, 352–9.

38. Baren JM, Nathanson PG. (2005) Recruitment and communication process for participation in the 2005 AEM Consensus Conference on the Ethical Conduct of Resuscitation Research: methodology, challenges, lessons learned. *Acad Emerg Med*. 12, 1027–30.

39. Mastroianni A, Kahn J. (2001) Swinging on the pendulum: shifting views of justice in human subjects research. *Hastings Cent Rep*. 31, 21–8.

Appendix: useful resources

Alexander Bracey

Clinical Research Assistant, Beth Israel Deaconess Medical Center, Boston, MA, USA

This section of the book includes resources that may be useful to those interested in learning more about the issues discussed here, as well as those that were not covered. There is a list of academic bioethics texts, and web addresses of bioethics news forums, academic journals, and government and independent organizations. Although this compilation represents only a small portion of the existing bioethics resources, it may serve as a foundation for further exploration into the field. There is also a comprehensive list of the major academic bioethics programs in the United States and Canada at the end of the section.

Books

Beauchamp TL, Childress JF. (2008) *Principles of Biomedical Ethics*, 6th ed. New York, NY: Oxford University Press. A comprehensive guide to the fundamentals of traditional and contemporary ethical issues.

Garrett TM, Baillie HM, Garrett RM. (2009) *Health Care Ethics: Principles and Problems*, 5th ed. Saddle River: Pearson Prentice Hall. A concise reference covering the range of contemporary issues in health care ethics.

Herring J. (2010) *Medical Law and Ethics*, 3rd ed. New York, NY: Oxford University Press. A comprehensive guide to the medical laws and ethics of healthcare.

Iserson KV, Sanders AB, Mathieu D. (1995) *Ethics in Emergency Medicine*, 2nd ed. Tucson: Galen Press. A comprehensive guide to understanding and approaching ethical issues in clinical emergency medicine.

Jonsen AR, Siegler M, Winslade WJ. (2006) *Clinical Ethics: A Practical Approach to Ethical Decisions in Clinical Medicine*, 6th ed. New York, NY: McGraw-Hill Medical. Guidelines for a systematic "four topics approach" to facing the challenges of clinical ethics.

Morrison EE. (2008) *Health Care Ethics: Critical Issues for the 21st Century*, 2nd ed. Sudbury: Jones & Barlett Publishers. A reference covering a range of ethical topics including contemporary issues.

Schears RM, Marco CA. (2006) Ethical issues in emergency medicine. *Emerg Med Clin North Am.* 24(3), 513–814. Issue of *Emergency Medicine Clinics of North America* dedicated to ethics in emergency medicine.

Singer PA, Viens AM. (2008) *Cambridge Textbook of Bioethics*. Cambridge: Cambridge University Press. A succinct, comprehensive guide to understanding clinical ethics.

Steinbock B, London AJ, Arras J. (2008) *Ethical Issues in Modern Medicine: Contemporary Readings in Bioethics*, 7th ed. New York, NY: McGraw-Hill.

Journals

Accountability in Research: www.tandf.co.uk/journals/titles/08989621.asp

American Journal of Bioethics: www.bioethics.net/journal

American Society of Law and Medicine and Ethics: www.aslme.org

Cambridge Quarterly of Healthcare Ethics: http://journals.cambridge.org/action/displayJournal?jid=CQH

Ethics & Behavior: www.tandf.co.uk/journals/titles/10508422.asp

Ethical Problems in Emergency Medicine: A Discussion-Based Review, First Edition. John Jesus, Shamai A. Grossman, Arthur R. Derse, James G. Adams, Richard Wolfe, and Peter Rosen.

© 2012 John Wiley & Sons, Ltd. Published 2012 by John Wiley & Sons, Ltd.

Hastings Center Report: www.thehastingscenter.org/
 Publications/HCRDefault.aspx
International Journal of Feminist Approaches to Bioethics:
 www.fabnet.org/ijfab.php
Journal of Clinical Ethics: www.clinicalethics.com
Journal of Empirical Research on Human Research Ethics:
 www.csueastbay.edu/JERHRE
Journal of Hospital Ethics: www.whcenter.org/body.cfm?id=
 556801
Journal of Medical Humanities: www.springer.com/new±%
 26±forthcoming±titles±%28default%29/journal/10912
Journal of Medicine and Philosophy: http://jmp.
 oxfordjournals.org
Kennedy Institute of Ethics Journal: http://muse.jhu.edu/
 journals/kennedy_institute_of_ethics_journal
Medical Law Review: http://medlaw.oxfordjournals.org
Perspectives in Biology and Medicine: http://muse.jhu.edu/
 journals/perspectives_in_biology_and_medicine
Public Health Ethics: http://phe.oxfordjournals.org

Resources for teaching bioethics

http://depts.washington.edu/bioethx/topics/index.html:
 Case-based bioethics topics from the Ethics in Medicine
 curriculum of the University of Washington.
http://wings.buffalo.edu/faculty/research/bioethics/osce.
 html: Standardized patient scenarios for teaching bioethics from the University of Toronto.
www.poynter.indiana.edu/tre/resources.shtml: Resources
 from the University of Indiana for teaching research
 ethics.

Government organizations

American Medical Association. Council on Ethical and Judicial Affairs: www.ama-assn.org/ama/pub/about-ama/our-
 people/ama-councils/council-ethical-judicial-
 affairs.page—Council that develops ethical policies for the
 American Medical Association.
Centers for Disease Control and Prevention (CDC): www.
 cdc.gov/about/ethics/—Program dedicated the interpreting ethical issues for the CDC with special regard to
 research ethics.
National Institutes of Health: http://bioethics.od.nih.gov—
 List of links to bioethics resources.
Office of Human Subjects Research: http://ohsr.od.nih.gov—
 Office to help National Institute of Health researchers to
 understand and comply with ethical standards.

Publications of the NIH Department of Bioethics:
 www.bioethics.nih.gov/research/index.shtml—Program
 that develops ethical policies for the NIH.
The Office of Research Integrity: http://ori.hhs.gov—Office
 that oversees public health service research integrity
 activities.
The President's Council on Bioethics: www.bioethics.gov—
 Commission that advises the president on emerging
 bioethical issues.
United Nations Educational, Scientific, and Cultural Organization: www.unesco.org/shs/bioethics—Organization
 dedicated to establishing bioethics dialog among the international community.
US Department of Health and Human Services regulations,
 with special regard to human research protections:
 www.hhs.gov—Primary United States government agency
 for protecting the health of American citizens and providing essential human services.
World Health Organization (WHO): www.who.int/ethics/
 en—WHO's ethics and health initiative policies and
 activities.

American academic bioethics programs

Albany Medical College Alden March Bioethics Program:
 www.amc.edu/Academic/bioethics/index.html
Albert Einstein College of Medicine Bioethics Program:
 www.einstein.yu.edu/masters-in-bioethics/home.aspx
 ?ekmensel=15074e5e_3686_3691_btnlink
Arizona State University Lincoln Center for Applied Ethics:
 www.lincolncenter.asu.edu/
Baylor College of Medicine Center for Medical Ethics &
 Health Policy: www.bcm.edu/ethics
Boston University Department of Health Law, Bioethics, and
 Human Rights: http://sph.bu.edu/Health-Law-Bioethics-
 a-Human-Rights/department-of-health-law-bioethics-a-
 human-rights/menu-id-90.html
Brown University Center for Biomedical Ethics: www.brown.edu/
 Departments/Center_for_Biomedical_Ethics/
Case Western Reserve University Department of Bioethics:
 www.case.edu/med/bioethics
Cleveland State University Bioethics Center: www.csuohio.
 edu/class/bioethics/
Creighton University Center for Health Policy and Ethics:
 http://chpe.creighton.edu/
Drew University Medical Humanities Program: www.drew.
 edu/graduate/academics/medical-humanities
Duquesne University Center for Healthcare Ethics: www.
 duq.edu/healthcare-ethics/
Emory University Center for Ethics: http://ethics.emory.edu/
 index.html

Georgetown University Center for Clinical Bioethics: http://clinicalbioethics.georgetown.edu

Georgia State University John Beer Blumenfeld Center for Ethics: www2.gsu.edu/~wwwcfe/index.html

Harvard University Edmond J. Safra Center for Ethics: www.ethics.harvard.edu/

Holy Apostles College and Seminary Pop John Paul II Bioethics Center: www.holyapostles.edu/bioethics

Indiana University Center for Bioethics: http://bioethics.iu.edu/

Johns Hopkins Berman Institute of Bioethics: www.bioethicsinstitute.org/

Kansas City University of Medicine and Biosciences Bioethics Program: www.kcumb.edu/Adm2/cob_acad_programs.asp

Loma Linda University Center for Christian Bioethics: www.llu.edu/central/bioethics

Loyola Marymount University Bioethics Institute: http://bellarmine.lmu.edu/bioethics.htm

Loyola University Neiswanger Institute for Bioethics and Health Policy: www.meddean.luc.edu/depts/bioethics

McGill University Biomedical Ethics: www.mcgill.ca/biomedicalethicsunit

Medical College of Wisconsin Center for the Study of Bioethics: www.mcw.edu/bioethics.htm

Michigan State University Center for Ethics and Humanities in the Life Sciences: www.bioethics.msu.edu

Midwestern University Bioethics: www.midwestern.edu/Programs_and_Admission/AZ_Bioethics.html

Mount Sinai School of Medicine, Union Graduate College Bioethics Program: www.bioethics.union.edu/

New York University Bioethics: http://bioethics.as.nyu.edu

Northwestern University Medical Humanities and Bioethics Program: http://bioethics.northwestern.edu

Rush University Health Ethics Program: www.rushu.rush.edu/catalog/acadprograms/chs/rhhv/rhhvdepartmentoverview.html

Santa Clark University Markkula Center for Applied Ethics: www.scu.edu/ethics

Saint Louis University Albert Gnaegi Center for Health Care Ethics: http://bioethics.slu.edu/

Stetson University Institute for Christian Ethics: www.stetson.edu/~ljguenth/group/

Stony Brook University Center for Medical Humanities, Compassionate Care, and Bioethics: www.stonybrook.edu/bioethics/index.shtml

Trinity International University Center for Bioethics and Human Dignity: www.tiu.edu/tiu/bioethics

Tuskegee University National Center for Bioethics in Research and Healthcare: http://tuskegee.edu/about_us/centers_of_excellence/bioethics_center.aspx

University of Alberta John Dossetor Health Ethics Health Ethics Centre: www.ualberta.ca/~bioethic/index.html

University of Buffalo Center for Clinical Ethics and Humanities in Health Care: http://wings.buffalo.edu/faculty/research/bioethics

University of California at Davis Center for Healthcare Policy and Research: www.ucdmc.ucdavis.edu/chsrpc/

University of California, San Francisco Philip R. Lee Institute for Health Policy Study: http://ihps.medschool.ucsf.edu/

University of Chicago MacLean Center for Clinical Medical Ethics: http://medicine.uchicago.edu/centers/ccme

University of Colorado at Boulder Center for Values and Social Policy: www.colorado.edu/philosophy/center/

University of Connecticut Department of Community Health and Healthcare: www.commed.uchc.edu/index.htm

University of Louisville Bioethics and Medical Humanities Program: http://louisville.edu/bioethicsma

University of Iowa Program in Bioethics and Humanities: www.medicine.uiowa.edu/bemh

University of Michigan Bioethics Program: www.med.umich.edu/bioethics/links.htm

University of Minnesota Center for Bioethics: www.ahc.umn.edu/bioethics

University of Montréal Bioethics Program: www.bioethique.umontreal.ca/en/index.shtml

University of Pennsylvania Center for Bioethics: www.bioethics.upenn.edu

University of Pittsburgh Center for Bioethics and Health Law: www.bioethics.pitt.edu

University of Princeton Center for Human Values: www.princeton.edu/~uchv/

University of Southern California Pacific Center for Health Policy and Ethics: http://lawweb.usc.edu/centers/paccenter/

University of South Florida Bioethics and Medical Humanities Program: http://hsc.usf.edu/medicine/internalmedicine/bioethics/index.htm

University of Texas Health Science Center at Tyler Bioethics Program: www.uthct.edu/research/bioethics

University of Texas Medical Branch Clinical Ethics Program: www.utmb.edu/imh/ethics/clinical.asp

University of Utah Medical Ethics and Humanities Division: http://medicine.utah.edu/internalmedicine/medicalethics

University of Virginia Bioethics Program: http://bioethics.virginia.edu

University of Washington Department of Bioethics and Humanities: https://depts.washington.edu/bhdept

Vanderbilt University Center for Ethics: www.vanderbilt.edu/CenterforEthics

Wake Forest University Center for Bioethics, Health, and Society: http://bioethics.wfu.edu/

Canadian academic bioethics programs

Columbia University Center for Bioethics: www.bioethicscolumbia.org

Saint Joseph's University Institute for Bioethics: www.sju.edu/academics/centers/bioethics/

University of British Columbia W. Maurice Young Centre for Applied Ethics: http://ethics.ubc.ca/

University of Calgary Office of Medical Bioethics: www.fp.ucalgary.ca/medbioethics/bioethic.html

University of Toronto Joint Centre for Bioethics: www.jointcentreforbioethics.ca

General and popular bioethics news

http://bioethics.com—Current bioethics news and issues.

http://bioethicsdiscussion.blogspot.com—Blog of Dr. Maurice Bernstein MD to discuss current topics in bioethics.

www.bioedge.org—Weekly newsletter about current bioethics topics and news.

www.msnbc.msn.com/id/3035344/ns/health-health_care—Current general bioethics news from MSNBC.com.

Additional resources

American College of Emergency Physicians: www.acep.org—The ethical policies of the American College of Emergency Physicians.

American College of Physicians: www.acponline.org/running_practice/ethics—Resources for ethics and professionalism.

American Medical Association: www.ama-assn.org/ama/pub/physician-resources/medical-ethics/about-ethics-group/ethics-resource-center.page?—Resources for ethics in healthcare.

American Medical Association Virtual Mentor: http://virtualmentor.ama-assn.org—The online ethics journal of the American Medical Association.

American Nurses Association: www.nursingworld.org/MainMenuCategories/EthicsStandards.aspx—Resources for ethical issues commonly encountered in nursing.

American Society for Bioethics and Humanities: www.asbh.org—Organization dedicated to promoting interdisciplinary discussions on bioethics.

Bioethics.net: www.bioethics.net—Bioethics news and resources.

Center for Bioethics & Human Dignity: http://cbhd.org—Judeo-Christian interpretation of ethical contemporary bioethical issues.

Council for International Organizations and Medical Sciences: www.cioms.ch/about/frame_bioethics.htm—International organization to promote international activities in biomedical sciences and its contribution to bioethics.

Dr. Faulk Schleisinger Institute for Medical-Halachic Research: www.medethics.org.il/—Jewish medical ethics resources.

Education in Palliative and End-of-Life Care: www.epec.net—Web resources of the Education in Palliative and End-of-life Care Organization.

Ethical and Religious Directives for Catholic Health Care Services: www.usccb.org/bishops/directives.shtml—Ethical and religious policies for Catholic health services.

Health Hippo: http://hippo.findlaw.com/hippohome.html—Collection of healthcare policy and regulatory materials.

Improving Palliative Care: Emergency Medicine—www.capc.org: Information on palliative care training and news.

Institutional Review Board: www.irbforum.org—Discussion and news forum for ethical, policy, and regulatory issues.

Intute Bioethicsweb- www.intute.ac.uk/healthandlifesciences/bioethicsweb—Resources for obtaining web-based biomedical ethics literature.

Islamic Medical Association of North America: www.imana.org/Ethics/ethics.html—Islamic medical ethics resources.

Kennedy Institute of Ethics: http://kennedyinstitute.georgetown.edu—Georgetown University's institute of ethics.

National Catholic Bioethics Center: www.ncbcenter.org—Catholic medical ethics resources and news.

National Reference Center for Bioethics Literature: http://bioethics.georgetown.edu/nrc—Bioethics research library.

Nuffield Council on Bioethics: www.nuffieldbioethics.org—Independent body that reviews reports on bioethical issues.

Public Responsibility in Medicine and Research: www.primr.org—Organization dedicated to advancing high ethical standards in research.

Society for Academic Emergency Medicine: www.saem.org/committees/ethics—Ethics committee of the Society for Academic Emergency Medicine.

The Park Ridge Center for Health, Faith, and Ethics: www.parkridgecenter.org—Organization dedicated to investigating the connection between health, faith, and ethics.

UK Clinical Ethics Network: www.ethics-network.org.uk—International ethical news and resources.

Website of the Hastings Center: www.thehastingscenter.org—Independent body that reviews reports on bioethical issues.

World Medical Association: www.wma.net/en/20activities/10ethics/—Resources on ethics policies.

Index

Page numbers in *italics* denote figures, those in **bold** denote tables.

Abu Ghraib 252, 253
ACE capacity tool 154
administrative interference 191–2
advanced directives 185
  see also do-not-resuscitate orders
adverse events 31
Advisory Committee on Immunization Practices
  (ACIP) 294
Affordable Care Act (2010) 107–8
against medical advice 94
age impairment in physicians 20
  management 23
alcohol abuse by physicians 16, 19
  management 21
alcohol testing 64
altered mental status 149–56
American College of Emergency Physicians 19, 31, 121
  code of ethics 42
  futility policy 122
  physician bystander guidelines 244
American Medical Association 19, 242
  Principles of Medical Ethics 31
Americans With Disabilities Act 23
anger management in physicians 16–17
  normative errors 17
antipsychotics
  atypical 145, 146
  classical 145, 146
antiviral drugs, allocation of 294
Aquinas, Thomas 42
assent to treatment 134
  refusal by minors 134–5
  see also consent
autonomy 4, 43–4, 76, 150, 152
  DNR orders 184
  emergency c-section 161–2
  non-medical observers 173–4
  organ donation 267
  see also consent
avian influenza A 291

battlefield triage 248, 254–6
  conditions of 254–5
  emergent wounded 254
  expectant wounded 254
  non-emergent wounded 254
Beauchamp, Tom, *Principles of Biomedical
  Ethics* 39
Beecher, Henry 248
Belmont Report 213
beneficence 44, 76
  DNR orders 184
  non-medical observers 175
Bentham, Jeremy 226, 227
benzodiazepines 145, 146
bereavement care 82
best interests 44
body-packing 64–5
body-stuffing 64–5
Botte v. *Pomeroy* 244
brain death 262, 267
Breithaput v. *Abram* 62–3, 64
Brody, Howard, *Ethics, the Medical Profession
  and the Pharmaceutical Industry* 192
burnout 19–20
bystander responsibility 237–45
  duty to act 238
  ethical aspects 240–1
    intervention 241–2
    non-intervention 242–3
  Good Samaritan laws 212, 217, 239, 244
  legal issues 244
  malpractice liability 33, 61, 237
  policies and guidelines 244

cadavers, practicing procedures on 301–10
Canada, Physicians' Achievement Review 23
Canadian Medical Association 242
Canadian Physician Review and Enhancement
  Program 23
cancer, end-of-life care 108–9

Ethical Problems in Emergency Medicine: A Discussion-Based Review, First Edition. John Jesus, Shamai A. Grossman,
Arthur R. Derse, James G. Adams, Richard Wolfe, and Peter Rosen.
© 2012 John Wiley & Sons, Ltd. Published 2012 by John Wiley & Sons, Ltd.

capacity *see* decisional capacity
cesarean section, perimortem 157–65
   clinical judgement 163
   familial consent 163
   fetal consent 162–3
   history 160–1
   maternal consent/autonomy 161–2
   maternal resuscitation 158
   mother-child precedence 161
   timing of 157–8
chemical restraint 145–6
   see also restraint
child abuse 276
Child Abuse and Neglect Data System (NCANDS) 276
Children's Health International Medical Project of
   Seattle (CHIMPS) 216
Childress, James, *Principles of Biomedical
   Ethics* 39
Christian Scientists 131
civil disobedience, mandatory reporting 282–3
clergy, role of 171–2
Colby v. *Schwartz* 244
colleagues, treatment of 3–14
   confidentiality 13
   emergency medicine 12–13
   refusal of care 4, 10–11
   risks and benefits
     to patient 8–9
     to physician 9–10
   special circumstances 11
combative patients 139–48
communicable disease reporting 276–9
communication 214–15
   disaster situations 290
*Community Strategy for Pandemic Influenza
   Mitigation* 294
compassion 50, 51
Confidential Enquiry into Maternal and Child Health
   (CEMACH) 161, 162
confidentiality 13, 62, 197–205
   legal issues 202–3
   mandatory reporting 203–4, 271–85
   presence of family members 204
conscience 42–3
consciousness, lapses of 281–2
consent 93, 152
   deferred 314
   emergency c-section 161–2
   emergency medical interventions 93–4
   fetus 162–3
   Final Rule 313–15

minors 133–4
   organ donation 267
   parental refusal 135
   research without 311–20
   see also decisional capacity
containment 145
contraception, postcoital 38–9
Council for International Ethical Guidelines for
   Biomedical Research Involving Human
   Subjects 213
cultural understanding 214–15
CURVES capacity tool 154

death 99–115
   determination of 265–6
     brain death 262, 267
   family's expectations 101
   imminent, patients' lack of awareness 99–100
   inappropriate treatment 100
   unpreventable 111–12
   see also end-of-life issues; palliative care
DECISION capacity tool 154
decisional capacity 89–97, 141, 144
   case discussion 155
   definition 149, 152
   determination of 95, 149–56, **153**
   documentation 155
   impaired 154–5
   minors 132
   sliding scale approach 154
   threats to 152–3
Declaration of Helsinki 213
defensive medicine 60–1
deferred consent 314
DeMay v. *Roberts* 175
diazepam 146
difficult patients 52
disability 103
disasters 227–9
   pandemics 287–98
disaster drills 291
disaster triage 221–36
   egalitarianism 226–7
   ethical issues 229–32
   inexperienced personnel 224
   necessity and self-preservation 232
   origins of 226
   public response 225
   societal value issues 230–2
   urgency and narratives of care 229–30
   utilitarianism 223, 226, 227

disclosure of information 95
disruptive behavior 20
    management 21–3
    restraint 139–48
distributive justice
    DNR orders 184
    non-medical observers 175
DNR orders *see* do-not-resuscitate orders
do-not-intubate orders 179–85
do-not-resuscitate orders 41, 83, 92, 110, 179–85
    autonomy 184
    beneficence 184
    distributive justice 184
    reversal of 182
    values and principles 183–5
doctor *see* physician
domestic violence 274, 280–1
duty of care 133
duty to warn 59–60, 280

egalitarianism 226–7, 228
elder abuse 280
Emergency Medical Treatment and Labor Act
        (1986) 107, 123
end-of-life issues 83
    challenges 94–5
    decision making *105*, **107**
    DNR orders 41, 83, 92, 110, 179–85
    ethical aspects 105, 109–10
    euthanasia 105, 113
    extubation 102
    futile treatments 103
    hospices 101
    patient preferences 110–11
    physician-assisted suicide 37–46, 105, 113
    symptomatic relief 100, 101, 105–7, *106*, 112
    treatment goals 101, 108
    treatment withdrawal *106*
    see also palliative care; refusal of care
equipoise 312, 313
error disclosure 27–35
    barriers to 33
    levels of 28
euthanasia 105, 113
Exception from Informed Consent Research (EFIC) 305
extubation of dying patients 102

fairness 53
families
    and confidentiality 204
    consent to emergency c-section 163

grief alleviation 72
    interference by 191–2
    teaching procedures in front of 72
family members, medical treatment of 3–14
    confidentiality 13
    emergency medicine 12
    refusal of care 4, 10–11
    risks and benefits
        to patient 8–9
        to physician 9–10
    special circumstances 11
family-witnessed resuscitation 69–77
    benefits of 74
    ethical aspects 75–6
    legal issues 71
fidelity 228
filming in emergency department 169–78
Final Rule 313–14
    guidelines 314–15
Flynn v. *United States* 244
force, use of 139–48
forensic medicine 60
friends, treatment of 3–14
    confidentiality 13
    emergency medicine 12
    refusal of care 4, 10–11
    risks and benefits
        to patient 8–9
        to physician 9–10
    special circumstances 11
futility *see* medical futility

Geneva Convention 249, 252
goals of care 84
Good Samaritan laws 212, 217, 239, 244
grief alleviation 72
guidelines
    Final Rule 314–15
    non-medical observers 176–7
    physician bystanders 244
    postmortem procedures 308–9

haloperidol 146
health emergency operations centers
        (HEOCs) 230
Health Insurance Portability and Accountability
        Act (HIPAA) (1996) 62, 63, 70, 170,
        201, 248
healthcare proxies 92–3
HEEAL mnemonic 30, 33–4
Higgins v. *Detroit Osteopathic Hospital Corp* 244

Hippocratic Oath 13, 62, 201
  disaster triage 221–2, 226, 228, 232
  treatment of prisoners 247, 248
HIV, mandatory reporting 279
hospice care 101
hypoxia 89–97

impaired physicians 15–26
  age impairment 20, 23
  alcohol abuse 16, 19, 21
  burnout 19–20
  definition and diagnosis 18–19
  disruptive behavior 20, 21–3
  legal and ethical responsibilities 23
  management 20–3
  psychiatric disorders 19–20, 21
  substance abuse 16, 18, 19, 21
impartiality 53
Improving Palliative Care in Emergency Medicine
    (IPAL-EM) 85
inexperienced personnel
  disaster triage 224
  international medical initiatives 217–18
informed consent see consent
informed refusal see refusal of care
institutional review boards 311, 318
International Code of Medical Ethics 242
international medical initiatives 209–20
  chronic care and elective surgery 216
  ethical issues 212–13
  lack of follow-up 210–11
  lack of time and resources 215
  language and culture 214–15
  non-licensed/inexperienced personnel 217–18
  Shoulder to Shoulder Model 217
  sustainability 216–17
  vulnerability of patients 214
interrogation of prisoners 252–4
intubation
  against patient's wishes 90
  palliative care 80
  practicing on cadavers 301–10
Iserson, Ken 303
Israeli Dying Patient Act (2005) 181, 182

Jehovah's Witnesses 38, 131, 132, 134, 151,
    182
judgement 5
judgemental attitudes/opinions 47–55
  difficult patients 52
  ethical considerations 52–3

  physician factors 52
  potential solutions 53–4
justice 44, 53

ketamine 146

Lacy v. Cooper Hospital/University Medical Center 308
language 214–15
Larrey, Dominique-Jean 226
legal issues
  bystander responsibility 244
  confidentiality 202–3
  ethical aspects 63–4
  family-witnessed resuscitation 71
  impaired physicians 23
  mandatory reporting 275–6
  medical futility 122–3
  non-medical observers 175–6
  police requests 62
  postmortem procedures 308
  privacy 201
legislation 62
  see also *individual laws and statutes*
life-saving interventions 85
litigation 57–66
lorazepam 146

McArthur Competence Assessment Tool (MacCAT) 154
malpractice liability 33, 61, 237
mandatory reporting 65, 203–4, 271–85
  civil disobedience 282–3
  communicable diseases 276–9
  confidentiality 203–4, 272
  domestic violence 274, 280–1
  duty to warn 280
  elder abuse 280
  ethical vs. legal considerations 275–6
  injuries and causes of death 279
  necessity for 276
  permissive reporting laws 282
  seizures and lapses of
      consciousness 281–2
  suspected/confirmed child abuse 276
  see also *police requests*
Mann, Thomas 71
medical errors 5
  definition of 31
  disclosure of 27–35
  HEEAL mnemonic 30, 33–4
  physician vs. patient attitudes 32
  vs. complications 30

medical futility 103, 117–25
  definition 119, 121
  determination of 124
  ethical issues 122
  legal issues 122–3
  professional guidance 122
  professional obligations 121–2
  prolongation of life 108, 119
  qualitative 121
  quantitative 121
  resuscitation 71, 118
  "slow codes" 120
midazolam 146
military personnel 247–58
  triage 248, 254–6
Mill, John Stuart 226, 227
Miller v. *NBC* 175
Mini-Mental State Examination 153–4, **153**
minors 129–38
  duty of care 133
  medical decision making by 132
  parental refusal of treatment 129–30, 135
  parental refusal of vaccinations 135–7
  refusal of assent to treatment 134–5

National Notifiable Diseases Surveillance System 277
National Pain Care Policy Act (2003) 107
National Vaccine Advisory Committee (NVAC) 294
National Vaccine Injury Compensation
      Program 136
non-governmental organizations 216
non-licensed personnel 217–18
non-maleficence 44, 53, 76
  non-medical observers 174–5
non-medical observers 169–78
  autonomy 173–4
  beneficence 175
  clergy 171–2
  distributive justice 175
  legal and regulatory aspects 175–6
  non-maleficence 174–5
  patient privacy 202
  policies, guidelines and best practices 176–7
  types of 174
non-physician influences 187–95
  administrative 191–2
  family 191–2
  pharmaceutical industry 192
  regulatory agencies 192–4
normative errors 17
Nuremberg Code 317

objectivity, loss of 5, 8
obstetric emergencies 157–65
Office for Human Research Protection (OHRP) 314
oligoanalgesia 193–4
organ donation 261–9
  determination of death 265–6
  donor care 267–8
  eligibility 264
  patient autonomy and consent 267
  public perception and trust 266–7
  temporary organ preservation 267–8
  Uniform Anatomical Gift Act 262, 264, 267
organ procurement organizations 262, 264
oseltamivir 294

pain management
  dying patients 100, 101, 105–7, *106*, 112
  palliative care 84–5
  regulatory interference 192–4
pain relief seeking 47–52
palliative care 79–87, 100
  clinical trials 109
  curable illness 80–1
  future directions 85–6
  goals of 84
  intubation 80
  life-saving interventions 85
  pain management 84–5
  place in course of illness 83
  prognostication 84
  risk-burden-benefit assessment 83–4
  sedation 112
  utilitarian aspects 82
  see also end-of-life issues
pandemics 287–98
  antiviral allocation 294
  healthcare service allocation 294–5
  professional duty of care 292
  resource allocation 293–4, **294**
  restrictions on personal liberty 292–3
  social distancing measures 293
  twenty-first century 296
  vaccine allocation 293–4
  see also disasters; disaster triage
parents
  belief systems of 131
  consent to treatment of minors 129–31
  refusal of childhood vaccinations 135–7
  refusal of consent 135
Patient Self Determination Act (1991) 110
patient- and family-centered care 135

patients
   autonomy 4, 43–4
   interests of 61–2
   requests from 37–46
   responsibilities of 59
   right to privacy 70
penicillin rationing 256
Percival, Thomas 13
permissive reporting laws 282
personal liberty, restrictions on 292–3
pharmaceutical industry, interference by 192
PHPs 21
physical restraint 144–5
   application of 145
   see also restraint
physical space 201–2
physician obligations 37–46
   beneficence 44
   conscience 42–3
   ethical issues 42
   justice 44
   non-maleficence 44
   respect for persons 43–4
physician-assisted suicide 37–46, 105, 113
physician-patient relationship 9, 76, 90
   confidentiality 13, 62, 197–205
physicians
   as agents of the state 57–66
   attitude to patients 250
   as bystanders 237–45
   impaired 15–26
   as patients 9
Physician's Order for Life-Sustaining Treatment
   (POLST) 91, 102, 110
Plato, *The Republic* 251
police requests 57–66
   alcohol testing 64
   case law 62–3
   drugs 64–5
   legal responsibilities 62
   mandatory reporting *see* mandatory reporting
   sexual assault kits 65
political pressures 187–95
Posey vest 145
positional asphyxia 145
postcoital contraception 38–9
postmortem procedures 301–10
   alternatives 306
   ethical arguments against 307
   ethical arguments for 306–7
   legal considerations 308

   policies and guidelines 308–9
   religious ethics 304
power of attorney 92
prescriptions 6–7
prima facie obligations 42
primum non nocere 33, 241
prioritization of life 230–2
prisoners, treatment of 247–58
   roles and duties 251–2
   torture and interrogation 252–4
   triage 248, 254–6
privacy 197–205
   desensitization to 202
   legal issues 201
   physical space 201–2
   presence of observers 202
professional behavior 18
professional code 201
professional obligations 121–2
prognostication 84
prolongation of life 108, 119
psychiatric disorders 19–20
   management 21
   restraint 139–48
psychotropic drugs 141

quality of life 84
Quarantine Act (1893) 277

racism 22
Rawls, John 228–9
   Political Liberalism 39
reasonable reliance 71
record keeping
   decisional capacity 155
   refusal of care 95
   see also mandatory reporting
refusal of care 4, 10–11, 89–97
   against medical advice 94
   capacity 91, 92
   DNR orders 41, 83, 92, 110, 179–85
   documentation of 95
   minors 133–4
regulatory agencies, interference by 192–4
religious ethics 183–4
reporting laws *see* mandatory reporting
research without informed consent 311–20
   ethical arguments for 315–17, *316*
   Final Rule 313–15
   resuscitation 317–18
   vulnerable populations 312

resource allocation 249, 321–4
  pandemics 293–4, **294**
respect for persons 43–4
restraint 139–48
  and capacity 144
  chemical 145–6
  controversy over 143–4
  how much 146
  physical 144–5
  reasons for 144
  tasers 140
resuscitation
  DNR orders 41, 83, 92, 110, 179–85
  family-witnessed 69–77
    benefits of 74
    ethical aspects 75–6
    legal issues 71
  futile, psychological value 71, 118
  research without informed consent 317–18
  stopping/not starting 112–13
  training 69–77
Richards, Gene, *The Knife and Gun Club* 171
risk-burden-benefit assessment 83–4
Rochin v. *California* 62–3

Sanchez-Scott v. *Alza Pharmaceuticals* 176
Schmerber v. *California* 62–3
secular ethics 183
sedation, palliative 112
seizures 281–2
self-determination 43–4
Sequential Organ Failure Assessment (SOFA) scoring
    system 295
sexual assault kits 65
sexual harassment 22
Shoulder to Shoulder Model 217
Shulman v. *Group W Productions* 175–6
sickle cell disease 47–52
sickness bias 8
"slow codes" 120
social distancing measures 293
societal responsibility 59–60
solidarity 223
stereotyping 53–4
stress 19
substance abuse 16, 18, 19
  management 21
suicide 151
  physician-assisted 37–46, 105, 113

SUPPORT trial 110
Surveillance, Epidemiology and End Results (SEER)
    Program 108

Tarasoff v. *Regents of University of California* 63, 280
tasers 140
teaching procedures
  on cadavers 301–10
  in front of families 72
  see also postmortem procedures
temporary organ preservation 267–8
Texas Advance Directive Act 123
To Err Is Human—Building a Safer Health System 31
torture 248, 252–4
training
  palliative care 85
  resuscitation 69–77
  see also teaching procedures
treatment withdrawal *106*
triage 227–9
  battlefield 248, 254–6
  disasters *see* disaster triage
  Sequential Organ Failure Assessment (SOFA) scoring
      system 295
trust 200–1
truth telling 27–35
Tuskegee Study of Untreated Syphilis 317

Uniform Anatomical Gift Act 262, 264, 267
utilitarianism 223, 226, 227, 228

vaccinations, parental refusal of 135–7
vaccines, allocation of 293–4
value of life 183–4
venereal disease 250–1
ventilation, non-invasive 91
VIP care 188

waiting times 47, 50, 51
wellness bias 8
Winslow, Gerald R 228–9
  Triage and Justice 228
Winston v. *Lee* 62–3
withdrawal of care 102, *106*
  minors 132
  see also end-of-life issues

zanamivir 294
ziprasidone 146